Adolescence isn't what it used to be! Even its definition has changed in recent years to encompass the preteen years through the early twenties. This extraordinary volume addresses problems old and new, and presents clear, concise information designed to make young people active participants in their health maintenance.

<u>WHAT DO YOU DO</u>

• when a teenager's growth is lagging behind his classmates'?
• at the first signs of risk-taking behaviors: smoking, drinking, drugs?
• throughout the dating years, when prevention of pregnancy and sexually transmitted diseases is paramount?
• when a girl has not menstruated or has irregular periods? What does this mean?
• when a sixteen-year-old repeatedly sleeps until noon? How much sleep is too much?

The answers to all your questions are here in the book no parent— or teen—can afford to overlook.

"I applaud Dr. Slap for her thorough and thoughtful explanation of health issues concerning adolescents and young adults. To ensure that these youth receive appropriate medical care, an understanding of what their health risks are and how to recognize their health problems when they develop is critical. Dr. Slap's book is a must read for parents, teachers, coaches, and health care providers."
—THE HONORABLE HARRIS WOFFORD,
United States Senate (Pennsylvania)

"At last, a book for the forgotten segment in our population. . . . The teen years are filled with great vulnerability and it is then that the seeds of future disease are sown. This is an enormously valuable, readable, understandable, and indeed enjoyable volume detailing the hows and whys of teenage health care."
—ISADORE ROSENFELD, M.D.,
author of *The Best Treatment*

TEENAGE
HEALTH
CARE

**THE FIRST COMPREHENSIVE
FAMILY GUIDE FOR
THE PRETEEN
TO YOUNG ADULT YEARS**

Gail B. Slap, M.D.
AND
Martha M. Jablow

Foreword by Dr. Benjamin Spock

POCKET BOOKS
New York   London   Toronto   Sydney   Tokyo   Singapore

The ideas, procedures, and suggestions in this book are intended to supplement, not replace, the medical and psychological advice of trained professionals. All matters regarding your health require medical supervision. Consult your physician before adopting the medical suggestions in this book, as well as about any condition that may require diagnosis or medical attention.

The authors and publishers disclaim any liability arising directly or indirectly from the use of this book.

An *Original* Publication of POCKET BOOKS

POCKET BOOKS, a division of Simon & Schuster Inc.
1230 Avenue of the Americas, New York, NY 10020

Slap, Gail B.
    Teenage health care : the first comprehensive family guide to
  promoting good health and understanding illness from the preteen to
  young adult years / Gail B. Slap and Martha M. Jablow.
        p.   cm.
    Includes index.
    ISBN 0-671-75412-2
    1. Teenagers—Health and hygiene. 2. Teenagers—Diseases.
I. Jablow, Martha Moraghan. II. Title.
RJ140.S58 1994
613'.0433—dc20   94-10427
                                                        CIP

First Pocket Books trade paperback printing September 1994

10 9 8 7 6 5 4 3 2 1

POCKET and colophon are registered trademarks of
Simon & Schuster Inc.

Cover design by Mike Stromberg
Cover photos by Superstock

Printed in the U.S.A.

To my husband, Albert, for his thoughtful guidance and steady encouragement, and to our sons, Matthew and Andrew, for their patience and understanding.

—G.B.S.

To my husband, Paul, for his good humor and support, and to our two wonderful teenagers, Cara and David.

—M.M.J.

CONTENTS

P A R T   I

AN OVERVIEW OF ADOLESCENCE

P A R T   I I

SPECIAL HEALTH ISSUES

P A R T   I I I

PSYCHOLOGICAL AND
BEHAVIORAL ISSUES

P A R T   V

MEDICAL CONDITIONS DURING ADOLESCENCE

FIGURES AND TABLES

HOW TO USE THIS BOOK

When you scan the Contents, you will notice that the scope of this book is quite wide—from general subjects, such as growth and development, to specific problems, such as infections. The book is divided into five parts:

- Part I discusses the physical changes of puberty and the basic health care needs of all teenagers.
- Part II deals with health issues that take on particular significance during adolescence, such as exercise, nutrition, and sleep.
- Part III focuses on psychological and behavioral problems, such as substance abuse and depression.
- Part IV addresses sexuality and reproduction.
- Part V contains information about medical disorders organized by the different systems of the body, such as the heart, digestive tract, and kidneys.

We suggest that you read Parts I through IV during a quiet time, when you do *not* face an illness or crisis. This book is not an emergency medical text to be shelved, unread, until a teenager is critically ill, seriously injured, or engaged in risky behaviors. You may decide to read a chapter in Part V when a particular problem arises. For example, if a teenager has knee pain, you would read Chapter 31, The Bones and Joints.

Teenage Health Care is not limited strictly to the teenage years, thirteen to nineteen. It is useful as early as age eight when the first signs of puberty may appear. The issues of health promotion and the diseases discussed are applicable for young adults into their twenties.

We have tried to make often-abstruse medical language as understandable as possible. Specific terms are defined within the context of each chapter. General medical terms that appear in several chapters are defined in the Glossary. The Index will help you find individual subjects, and cross-references are used throughout

the book to help locate related information in other chapters. A
Resources list provides sources of additional information or help in
particular areas.

We hope that you will use this book to understand an adolescent's concern, to clarify the seriousness of a problem, and to
decide when to seek medical help. We encourage parents and teenagers to read the book together and to use it as a forum for sharing
and open discussion.

FOREWORD

By Dr. Benjamin Spock

Earlier in my career, I learned how important it is to give teenagers clear information. I was a physician in a girls' school, an hour a day for ten years, and I saw how self-conscious young people can be as their bodies change during puberty. Some worried because they were growing and developing way ahead of their classmates. Others, with slower growth and sexual maturation, worried that they would never catch up. I found that early and late developers alike welcomed my explanations and were relieved to learn that their differences in growth would even out with time.

Teenagers deserve solid information both for reassurance and to learn how to take care of themselves. Unfortunately, self-consciousness about their changing bodies often keeps them from voicing their concerns to parents or family physicians. Whether they're worried about growth, fatigue, headaches, or menstrual irregularity, teenagers can easily get confused about a problem's cause and significance. This confusion—especially if it's tied to self-consciousness—can block much needed discussion and even treatment.

That's where *Teenage Health Care* comes in. This book will be extraordinarily valuable for *both* parents and teenagers, because it reassures and informs at the same time. It's truly an encyclopedia of the physical changes and problems that affect teenagers—acne, AIDS, eating disorders, sexually transmitted diseases, sports injuries . . . The list is long. This book tells you what causes different problems, how they are diagnosed, how they may be treated.

Some conditions are common. Some are rare. It is good to have them all covered in one easy-to-use book. You'll learn when symptoms point to certain conditions, which diseases are dangerous and which aren't, which symptoms need quick medical attention, and which can be watched or even ignored. Most of the book deals with physical health, but emotional issues are also included. *Teenage Health Care* is a breakthrough book, one that is especially timely because of the staggering health issues facing teenagers today.

When I wrote *Baby and Child Care* a half-century ago, adolescence was a simpler time. As I updated the book over the years, new problems arose, like drug use in the 1960s. Today, adolescence is more challenging for teenagers, parents, and health professionals than at any time in my life.

Today's teenagers have to deal with the physical changes of puberty in a social environment that is much different from earlier generations. They're growing up with many unprecedented strains: single-parent households; two parents working outside the home; competitiveness that pressures parents to pressure their children; materialism that eclipses life's higher values; the threat of AIDS. Violence has become so common on TV and in the movies that it numbs many into accepting it as a routine way to settle conflicts. Advertising uses sexual content to glamorize smoking cigarettes and drinking alcohol. All of these factors strongly influence teenagers' health and well-being.

Millions of teenagers have early sexual intercourse, practice unsafe sex, and contract sexually transmitted diseases. Over a million teenagers become pregnant each year. Eating disorders are common. Nearly ninety percent of teenagers experiment with alcohol, and one in three tries illegal drugs. Teenage suicide has nearly tripled in recent years. These are not just social problems. They are vital health issues, too, and they are addressed here.

Faced with these scary figures and trends, some families want to throw up their hands in despair and discouragement. They can take heart that *Teenage Health Care* will answer their questions, help them prevent many problems, recognize early signs, and find treatment. By explaining how teenagers' decisions and actions can affect their health, Dr. Slap boosts their ability to live healthier lives in these challenging times.

In *Baby and Child Care,* I told parents, "Love and enjoy your child for what he is," because the child who feels accepted becomes happy and confident. The same can be said to parents of teenagers, and *Teenage Health Care* can help families reach that goal. Parents who dread adolescent storm and stress will discover that many teenagers experience no major turbulence. When problems do arise, the book guides you through the shoals, offering sound advice and reliable resources.

I want to make a special point about one subject that Dr. Slap addresses in Chapters 11 and 12. Teenagers have always wanted to sample the dangerous aspects of their society, as we remember from our own youth. But alcohol and drug use, which can take root in adolescence, can wreck promising careers and families. Alcohol and driving are a deadly combination. I firmly believe that all parents should ask their teenagers to promise that they will *never,* under any circumstance, ride with drivers who have been drinking. This includes beer, which some teenagers and even parents mistakenly consider only mildly intoxicating. They also need to face the fact that alcohol can impair judgment and lead to unsafe sex.

I urge parents to be open and honest in talking with teenagers about their own beliefs, ideas, and values. I say this because many good parents these days avoid such conversations for fear that their children will find them old-fashioned. Actually, most teenagers and preteens are really eager to hear and test the views of parents, as well as teachers and other adults they like or admire. But teenagers find it irritating when parents act as if they are always right because they are older. Eyes will roll if parents preach or talk too much. Instead, parents can listen to teenagers and nod in a way that says, "I see what you mean." Parents can best offer their ideals as "This is what I believe."

It's particularly important to hold these conversations just before the teen years, before adolescents have firmly decided that their friends possess the ultimate truth. If those years have passed, don't give up. It's never too late to start talking—and keep talking—about values and experiences. Many of the subjects in this book can be a jumping-off point to begin discussions. Even if the first conversations are halting or awkward, they may clear the way for future talks that help teenagers choose safer, healthier paths to adulthood.

I've always encouraged parents to trust their instincts and common sense in caring for babies and young children. I've said, "You know more than you think you do." This still holds true when children become teenagers. In that spirit, *Teenage Health Care* carries on the tradition of *Baby and Child Care*. Instincts and common sense can be strengthened, of course, by knowledge. The information in these pages gives families confidence to trust themselves. The more informed teenagers and parents become about health matters, the stronger a partnership they can build with their doctor to ensure good health care.

One of the things I like most about this book is Dr. Slap's respect for teenagers. She encourages parents to give teenagers gradually increasing responsibility for their own well-being. Most teenagers want—and deserve—to know about their health and development. *Teenage Health Care* presents that information in a useful way and speaks in a positive, supportive voice. Teenagers will find no scolding or "talking down" in this book. The reader, regardless of age, is assumed to be a sensible person entitled to truthful, straight talk.

I highly recommend *Teenage Health Care*. It is a wonderful resource that should remain on family bookshelves for years to come, serving as a ready, comprehensive companion. I hope you read it often, share it, and discuss it with each other.

ACKNOWLEDGMENTS

We are grateful to our editor, Paul D. McCarthy. From the beginning, he believed that this book would help families promote the health and well-being of all adolescents. His guidance and encouragement have been steadfast. We also thank our agent, Philippa Brophy, for bringing us to Paul and Pocket Books, and for her ongoing support.

INTRODUCTION

First it was colic during infancy. Then a toddler's earache at 2:00 A.M. Or an eye tightly glued shut . . . chicken pox . . . countless colds and fevers . . . bee stings . . . cuts and stitches . . . an arm fractured in a skateboard spill . . .

By the time children reach adolescence, families have become seasoned veterans of many illnesses and injuries, major and minor. Now those dashes to the emergency room and late-night calls to the doctor have all but disappeared, along with the Mickey Mouse Band-Aids. The vaporizer, which kept a sniffly child company through many long nights, has been pushed to the back of the closet, forgotten. The family has managed to survive the childhood medical wars.

Adolescence would seem to offer a welcome respite between the frequent colds and cuts of childhood and the chronic conditions of older adulthood. Families anticipate fewer illnesses, infrequent visits to the doctor, less worry about medical problems. Teenagers are expected to be strong and healthy, free of serious disease and disability. It is assumed that their bodies will grow from child-size to adult proportions smoothly, on schedule, without complications.

These assumptions are generally true. Most children do enter their teenage years sound and resilient. But if families define health narrowly—as simply an absence of disease—they may be lulled into a false sense of security. The leading causes of adolescent death are not physical disease but rather injury, homicide, and suicide. Consequently, a definition of adolescent health must include the *maintenance* of well-being as well as the *prevention* of injury and illness. This broad definition implies that families can actively promote adolescent health rather than passively accept it as just an absence of disease.

Each stage of human development has specific health needs. Adolescence is no exception. The health issues of teenagers differ from those of children and adults. A severe illness in early adolescence, for instance, may delay puberty and sexual maturation. Optimal health during adolescence requires that parents and teenagers learn together about growth, development, behavior, and prevention.

Too often other factors stand in the way of this knowledge. For example, when parents and teenagers hear the alarming statistics about adolescent injury, homicide, suicide, substance abuse, pregnancy, sexually transmitted disease, and HIV infection, they want to believe, "It won't happen to us . . . That applies to other teenagers, other families." These problems often are regarded as completely avoidable—"If they hadn't been drinking and driving . . ." "If they hadn't been sexually active so young . . ." Many teenage tragedies can and should be prevented, but prevention requires education, skill, and foresight on the part of parents, teenagers, health professionals, and communities.

Good health also may be inhibited when adolescents and adults are not on the same wavelength. A teenager's perception and understanding often differ from an adult's. Parents may underestimate the emotional effect of a seemingly minor issue. An extra few pounds or mild acne may seem trivial to a parent but can become a constant worry to a sixteen-year-old. Parents may assume that their teenager understands that an ache or pain is not serious when, in fact, the teenager is too frightened or embarrassed to discuss it.

Some of the gaps between parents and teenagers reflect their different ways of seeing the world. Cognitive ability is still evolving during adolescence. Most young teenagers (ages eleven to fourteen) think concretely. If a problem can be named, if the cause is identified, and if the treatment is clear, a younger teenager can get a handle on it. Abstract thinking—the ability to make complex associations or to link past events with current or future outcomes— may not develop until mid- or late adolescence. It is not unusual for some teenagers to seek help only for the most immediate, visible, or clear-cut symptoms. They may not recognize or discuss problems that they cannot articulate. They may not grasp the connection between behavior and consequence or cause and effect (such as the association between smoking today and lung cancer tomorrow).

Even when communication and health awareness are excellent, there are times when an adolescent's symptom or complaint results in anxiety for both teenager and parent:

"Are the headaches serious? Could it be a brain tumor? Is it just tension because of final exams?"

"What is that breast lump? Do teenagers get breast cancer?"

"Why does he always seem tired? How much sleep does a teenager really need?"

We have written this book to provide readily available information about medical issues during adolescence. It should not be used to make a final diagnosis or to decide on treatment. This is the job of health professionals, teenagers, and parents together. The book is intended to help families anticipate and recognize the normal events of adolescence, as well as interpret signs and symptoms that require further medical care.

Decisions about when to evaluate, test, and treat can be difficult, and the procedures are often costly. The teenager's well-being is always foremost, but there are times when the balance between cost, risk, and benefit is questionable. Families must discuss all of these issues with their doctors. More is not always better. Good health care weighs all the issues facing the family—well-being, financial burden, and peace of mind.

The subjects covered in this book are broad, from fairly clear-cut problems, like sunburn, to the more complex and societal, like HIV and AIDS. Emphasis is on the physical rather than the psychological dimensions of the issues. That is not meant to diminish the importance of psychological health during adolescence. The causes and consequences of many physical conditions, such as anorexia nervosa, sexually transmitted disease, and unplanned pregnancy, are tightly interwoven with psychological threads. Even a problem such as mild acne has a psychological impact on a teenager. Throughout the book, we incorporate mental health and psychological dimensions as they affect the adolescent's physical well-being. For more detailed information about the psychology of adolescence, readers may turn to the many excellent resources on the shelves of libraries and bookstores. At the end of this book, the Resources list includes books about the psychology and culture of adolescence.

We hope that *Teenage Health Care* will help families experience the joy and wonder of adolescence. Too often these years suffer a bad rap. Jokes about raging hormones and "storm and stress" lead parents and other adults to assume that adolescence must be an adversarial period, to be lived in the trenches, to be dreaded as intolerable years that will try even the most patient parental soul. Adolescence is a time of change and challenge, but with change comes healthy growth and a new respect for the adolescent as a responsible individual.

We hope that this book will be used collaboratively by families as questions and problems arise. Any issue, large or small, is more manageable when it is discussed and shared by adolescents and caring adults working together. Decisions that are made jointly can enhance maturation and can make adolescence a richer experience for both teenagers and parents.

The family, as the basic unit in our society, has a major influence on the health of youth. During childhood, the parent is the active guardian of health, taking temperatures and scheduling doctors' appointments. Adolescence offers a special opportunity for a gradual shifting of this responsibility within the family unit. As the bridge from childhood to adulthood, adolescence gives young people a chance to assume more independence in their decision making and to take increasing control of their health. Parents may remain at the front line, but they now can share the responsibility with their teenagers.

Most adolescents are no longer open-mouthed children passively taking their spoonfuls of medicine. They want to participate actively in their health maintenance. If they are to become well-informed, healthy adults and if the coming generations of young adults are to become savvy health care consumers, teenagers must be given the opportunity to take the reins of their medical care.

The book also was written to help teenagers and parents navigate the health care system. Information about adolescent health care can diminish anxiety about the office visit, promote better use of health services, and decrease the need for emergency or crisis intervention. Improved health and better access to medical care require a partnership between health providers and informed consumers. Biotechnical advances are not enough to improve health in contemporary society. We need a better collective knowledge of what constitutes good health and how to attain it. For the adolescent, this knowledge, access, and utilization are best achieved through a team effort involving the family, school, and medical profession. The overriding goal is good health and quality care for all young people. They are our most precious resource and our future.

I

AN
OVERVIEW
OF
ADOLESCENCE

1

The Concept of Adolescence

Our current-day concept of adolescence has evolved over thousands of years. The word "adolescence," from the Latin *adolescere* ("to grow up"), has been used in the English language since the fifteenth century. The idea that adolescence is a transition between childhood and adulthood, however, probably dates back to prehistoric times. Society's changing definition and expectation of adolescence help explain some of the health issues confronting youth today.

Every early society had to incorporate each new generation of youth into its culture in order for the community to survive. In primitive or ancient societies, dramatic rites of passage marked a child's transition to adulthood. Some cultures prescribed initiation ceremonies that required a youth to sacrifice some blood or teeth in order to enter the adult world—a world where his or her role was clearly defined and usually followed the parental position or occupation. Transition to adulthood was quick and clean in these early cultures. The essential message was: "Now that your body can do an adult's job and can reproduce, get to work. Go out and hunt an animal for supper or forage for nuts and berries."

In the fifth to second centuries B.C., the Sumerian civilization flourished in the Near East as the first "high civilization" in human history. The Sumerians were the first to write and the first to socialize their young people through a school system. Sumerian clay tablets, discovered by twentieth-century archaeologists, were an ancient version of today's three-ring notebooks. One tablet records a dialogue between a Sumerian teenager and his father that sounds uncannily familiar:

> "Where did you go?"
> "I did not go anywhere."
> "If you did not go anywhere, why do you idle about? Go to school
> . . . it will be of benefit to you."[1]

In classical Greece, Plato, Aristotle, and other philosophers began to divide human life into distinct stages. Plato thought that adolescence was the period for developing rational and critical thought and, therefore, should be the time to study math and science. Aristotle wrote that adolescents are

> . . . prone to desire and ready to carry any desire that may have formed into action. . . . They are changeful, too, and fickle in their desires, which are as transitory as they are vehement. . . . They are passionate, irascible, and apt to be carried away by their impulses. . . . If the young commit a fault, it is always on the side of excess and exaggeration. . . . They regard themselves as omniscient and are positive in their assertions; this is, in fact, the reason of their carrying everything too far."[2]

In the Middle Ages, children were seen as miniature adults. From the time of conception, a tiny man or woman was thought to exist in the sperm. Growing up simply meant growing larger. This belief was challenged during the Renaissance as new ideas about human development blossomed.

Philosopher John Locke proposed that the human mind was a *tabula rasa,* a blank slate, upon which experience and learning are imprinted over time. This was quite a different notion than the Middle Ages idea of child as mini-adult. To Locke, a young person began life without inborn ideas and proceeded from the passive mind of childhood to the active rationality of adolescence as increasing experiences were imprinted on the mind's slate. Later, in the Age of Reason, Jean-Jacques Rousseau went a step further. He divided life into stages that paralleled the development of the human race from primitive to civilized. He thought of the period from age five to twelve as "savage." Rousseau believed that rational thinking developed during "youth," age twelve to fifteen, while emotional maturity and social responsibility developed in "adolescence," age fifteen to twenty.

These concepts of adolescence prevailed in Western thought until the nineteenth century. Families were large and children were spaced closely together during the 1800s. Life expectancy was much shorter than it is today. The average age of the American population in 1800 was only sixteen. In a predominantly agricultural society, young people were pushed quickly into adult roles for economic reasons. Boys plowed and planted alongside their fathers; girls cooked, sewed, and harvested alongside their mothers. Young people eased into familiar adult roles and responsibilities. As they grew older, expectations were clear—they had only to look at their parents and grandparents to glimpse their own futures. As soon as they were physically able, youth of the past were expected to do adult work and to keep doing it generation after generation.

Not everyone in pre-industrial America lived on a farm, of course. Children of nonfarmers were assigned defined roles leading to adult occupations. Wealthy shipping merchants sent sons, sometimes as young as nine years old, to become cabin boys in preparation for eventually entering papa's business. Other boys left home at twelve or thirteen to become plowboys, errand boys, or apprentices to craftsmen, particularly when their parents had younger mouths to feed. Boys could begin apprenticeships to lawyers or doctors by age sixteen, and many began to practice their professions by seventeen or eighteen.

Girls, too, left home for economic reasons. According to the 1830 census, there were more fifteen- to nineteen-year-old girls than boys in the cities of New England. Because the predominantly agricultural economy valued boys more highly than girls, young women moved to towns and cities to work as teachers, factory workers, or shop clerks.[3]

As America rapidly industrialized in the second half of the 1800s, thousands of youth migrated to cities in search of new occupations and more education. But urban migration was disruptive. It left young people without role models or family structure and caused rifts between generations. Until this time, most young people grew up in multigenerational families. Once on their own in the cities, they relied on their contemporaries more than on their parents and grandparents. By 1900, even younger children who remained on the farm were spending more time in school with their peers. All of these changes led to a greater segregation of youth and diminished communication between generations.

As young people became less dependent on their families, adults other than parents began to organize activities to mold character and "keep them out of trouble." Youth groups, clubs, and religious organizations sprung up to occupy adolescents' time. Most were run by adults who imparted religious or moral values and tried to protect youth "from the alien culture of big cities."[4]

Twentieth-Century Adolescence

With the dawn of the twentieth century, adolescence began to take on a different meaning. Educators, social workers, psychologists, and urban reformers reconstructed the concept of adolescence. The leading architect of a modern view of adolescence was Granville Stanley Hall, a psychologist and educator who in 1904 published a two-volume text on adolescence. Strongly influenced by Charles Darwin, Hall believed that each individual goes through all evolutionary stages since time began. In other words, the human embryo passes through amphibian and reptilian phases before becoming mammalian. Hall proposed a parallel for psychological development: each human goes through stages that correspond to all of human history. He believed that adolescence corresponds to the era of savagery and adulthood to the era of civilization.

Hall's belief that behavior was biologically determined was discredited by social scientists of the 1920s who emphasized the roles of environment and culture. Despite this, one of Hall's ideas endured for most of this century. That was the characterization of adolescence as a turbulent period, a time of particular sensitivity and inner turmoil. Hall was not the originator of this idea. He extrapolated it from German writers like Goethe and Schiller who led an eighteenth-century literary movement called Sturm und Drang (Storm and Stress), which emphasized romantic, youthful idealism and rebellion against tradition.

Hall's view of adolescent storm and stress was supported by many influential psychoanalysts such as Anna Freud and Erik Erikson. It was countered, however, by anthropologist Margaret Mead, who published a landmark study on adolescence in 1928. Dr. Mead spent three years in Samoa addressing the questions, "Are the disturbances which vex our (American) adolescents due to the nature of adolescence itself or to the civilisation? Under different conditions does adolescence present a different picture?"[5] She concluded that "adolescence is not necessarily a time of stress and strain, but that cultural conditions make it so. . . . The stress is in our civilisation, not in the physical changes through which our children pass."[6]

Adolescence in the 1990's

Recent research suggests that up to 40 percent of American youth progress through adolescence smoothly, without much storm and stress. The other 60 percent experience varying degrees of confusion, frustration, and uneasy change.

Every stage of life brings change, but why is adolescence often a more difficult transition than other stages? What makes it uniquely challenging and risky? Some answers lie in the fact that adolescents today confront a new set of health problems, distinct from those of earlier generations. The advent of antibiotics and improved medical technology has shifted the balance from traditional medical problems, such as infections and cancer, to problems with a social basis. The traditional medical problems certainly have not disappeared— up to two million adolescents continue to have serious medical or psychiatric illnesses—but many more teenagers experience health problems that are the result of their environment or their behavior. The most serious problems of youth today fall into the following categories:

Injury and violence. Nearly 80 percent of deaths among youth ages fifteen to twenty-four are caused by injury and violence. Motor vehicle injuries alone are the leading cause of death among adolescents, and half of these incidents involve drinking and driving. The homicide rate has tripled among fifteen- to twenty-four-year-olds in the past thirty years and has doubled among younger teenagers (ages ten to fourteen) in the past twenty years.

Depression and suicide. Mental health problems affect over 600,000 American adolescents. Of all the disabilities among ten- to eighteen-year-olds, one-third are due to mental disorders. In the past twenty years, the suicide rate has tripled among ten- to fourteen-year-olds and has doubled among fifteen- to nineteen-year-olds. For every adolescent who commits suicide, an estimated 50 to 200 adolescents attempt it.

Alcohol and drug use. Nearly 90 percent of high school seniors report some experimentation with alcohol. Over a quarter of these seniors report binge drinking (at least five drinks at one time) within the past two weeks. A 1991 Report of the Surgeon General revealed that more than half of junior and senior high school students (10.6 to 20.7 million seventh through twelfth graders) drink alcohol. Eight million of them drink weekly; three million drink alone; and four million drink when they are upset. The Report also showed that teenagers know very little about alcohol. Almost 80 percent do not know that a twelve-ounce can of beer contains as much alcohol as a shot of whiskey. One in three does not know that a wine cooler contains alcohol. Over five million are unsure about the age at which it is legal to buy alcohol.

Over 40 percent of seniors have used marijuana or another illicit drug at some time in their lives. Despite a decline in cigarette smoking among adults, there has been little or no decline in smoking among adolescents in the past decade. Nearly 30 percent of high school seniors said they had smoked in the past month, and 19 percent reported smoking every day.

Pregnancy. One million teenagers become pregnant each year. Four of every ten girls who turn fourteen this year will be pregnant before they turn twenty. Pregnancy is the most common reason for school dropout among girls. Perhaps because of their limited education, adolescent mothers are seven times more likely to live below the poverty level than are older mothers. Although 80 percent of adolescent pregnancies are unintended, 70 percent of sexually active adolescent girls do not use contraception regularly.

Sexually transmitted disease. Over half of all adolescents aged fifteen to nineteen have had sexual intercourse and one-quarter of these youth have at least one sexually transmitted disease before leaving high school. In the past thirty years, gonorrhea has increased fourfold among ten- to fourteen-year-olds and threefold among fifteen- to nineteen-year-olds. Of greatest concern is the rate of infection with HIV (human immunodeficiency virus). Although AIDS (acquired immunodeficiency syndrome) is far less common among teenagers than adults, the long period of time between infection and illness makes it likely that many adults with AIDS were infected during adolescence.

These problems have enormous ramifications both for the individual adolescent and for society as a whole. With appropriate health care and education, some of these problems are preventable. Unfortunately, many teenagers face serious barriers to care, including concerns about confidentiality and payment, unavailability of age-appropriate services, and confusion about how to coordinate various components of health service, such as family planning, general medical care, and counseling. Increased awareness of these barriers is resulting in a growing number of programs for adolescent health at many levels: schools, communities, federal and state legislation, and organized medicine. As we approach the twenty-first century, these efforts may help reverse the disturbing statistics reported above.

New Survivors and Longer Adolescence

Against this background, two other issues set today's concept of adolescence apart from that of earlier generations:

Chronic disease and disability. Some 84 percent of children with chronic disease or disability now survive at least to young adulthood. This is a radical change from a generation ago. Modern medical science has increased the survival rate and has helped to improve the quality of life for thousands of young people who might have died in infancy or childhood if they had been born twenty years earlier. These survivors enter young adulthood with unique health needs. As the first generation to conquer previously fatal conditions, these brave young people are traveling uncharted territory. Some may struggle with delayed growth, others with the long-term side efects of their treatment, others with relapse of their disease. All must adjust to an adult world in which there are few role models.

Duration of adolescence. The teenage years now encompass more than ages thirteen to nineteen. Adolescence begins earlier and lasts longer than it did in other times. In developed countries like the United States, improved nutrition and higher economic standards have contributed to earlier physical development. The average age when puberty begins in both girls and boys has decreased since the turn of the century. "Puberty" is a biological term referring to sexual maturation: the start of menstruation, breast development, genital growth, and secondary sex characteristics such as facial, axillary (underarm), and pubic hair. "Adolescence" is a broader term that incorporates biology with social, psychological, and cultural factors. It may begin as early as age eight and last into the twenties.

The average age of menarche, when a girl begins to menstruate, has fallen about two months each decade in the United States. In 1877, the average age was 14.75 years. By 1900, it was fourteen years, and in 1947 it was 12.8 years. The downward trend has leveled off since then, with recent estimates between 12.5 and 12.8 years.

In the eighteenth century, the voices of teenage boys in Bach choirs changed at about age eighteen. Today the average age is 13.3. As with girls, the age of puberty in boys has stabilized as better nutrition has become more widely available.

The earlier onset of puberty has meant that society places heavier responsibilities on youth at a younger age. Children now learn about drugs, sex, and AIDS in elementary school. Culturally, they are growing up faster than ever—fourth-grade girls are wearing makeup and many, despite normal weights, are dieting.

At the other end of the spectrum, adolescence has been stretched well beyond age twenty-one. Countless young adults in college and graduate or professional schools remain economically dependent on their parents. Relying on Mom and Dad for tuition, room, and board may entail more than just financial support. If Dad's car is borrowed, Dad may well expect to know where the twenty-five-year-old is going, with whom, for how long. Mom may still be doing the laundry, straightening the collar, reminding her adult child to eat regularly. The adult child may chafe at this "interference." As long as there is economic dependency, whether living with or without parents, the child is still trying to carve out personal identity and autonomy.

The gradual lengthening of adolescence has been going on for much of this century, but a new twist has been noticed recently: more and more adults in their mid-twenties to early thirties are living with their parents. According to a 1990 Census Bureau survey, 32 percent of single men and 20 percent of single women between the ages of twenty-five and thirty-four were living with their parents. Between 1970 and 1990, the proportion of both married and single individuals in this age bracket increased markedly: from 9.5 percent to 15 percent for men and 6.6 percent to 8.1 percent for women.

Young adults may decide to live with parents because they cannot find jobs, because they cannot afford homes of their own, or because their parents are elderly, widowed, or divorced. Older mothers, who would otherwise live alone, may enjoy the adult child's companionship and the security of having another person at home. For the young adult, living costs might be lower and day-to-day needs, such as shopping, cooking, and laundry, may be taken care of by the parent.

What is the significance of this trend? In a psychological sense, although puberty is long completed, adolescence is prolonged. From the perspective of health, parents may still be responsible for the young adult's medical bills and may continue to worry that their grown child eats well, gets enough sleep, exercises, and prevents disease. Parents, in a sense, remain the gatekeepers of their adult child's health.

In a highly technical society like ours, where there are enough workers to go around and where a surplus often exists, adolescence can become a holding pattern. Unlike an agrarian society, where every individual is needed in the field, an industrial/technological society tends to reward more education. As a result, employment is delayed. Young people today often remain in school longer, dependent on parental help well beyond the teenage years.

The worldwide social impact of a longer adolescence may become immense in the twenty-first century. In the past twenty years, the fifteen- to twenty-four-year-old population rose by 66 percent, compared to a 46 percent increase across all age groups. By the year 2000, an estimated 84 percent of the world's 1.2 billion youth will live in developing countries. These young people will constitute both the greatest resource and the greatest risk for the developing world in the twenty-first century. Problems now common in industrialized nations may reach a vast global population. It will be a tremendous challenge to governments and individuals to monitor development, treat and prevent disease, and smooth the transition from childhood to adulthood.

The Tasks of Adolescence

The markers of adult status are imprecise, but experts who study adolescence generally agree that the passage from childhood to adulthood encompasses several psychological and social tasks. When the teenager has mastered these tasks, he or she has graduated from adolescence:

Establishment of autonomy. This task requires that adolescents become emotionally and economically independent of their parents. Some children seem to assert their independence from infancy, but most begin to struggle for autonomy at ages twelve to fourteen. Early adolescents may show less interest in family activities and more resistance to parents' advice. By mid-adolescence (ages fifteen to seventeen), the peer group assumes primary social importance in a teenager's life and family conflict is likely to be at its peak. This diminishes in late adolescence as the eighteen- to twenty-one-year-old establishes independence and an identity apart from the family.

Psychosocial and psychosexual development. This task is really made up of four parts: the acceptance of physical change, the establishment of peer relationships, the development of responsible behavior, and the evolution of a personal value system consistent with the social environment.

The rapid physical changes of puberty—breast development, menarche, growth spurt, secondary sex characteristics—usually produce a preoccupation with self. Teenagers are concerned about normalcy—"Is what's happening to my body normal?" And they closely compare their own physical development with that of other teenagers.

In early adolescence, peer group involvement tends to be same-sex, with strong, often idealized, friendships. As they reach the end of puberty—that is, when they have reached sexual maturity—teenagers are less preoccupied with bodily changes and more interested in the dress and social codes of their peers. Dating and sexual experimentation start to replace the larger, same-sex networks of early adolescence.

The timing of physical changes (which will be discussed in detail in the next chapter) may affect social performance during early and mid-puberty. Boys who mature early tend to be taller, stronger, better at team sports, and judged "older" than boys who mature more gradually but who eventually catch up. For some girls, early maturation can be a social disadvantage. Their onset of puberty may be perfectly within the normal range, but they may need more reassurance about their development than do girls who mature later.

While physical changes affect a teenager's social performance, cognitive changes during puberty may affect school performance. The concrete thinking of childhood decreases as the young adolescent begins to deal with more abstract concepts. High schools rely on the development of abstract thinking when they introduce subjects such as algebra, geometry, and physics. Young teenagers who remain at the level of concrete thinking may have unexpected difficulty with these subjects until the ability to reason abstractly develops.

Daydreaming is common and normal during adolescence. The new ability to think in the abstract produces an array of insights and cognitive innovations. Daydreaming is just as important in adolescence as fantasy play is in childhood.

The capacity for future orientation. This final task usually occurs in late adolescence when self-consciousness about physical changes has passed and when skirmishes for independence are waning. Cognitive maturity brings an adult perspective of time so that older teenagers are now able to think about setting realistic goals: "What do I want to do with my life? What career and life-style choices shall I make?"

With this new ability to look toward the future, older adolescents begin to make vocational and life-style decisions that will establish them as contributing members of society. They expect to be treated as adults and usually are capable of managing adult responsibilities.

Today's young people have more time and space to master these tasks because adolescence has become longer. With more time comes more opportunity to interact with parents and to wrestle with their own inner struggles. Ironically, the legal age of majority has dropped even as adolescence has stretched into the adult years. In most American states, Canadian provinces, and European countries, the legal age has dropped from twenty-one to eighteen or nineteen. This can be confusing and frustrating to a teenager: "I can drive a car at sixteen (in most states), vote and serve in the military at eighteen, but I can't buy alcohol until I'm twenty-one! Just when am I considered an adult, anyway?"

It is helpful for parents and teenagers to keep in mind that the transition to adulthood will not be perfectly smooth for any individual. By recognizing that the biological, psychological, and social aspects of an adolescent's life are interwoven, we can help to integrate these threads into a smoother whole. Adults can support teenagers by providing resources that ease adjustment. In particular, parents and teenagers can approach health professionals for guidance in understanding the biological changes of puberty and in managing the health concerns associated with maturation. A place to begin is the next chapter, which discusses normal growth and development during adolescence.

2
Normal Growth and Development

The human body is in transition at every age, but adolescence stands apart because of the rapidity and magnitude of the physical changes that occur during these years. Puberty, the biological process of reproductive maturation, affects virtually every tissue in the body. Consider the following:

• Forty percent of an adult's ideal weight and 25 percent of height are achieved during adolescence.

• In boys, the weight of the heart doubles and blood pressure increases during puberty. In girls, heart weight and blood pressure increase less and stabilize earlier.

• In boys and girls, the filling capacity of the lung increases and the rate of breathing decreases.

• The brain reaches its adult size by early adolescence, but there is a slow evolution from the low-frequency brain waves of childhood to the more rapid waves of adulthood.

• The lymphoid system grows rapidly during late childhood and early adolescence. This network of small vessels flushes fluid from the tissues into small bean-shaped nodes located throughout the body. By age twelve, these lymph nodes are twice as large as they will be at age twenty. It is not uncommon, therefore, for teenagers to feel pea-sized lymph nodes in the neck, groin, or under the arms. Any node that is persistently larger than pea-size should be examined by a doctor.

"How Much Will I Grow?"

Growth is influenced by genes, hormones, nutrition, and environmental factors such as climate and season. All interact in a complex dance within every individual. Genes and environment vary from one teenager to another, whereas hormones are fairly similar. A basic knowledge of hormones is necessary to understand the mysteries and magic of adolescent growth and development.

Hormones are chemicals secreted into the bloodstream by the endocrine, or ductless, glands. Like an agent on a mission, each hormone has a designated job and specific targets. Two types of hormones, called growth hormone and thyroid hormone, regulate growth throughout childhood. During adolescence, these two hormones take a backseat to the sex hormones in determining growth. The sex hormones—androgens, estrogens, and progesterone—are produced in both sexes but in different sites and concentrations. In late childhood, the brain sends a hormonal message to the ovaries, the testes, and the adrenal glands that it is time to wake up and produce sex hormones. This is the beginning of puberty.

Once it begins, puberty progresses in a very predictable way on a population-wide basis. That is, the stages follow each other in a consistent sequence when large numbers of teenagers are studied. However, for the *individual* teenager, the sequence and timing may differ from that of the population. In other words, the onset and progression of puberty vary from one teenager to another. The most visible proof can be found in any eighth- or ninth-grade classroom. Some boys may be pushing five feet and 100 pounds. Others have already hit six feet and are as thin as beanpoles or as hefty as linebackers. Those in the middle height range differ in weight, muscle development, and secondary sex characteristics. During these years, girls tend to appear more mature than boys. But they too will vary widely in the stage of puberty. Some still look childlike while others look like young adults.

The common denominator is that all teenagers in early adolescence are concerned about their growth and development in comparison with their peers—"Do I look like my friends?" The tendency to compare self with peers can produce confusion and, at times, unnecessary alarm. Parents and other adults can reassure adolescents by pointing out that while there is a broad range, 90 to 95 percent of all teenagers fall within normal growth patterns.

Adolescents who are developing more slowly than their friends will catch up. Those who shoot up early will slow down. Another way to consider it is this: during adolescence, an individual's age in years or grade in school may not correlate with his or her height, weight, or sexual maturity.

Growth Curves

Ever since the child's first visit to a physician, many parents have been shown growth curves with their child's height and weight plotted along them. Growth curves pool all American children and come up with a distribution in height and weight from birth to age eighteen (Figures 2.1 and 2.2). Only 5 percent of children at each end of the spectrum—the smallest children, below the fifth percentile, and the largest children, above the ninety-five percentile—are considered to be outside the normal range. In other words, out of every 100 children, five are considered smaller than normal and five are considered larger than normal. The remaining ninety children, between the fifth and ninety-fifth percentiles, are considered to be normal in height and weight. This normal range, however, is filled with individual variation.

Throughout childhood, most youngsters grow steadily along the same growth curve. Because there is little spread between the curves in early childhood and little difference in the growth of boys compared to girls, a three-year-old who falls in the twenty-fifth percentile for height or weight does not look very different than a three-year-old who falls in the seventy-fifth percentile. But in adolescence, there is a much wider spread between the curves and much more difference by gender. Jennifer, a seventeen-year-old girl in the twenty-fifty percentile for height and weight, is three and a half inches shorter and twenty-six pounds lighter than Lisa, also seventeen, who is in the seventy-fifty percentile. Jennifer is also five inches shorter and twenty pounds lighter than Daniel, a seventeen-year-old boy who is also in the twenty-fifth percentile.

Consider another three friends, all within six months of each other in age: Ben is at the tenth percentile for height. Charlie is at the ninetieth. Josh is smack in the middle, at the fiftieth percentile. Josh may feel the most normal, but Ben and Charlie are equally normal. Just as adults vary widely in height, so do teenagers. While the adult's stature is constant, the adolescent's is rapidly changing. This change can confuse or complicate the adolescent's tendency to compare his or her development with that of friends.

GROWTH CURVES, FEMALE

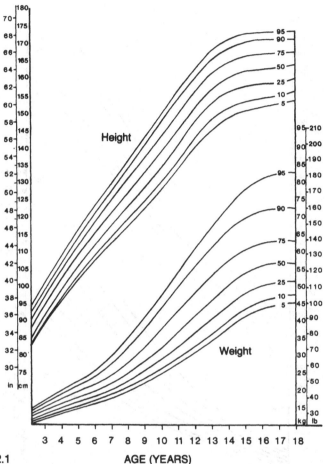

Figure 2.1   AGE (YEARS)

Growth curves show the normal range of height and weight. The National Center for Health Statistics constructed growth charts by pooling height and weight data of American children between ages 2 and 18. The seven curved lines for height and the other seven curved lines for weight represent *percentiles,* or statistical measurements based on 100 individuals.

To plot her percentile in height, a girl should find her age along the bottom of the chart and her height (inches or centimeters) along the left side of the chart. She should draw a vertical line up from her age and a horizontal line from her height to the right until it meets the vertical line. The point where the lines meet shows her percentile ranking. For example, a 15-year-old girl who is 62 inches (157 cm) tall is at the 25th percentile for height. This means that among 100 15-year-old girls, she is taller than 24 and shorter than 75 girls. She can plot her weight percentile in the same way by drawing a vertical line from her age and a horizontal line from her weight (kilograms or pounds) on the right side of the chart.

Measurements taken over the years and recorded on the growth curve chart will show an individual's growth pattern.

GROWTH CURVES, MALE

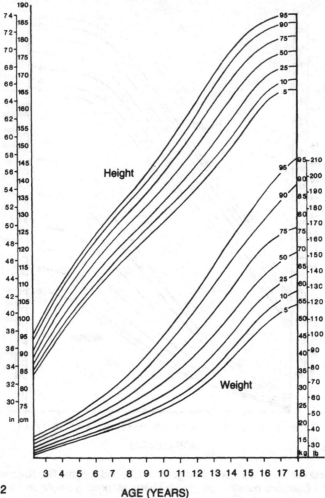

Figure 2.2   AGE (YEARS)

Growth curves show the normal range of height and weight. The National Center for Health Statistics constructed growth charts by pooling height and weight data of American children between ages 2 and 18. The seven curved lines for height and the other seven curved lines for weight represent *percentiles*, or statistical measurements based on 100 individuals.

To plot his percentile in height, a boy should find his age along the bottom of the chart and his height (inches or centimeters) along the left side of the chart. He should draw a vertical line up from his age and a horizontal line from his height to the right until it meets the vertical line. The point where the lines meet shows his percentile ranking. For example, a 14-year-old boy who is 68 inches (173 cm) tall is at the 90th percentile for height. This means that among 100 14-year-old boys, he is taller than 89 and shorter than 10 boys. He can plot his weight percentile in the same way by drawing a vertical line from his age and a horizontal line from his weight (kilograms or pounds) on the right side of the chart.

Measurements taken over the years and recorded on the growth curve chart will show an individual's growth pattern.

Stages of Sexual Maturity

The hallmark of adolescence is sexual maturation. This involves breast development, genital development, secondary sexual characteristics (such as change in voice or growth of facial hair), and the ability to reproduce. The many facets of sexual maturation make it difficult to determine how far into puberty a teenager is. And the stage of puberty is an important part of an adolescent's overall assessment because it determines how much time remains for growth. Once sexual maturation is complete, growth in height ceases.

A useful method for assessing sexual maturation was developed by Dr. James M. Tanner and his colleagues. Dr. Tanner identified five stages that could be rated by physical examination. These sexual maturity ratings, or Tanner stages, occur in a predictable sequence. It is important to keep in mind that the age of onset and the rate of progression from one stage to the next—the "tempo," as Dr. Tanner called them—are highly variable from one teenager to another, even within the same family.

Tanner stages may sound simple and straightforward, but interpreting them accurately for any individual can be difficult even for a health professional. It may be helpful for parents and teenagers to know the sequence of the Tanner stages, but they should not attempt to interpret the stages rigidly. It is wiser to discuss them with a health care professional who has examined many adolescents and is experienced at interpreting the standards.

GIRLS

When the physician or nurse examines an adolescent girl, two ratings of sexual maturity are noted. One rating applies to breast development (Figure 2.3). The second rating applies to pubic hair development (Figure 2.4). These two aspects of development are rated separately rather than averaged because they may proceed differently.

The breast stage is based on breast contour, not on breast size. The contour refers to the shape of the breast, the areola (the pigmented ring surrounding the nipple), and the nipple. The five Tanner stages for breast development are as follows:

THE STAGES OF BREAST DEVELOPMENT IN FEMALES

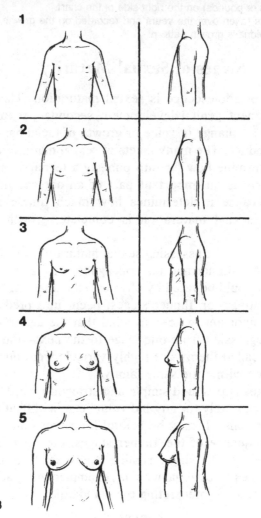

Figure 2.3

1. The first stage for girls is called prepubertal because there are no signs of breast development.
2. The second stage consists of early breast budding.
3. The third stage brings an elevation of the breast and the areola.
4. The fourth stage is marked by the projection of the areola and nipple above the breast itself.
5. By the fifth stage, the breasts are mature. The areola has flattened to the level of the breast and only the nipple projects.

Sexual maturity ratings based on pubic hair development for girls are as follows:

THE STAGES OF PUBIC HAIR DEVELOPMENT IN FEMALES

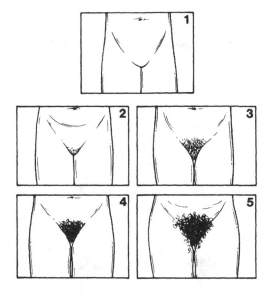

Figure 2.4

1. There is no pubic hair.
2. A few straight or slightly curled hairs appear, usually over the labia.
3. Pubic hair becomes darker, more curled, and coarser.
4. Moderate to abundant pubic hair now extends above the labia.
5. The hair is adult in appearance, with extension to the thighs.

Puberty in girls begins with breast development between ages eight and thirteen. The growth spurt, when height increases most rapidly, usually occurs about one year before her first menstrual period (called menarche). A girl may reach nearly her full height before menarche, and most girls stop growing within two years after menarche. The average age of menarche in America is 12.8 years, but the normal range for American girls falls between 10.8 and 14.6 years of age.

The average length of puberty in girls is four years, though it can be as short as one and a half years or as long as five years and still be considered normal.

BOYS

Tanner stages for boys are also divided into two separate sexual maturity ratings, one based on genitalia (Figure 2.5) and the second on pubic hair development (Figure 2.6). First, the sequence of genital maturation:

THE STAGES OF GENITAL DEVELOPMENT IN MALES

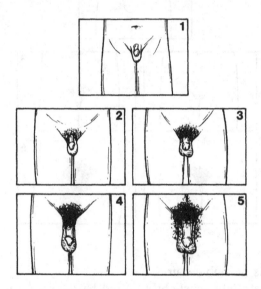

Figure 2.5

1. The first Tanner stage for boys is prepubertal. The penis, testes, and scrotum are of childhood size.
2. The second stage is marked by an enlargement of the scrotum and testes, with reddening of the scrotal skin.
3. The third stage brings lengthening of the penis and further enlargement of the testes and scrotum.
4. In the fourth stage, the scrotum and testes continue to grow. The size of the penis increases in both length and breadth.
5. In the fifth stage, the genitalia are adult in size and shape.

The five Tanner stages based on pubic hair development in boys include:

THE STAGES OF PUBIC HAIR DEVELOPMENT IN MALES

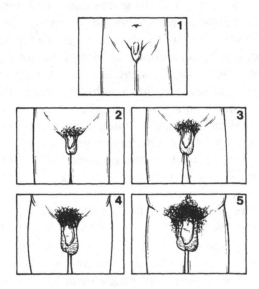

Figure 2.6

1. There is no pubic hair.
2. Straight or slightly curled hair appears at the base of the penis.
3. Pubic hair becomes darker, more curled, and coarser.
4. Pubic hair is now adultlike, though it covers a smaller area than in the adult.
5. Pubic hair now extends to the thighs.

Puberty for boys usually begins with testicular enlargement between ages 9.5 and 13.5. As puberty progresses, sperm are produced. A boy generally experiences his first ejaculation between ages twelve and fourteen. For most boys, the growth spurt occurs between ten and sixteen, and the full height is reached by seventeen or eighteen. The average duration of puberty in boys is three years, but can range from two to five years. While puberty begins later in boys than in girls, its shorter time span in boys results in similar ages at which both sexes complete puberty.

Sexual Maturation and Height

The sexual maturity ratings, or Tanner stages, are closely corre-lated with other pubertal events, such as menarche and the growth spurt. Tanner stages can help to gauge how much more time an adolescent has to grow. A teenage boy, for example, who is worried about being too short and who is Tanner stage two for both gentalia and pubic hair, can be reassured that he still has time to grow. In contrast, a boy who is Tanner stage five has already experienced his growth spurt and probably has reached his final adult height.

For girls, the height spurt tends to occur at Tanner stage two or three. At the peak of her growth spurt, a girl may grow 2.4 to 4.2 inches (6 to 10.5 cm, or centimeters) a year. In 95 percent of all girls, the most rapid growth occurs between 9.7 and 13.3 years of age, at an average age of 11.5 years. Most girls reach their final adult height by age sixteen.

For boys, the growth spurt for height comes later, usually at Tanner stage four. A boy may grow 2.8 to 4.8 inches (7 to 12 cm) a year during his growth spurt. In 95 percent of all boys, this occurs between 11.7 and 15.3 years of age, at an average age of 13.5 years. Most boys reach their final adult height by age eighteen.

It is important to remember that the timing of the growth spurt does not predict the final adult height. Teenagers who enter the growth spurt earlier than their peers usually stop growing earlier. Teenagers who enter the growth spurt later tend to grow more quickly over a shorter period of time. Consequently, the average adult height for early and late maturers is the same. Two other relevant points about growth spurts:

• For both boys and girls, these periods of rapid growth last an average of two to three years.
• Many factors affect the tempo of growth. For example, in tem-perate climates, children grow more quickly in spring and summer than in winter. Because of the many factors that can affect growth, it is not unusual to see little change in height over a two- or three-month period, followed by a large change over the next few months. It is incorrect to decide that an adolescent is growing too slowly just because his or her height did not change between December and February. The rate of growth should be determined over at least a six- to twelve-month interval.

Predicting the final adult height that an adolescent will reach is difficult and inexact. A doctor can use the adolescent's age, sexual maturity rating, and current height to make some estimation. The parents' height also is somewhat predictive of the teenager's final height. The most accurate method requires an X-ray study of the adolescent's hand and wrist to determine the *bone age*. Standards have been developed that describe the way in which the bones grow at any given age. By comparing the adolescent's X-ray with the set of standards, the adolescent's bone age can be determined.

The most accurate method for predicting adult height is based on the adolescent's current height, bone age, and chronological age. For the vast majority of teenagers, however, assessing the bone age is unnecessary. The bone age is most useful when growth is not following a normal pattern.

Weight Gain

Weight gain normally peaks during the height spurt. The weight that is gained during the teenage years accounts for over 40 percent of the ideal adult weight for both sexes. But the pattern and composition of the weight gain differ in girls and boys.

When a girl enters puberty, approximately 16 percent of her body is adipose tissue, or fat. By adulthood, nearly 27 percent of her body mass is fat. This does not mean that a normal-weight little girl becomes an overweight adult woman. Rather, during puberty the composition of her body mass changes: lean body tissue, or muscle, increases less dramatically than does adipose tissue. Because of this shift in the relative proportions of fat and muscle, a girl's lean body mass actually decreases during puberty. She is *not* losing muscle; rather, she is gaining muscle less quickly than she is gaining fat. The increased proportion of fat is very important for normal reproductive development. A certain minimum proportion of the body must be adipose tissue in order for menarche to occur. When a young girl's body fat reaches this critical level, her menstrual periods begin. She then must maintain a certain amount of fat for regular cycles to continue.

For boys, lean body mass increases during puberty. Boys enter puberty with 14 percent body fat. It decreases to 11 percent early in puberty and, if an ideal body weight is maintained, remains constant in adulthood.

Muscle mass peaks for both boys and girls about three months after the height spurt. The increase is twice as great in boys as in girls. Muscle strength generally lags behind muscle mass until boys reach Tanner stage five.

Some Causes of Concern

Almost every teenager wonders from time to time about his or her place along the growth and development path. Many worry about being too tall or too short, too heavy or too thin. As explained earlier, 90 to 95 percent of all teenagers fall within the normal range for height and weight. Yet each proceeds at an individual tempo depending on genetic, environmental, and hormonal factors.

If a teenager is worried about growing too slowly or too fast, it is helpful to look again at his or her growth curves for height and weight since childhood. The growth curves can be constructed from dated notes in the adolescent's childhood medical records, or even from dated scratches or pencil marks on the kitchen doorframe. Take these measurements along to a health care visit. They provide important information for the physician when evaluating an adolescent's concern about growth.

Parents often worry if they notice that a teenager falls off his or her childhood curve. This is not unusual, however, and it is one more bit of evidence that shows how different childhood and adolescence can be. For example, a healthy teenage boy who followed a fiftieth percentile curve steadily through childhood may drop down to the fortieth percentile in early adolescence. This does not mean that his growth is stunted or that he will be a shorter adult than expected. It usually means that puberty and the growth spurt are happening a bit later for him than for the average fiftieth percentile boy. If this is the case, the adolescent will catch up and will be a fiftieth percentile adult.

Another teenager who develops early, with a growth spurt sooner than his peers, will leap above his childhood curve. In two or three years, as the rest of his peers catch up, he will fall back to his earlier percentile.

Deviation from a growth curve need not mean that something is wrong. Teenagers accept this more easily when they understand that the most common reason for the deviation is the timing of puberty—both its onset and its progression. Because growth is so important, however, it is best to discuss concerns about height, weight, and sexual maturation with an experienced physician or nurse.

The media have written and broadcast a great deal of information about hormone therapy to promote growth. Some three million children are born in this country each year and, by definition, 90,000 of them will fall below the third percentile for height. Some children will always be the shortest of the group.

The decision about whether to use hormonal therapy to boost a child's growth is often a difficult one for both parents and physicians. Because growth hormone can now be produced synthetically, availability is no longer an issue. But it is a costly form of therapy whose long-term effects are unclear.

For the vast majority of teenagers, treatment with growth hormone will not alter height and should not be prescribed. On the other hand, the treatment is indicated for children with documented deficiency of growth hormone. Most of these children are recognized and treated long before puberty.

Other types of hormonal therapy may be indicated for some teenagers. For example, growth may be delayed because of hypothyroidism, or a deficiency of thyroid hormone. This is treated easily with a synthetic thyroid hormone in pill form. In another situation, called *constitutional delay* of puberty, a short course of androgen therapy may be indicated. Constitutional delay means that there is no identified reason for the delay in the onset of puberty. A physician has fully evaluated the teenager and has excluded disease, short familial stature, malnutrition, or any other reason that could interfere with growth. Constitutional delay does *not* apply to the teenager who grew along the fifth percentile throughout childhood and is still at the fifth percentile as an adolescent. Rather it may apply to the adolescent who grew along a given curve, has now slowed down substantially, and has drifted further and further from that curve.

For some adolescents with constitutional delay, physicians may give a short (about three months) course of hormone therapy to stimulate puberty and the growth spurt. The hormone that is most commonly used in both boys and girls is an androgen. Short-term androgen therapy is considered safe and effective, and it often helps a teenager whose self-image is seriously impaired by delayed growth. Growth disorders are discussed in greater detail in Chapter 33.

A common concern of teenage boys in *gynecomastia,* or male breast swelling. This typically occurs in young adolescent boys who are at Tanner stage two or three. The area around the nipples may feel tender or lumpy. For the vast majority of boys, gynecomastia does not indicate disease, though it can cause significant embarrassment and worry. Young teenage boys concerned about their sexual identity and development may become confused and frightened by the appearance of breast tissue. Boys should be reassured by a few facts: gynecomastia is very common; it usually disappears without treatment; and there is no relationship between gynecomastia and breast cancer in males.

Over 60 percent of teenage boys experience gynecomastia. It disappears within a year in nearly two out of three boys and lasts over two years in less than 8 percent. When gynecomastia persists into young adulthood, surgery can be considered. Hormonal therapy is not recommended.

The exact cause of gynecomastia is unknown, but it probably is related to the hormonal changes that occur during puberty. The levels of both estrogens ("female" hormones) and androgens ("male" hormones) increase in boys and girls. As the ratios of these hormones adjust, some female characteristics, such as gynecomastia, may appear in males and some male charateristics, such as increased body hair, may appear in females. Gynecomastia may be related to some medications. If a boy with gynecomastia is on medication, or if gynecomastia appears before puberty begins or after it has been completed, a doctor should be consulted.

Most adolescents have some questions or concerns about their own growth and development. It is always best to talk about these issues with a knowledgeable doctor or nurse. Routine health visits, described in the next chapter, are the perfect time to reassess and clarify the adolescent's progress.

3

The Routine Health Examination

Two complementary principles are required to maintain wellness: disease prevention and health promotion. *Prevention* involves avoiding harmful behaviors, substances, foods, and environments. *Promotion* calls for appropriate exercise, hygiene, good nutrition, adequate sleep, regular health examinations, and up-to-date immunizations. Prevention and promotion are two sides of the same coin. Prevention may be viewed as the more passive side—avoiding harm—while promotion demands more active involvement. Both require decision making. Deciding not to smoke a cigarette (disease prevention) is every bit as important as deciding to exercise (health promotion).

Teenagers want to be healthy and strong, active and attractive. Adolescence can be a prime time to learn how to prevent illness and promote optimal health. With support from parents, school personnel, and health professionals, teenagers can begin to develop lifelong health values and practices.

An early step toward health promotion is a visit to a doctor or nurse. "But why? There's nothing wrong with me," a teenager might object. During early childhood, routine physical examinations were accepted as yearly events, but as children become teenagers, they tend to question the reason for these visits unless they are ill. Parents may begin to agree. The physical examination required for school, camp, sports, or employment may seem an unnecessary nuisance for most adolescents. These health care visits, however, provide an opportunity to detect disease or dysfunction and to pre-

29

vent future problems. It is a time to discuss issues that seem too small to warrant an appointment yet worry the teenager or parent. Perhaps most importantly, these visits help to build a relationship between teenager and physician. This relationship makes health promotion more enjoyable and diminishes discomfort and anxiety at times of illness.

An annual checkup gives the physician or nurse an opportunity to keep an eye on the fast-moving changes of the adolescent body. It is a chance to discuss exercise, nutrition, sexuality, and other health issues. The doctor should take some time to talk with the teenager about the reasons to avoid cigarettes, alcohol, and drugs; pregnancy prevention and sexually transmitted disease; seat belts, bicycle helmets, and other injury-prevention measures. Such conversations can help teenagers understand the range of available services and put them at ease when using the health care system.

What Type of Doctor to See

When children reach their teenage years, they and their parents may wonder what type of doctor is most appropriate: a pediatrician? an internist? a family practice physician? a gynecologist?

Many teenagers want to remain with the pediatrician or family physician whom they saw throughout childhood. If the physician sees adolescent-aged patients, there is no reason to suggest a change. The trust and rapport developed over the years can provide important continuity for the adolescent.

Other teenagers may resent seeing a doctor who cares for babies. This is exacerbated when the waiting room is full of toddlers, Dr. Seuss books, and Sesame Street pictures. Many pediatricians in recent years have begun to separate the adolescent medicine component of their practices. Some try to schedule teenagers' appointments close together, after school, or in the early evening. If the teenager expresses discomfort in a pediatric setting, though, it may be time to move on to a physician specializing in adolescent medicine or to an adult-care provider, such as an internist or family practice physician. Teenagers and parents should feel comfortable and confident about the physician's knowledge of the medical, emotional, and social concerns of adolescents.

If all members of the family have visited the same internist or family practitioner for many years, an adolescent may suddenly express the desire to see another physician. The adolescent may feel awkward about talking to the same doctor who sees Mom or Dad. Confidentiality and trust are very important to a teenager. The request to see another health professional is understandable and should be discussed, not discouraged. The family physician can be very helpful in this situation and may suggest that the teenager see a partner in the same medical practice or may recommend another colleague across town.

With girls, the question arises, "When should I see a gynecologist?" An adolescent girl begins to receive gynecological care when she has a gynecological problem or when she becomes sexually active. The term "sexually active" may be unclear to some teenagers. They may not consider themselves sexually active, for example, if they have engaged in sexual intercourse only once. That is incorrect. The term refers to sexual intercourse *ever* (even once) regardless of frequency.

Many pediatricians, internists, and family practitioners are skilled at providing routine gynecological care. They may offer such care, they may suggest that the teenager see a gynecologist, or the teenager herself may want to see a gynecologist. The important factor is that she gets the care she needs.

In our highly mobile society, another question often arises: "How do we find a doctor when we move to a new city or town?" Although adolescent medicine is emerging as a subspecialty in health care, there are still few doctors across the country whose primary practice is the care of teenagers. In many states, there are adolescent clinics, often affiliated with teaching hospitals or medical schools. If you live near a medical school, you may wish to call its hospital and inquire about a specialist in adolescent medicine.

Many communities have established school-based clinics in middle schools and high schools where adolescents can receive comprehensive medical care. The Society for Adolescent Medicine (phone: 816/795-TEEN) can provide the names of its members in your area. The local county medical society can also be helpful in locating a clinic or a physician who provides adolescent care.

"Does Mom or Dad Come with Me to the Doctor?"

Once a physician has been found and an appointment has been scheduled, a teenager or parent may raise a difficult question: "What is the parent's role now?" When the child was younger, Mom or Dad was present throughout every visit. The parent answered the doctor's inquiries, held the child's hand, stayed in the room during the physical examination, dried the tears after an inoculation, and asked questions about the child's health. The child played a more passive part in the medical process.

With increased education and sophistication, the teenager now has the opportunity to become an active health care consumer. For that to happen, parents need to take a smaller role. Specifically, they need to give their teenager time alone with the doctor. Confidentiality becomes very important when an adolescent visits the doctor. A teenager may want to ask the physician questions without a parent present. The physician, as well, may receive more detailed or honest information when the adolescent is alone. No matter how open and loving a parent–teen relationship is, most teenagers do not want Mom in the room when the doctor asks, "Do you smoke cigarettes, drink alcohol, use drugs? Have you had sexual intercourse? Do you always use condoms? Let's spend a few minutes talking about how to prevent pregnancy and sexually transmitted disease."

Some physicians find that one way to handle this situation is to ask parents at the beginning of the visit whether they have any questions or concerns about the teenager's health. The doctor then explains that it is his or her practice to talk with the teenager alone and to do the physical examination while parents wait in the reception room. Later, the parent will be invited to join the adolescent in the doctor's office to discuss any findings or concerns. Most doctors who care for adolescents also assure their patients that any questions or problems will remain confidential, without disclosure to parents, unless the problems are life-threatening or the adolescent has agreed to involve parents.

If a teenager asks to have a parent present during the examination, that is fine. But the teenager, rather than the parent, should answer the doctor's questions. The point of routine health screening during adolescence is not only to prevent disease and promote well-being—it is also to encourage the teenager to become a responsible health care consumer.

Some teenagers may be sensitive to the doctor's gender. A boy may want to see a male physician, or a girl may prefer a female physician. Those preferences should be respected whenever possible. Adolescent females who are anxious about seeing male doctors for gynecologic examinations should be told that a woman (a nurse, receptionist, or her mother) will be present throughout the examination.

What to Expect During a Doctor's Visit

Teenagers about to walk through the physician's door expect to stand on a scale and to be measured for height. They expect the ear checks of childhood, the stethoscope to listen to the heart and lungs, and the reflex hammer to tap the knees. But what else? "What questions will I be asked?" "Will I need to undress?" "What parts of me will be examined?" Adolescent health screening—whether a first visit to a new physician or a return visit to a familiar pediatrician or family doctor—consists of four parts: the medical history, the physical examination, laboratory tests, and the assessment and plan.

The Medical History

On a first visit, a complete medical history should be taken. On subsequent visits, the history will be updated. Some doctors ask a teenage patient to fill out a standard form in the waiting room. The written answers are then followed up verbally when the physician meets with the adolescent. A parent's help usually is needed on questions pertaining to family medical history and the teenager's immunization record. When seeing a new doctor, it is important to bring along past health records. If the adolescent's medical history is complicated, time can be saved if the physicians who previously provided care send copies of their records to the new physician before the first visit.

The medical history includes gathering information about all aspects of the adolescent's health and development—both physical and psychological. It begins with the chief complaint, or the major reason for the visit. If there is a problem, much of the time will be spent discussing the symptoms, when they began, what makes them better or worse, what treatment has been used, etc. The adolescent's past medical history, separate from the chief complaint, then will be discussed. This history includes growth and development, childhood illnesses, hospitalizations, allergies, immunizations, and current medications. The family medical history typically focuses on the ages and health of the adolescent's parents, siblings, and grandparents. The doctor usually will ask if these relatives have had heart disease, high blood pressure, diabetes, high cholesterol, or cancer. Any other diseases in the family also should be noted at this time.

The teenager and doctor will spend time going through a general review of systems, which involves a series of quick questions about any problems with any system of the body. For example: Trouble seeing the blackboard? decreased hearing? rashes? chest pain? trouble breathing? etc. The health form completed by the adolescent before the visit may help the physician identify areas that need to be discussed. This may also be the time to talk about nutrition, exercise, sleep, and dental care. Depending on the physician's style and the adolescent's comfort, nonmedical issues will be discussed. These include some straightforward questions about family, school, activities, and friends. They also include some sensitive questions about family relationships, school performance, self-image, mood, dating, sexual activity, smoking, drinking, and drug use. This discussion should almost always occur when the parent is out of the room.

Certain aspects of a teenager's medical history differ from the history taken during childhood or adulthood. These areas include the following:

GROWTH AND DEVELOPMENT

The history will begin with questions about events before the teenager was even born. The doctor may ask about the mother's health during pregnancy. Is there any possibility that the teenager had been exposed before birth to synthetic hormones taken by the mother? Was the mother's delivery normal?

Questions may be asked about the teenager's infancy: birth weight, feeding history, landmarks of development such as the age at which he or she first talked and walked. The developmental history during childhood includes questions about both physical growth and psychological growth. School history is especially important. The doctor may ask about absenteeism, special classes, grade repetition, testing, academic performance, and peer relationships. Questions about pubertal development will be asked: Age of beginning breast development, genital growth, pubic hair? Age of menarche? Menstrual pattern or pain? Increase in height and weight throughout childhood?

IMMUNIZATIONS

The history will determine if immunizations are up to date. Surveys indicate that many teenagers in the United States are not adequately immunized against infections such as measles, German measles, mumps, and tetanus. Measles outbreaks in schools and on college campuses draw attention to this fact each year. Relying on parents' memory about childhood illnesses or immunizations is not adequate—physicians need dated records. All immunizations should be checked and updated by age fourteen. Specifically:

Tetanus and diphtheria. Adolescents who have never been immunized against tetanus and diphtheria or whose immunization history is questionable should receive three adult-type tetanus–diphtheria (Td) injections. This Td preparation is less likely to cause reactions than the DT or DPT (diphtheria–pertussis–tetanus) preparations used in childhood. The lower case "d" in the Td formulation indicates a smaller dose of the diphtheria vaccine than in the DT or DPT formulation. The first two Td doses for the adolescent who has never been immunized are given one to two months apart and the third is given six to twelve months later. All teenagers and adults who have been fully immunized for tetanus and diphtheria, either in childhood or via this regime, then should receive Td booster shots every ten years throughout life. Most children have completed the primary Td series between ages four and six, so the booster would be given between fourteen and sixteen. If a child has received an extra Td shot because of a cut or wound, the booster should come ten years after that time.

In young children, pertussis vaccine is usually given along with tetanus–diphtheria, but a pertussis shot is not recommended as part of primary immunization after seven years of age because the disease is less common and less severe after this age. Adolescents, therefore, need not receive pertussis boosters.

Measles, mumps, rubella (German measles). Most American teenagers received a measles–mumps–rubella (MMR) shot in childhood, usually between twelve and fifteen months of age. Parents whose children were immunized before the late 1980s often were told that this single MMR injection would provide lifelong immunity. The sporadic outbreaks of measles in the last five to ten years have necessitated a change in that outlook. It now appears that a single measles shot does not provide adequate protection. Adolescents, therefore, should receive a second measles immunization. It is less clear if the mumps and rubella portions of the MMR provide lifelong immunity. Because the combination shot is safe and effective, the MMR generally is given rather than the measles vaccine alone.

Adolescents who were never immunized against measles, and who do not have written confirmation from a doctor that they had the disease measles, must either have a measles (or MMR) shot or have a blood test that confirms that they are immune.

This same recommendation holds for mumps. Parents often consider mumps an uncomfortable but not very serious disease. Complications *do* occur, though, including infection of the brain or spinal fluid (meningoencephalitis). In addition, a common complication of mumps after puberty is orchitis, a painful inflammation of the testes. After the infection has cleared, testicular scarring and infertility may result. Because of these and other complications, all adolescents—male and female—must have a doctor's notation of either having received a mumps shot or having had the disease.

Rubella (commonly called German measles) is usually a mild disease in children and adolescents. But if a pregnant woman contracts rubella, especially during the first three months of pregnancy, serious birth defects can result. To decrease this risk, all children and adolescents—male and female—should be immunized against rubella. A history of the disease is *not* proof of immunity because other infections can mimic rubella. There are only two ways to prove immunity: a doctor's note documenting that a rubella shot (or MMR) was given or a blood test that confirms immunity.

If a teenager's rubella immunization is uncertain and she is pregnant or at risk of soon becoming pregnant, a doctor usually will do the blood test. If reimmunization is warranted, it will not be done until the doctor is certain that the adolescent is not pregnant. The shot will then be given after a normal menstrual period, and the young woman will be advised not to become pregnant for at least three months after the immunization.

Polio. If a teenager under age eighteen has never been vaccinated against polio, or if the immunization is questionable, a three-dose series of oral polio vaccine is recommended. Like the Td series, the first is followed by another after two months and a final dose is given six to twelve months later. If a teenager's immunization was never completed, the missing doses should be given. The oral polio vaccine should not be given to adolescents with immunodeficiency diseases (such as leukemia, cancer, AIDS) or to teenagers who are receiving therapy that impairs the immune system (such as corticosteroids, radiation, chemotherapy).

Tuberculosis. Control of tuberculosis depends in part on a simple skin test to identify infected individuals. The skin test is usually performed in babies at twelve to fifteen months of age, in children about to enter elementary school (ages four to six), and again in adolescence (ages fourteen to sixteen).

If a doctor or nurse determines that a skin test is positive, a chest X-ray will be done. In most cases, the chest X-ray will not show signs of active disease. It usually is recommended that adolescents who have a positive test but no other evidence of disease take a medication called isoniazid (INH) to prevent activation of the infection. The medication usually is given once daily for nine months.

Other vaccines. The influenza vaccine, or "flu shot," is recommended for adolescents with chronic lung disease (including moderate asthma), diabetes, significant heart disease, immunodeficiency due to illness or medication, and chronic kidney disease. It is also given to adolescents with diseases that require long-term aspirin, such as juvenile rheumatoid arthritis, because the aspirin increases the risk of Reye syndrome, a life-threatening liver and brain disease, (Chapters 29 and 34) following influenza infection. The flu shot must be repeated in the early fall of each year, before the flu season begins.

The flu shot generally is not recommended for healthy adolescents. It may be considered, however, for adolescents living in institutions or dormitories where the control of the spread of infection is difficult.

The pneumococcal vaccine is not recommended for healthy adolescents living in the United States. It is recommended for adolescents with diseases that impair their ability to handle infections caused by the pneumococcus bacteria. These diseases include sickle cell disease, absence of a spleen, cancer of the lymph glands, and HIV infection.

The hepatitis B vaccine now is recommended for all children and adolescents. Hepatitis B is a virus that can cause severe liver disease (Chapter 29). The vaccine consists of three injections given over a period of six months.

EXERCISE AND NUTRITION

Exercise and nutrition are also discussed as part of the teenager's medical history. Most adolescents are concerned about their developing bodies and want to know which foods are healthy and which to avoid. In inquiring about a typical day's food intake, the doctor may explain that teenagers require more calories than adults. The average teenage girl consumes approximately 2,200 calories a day and the average boy 2,800, but each person's caloric needs differ, depending on age, size, and physical activity. An early discussion of nutrition and exercise may help prepare the adolescent for dietary adjustments if body weight is too high or low, or if the cholesterol is too high. (More about exercise in Chapter 4 and nutrition in Chapter 5.)

FAMILY HISTORY

The comprehensive medical history includes the history of the adolescent's family. If there is concern about the adolescent's growth or development, the physician may ask about the height, weight, or ages at puberty of the parents, siblings, or grandparents. As noted earlier, family history always includes questions about diseases within the family. In particular, the doctor may ask about heart disease, high blood pressure, and high cholesterol in family members because these problems tend to run in families and, in some cases, can be prevented if the risk is detected early (Chapter 28).

PSYCHOLOGICAL, SOCIAL, AND SEXUAL HISTORY

The information discussed so far has been medical. Most adolescents will readily answer questions about diet, exercise, and family medical history. Other parts of the medical history may surprise some teenagers unless they understand that physicians must go beyond strictly medical questions to assess overall health.

A comprehensive medical history includes questions about school, family relationships, emotions, sexual activity, and drug use. Such questions are not intended to be "nosy." They are part of routine health screening for *all* teenagers. When doctors ask these questions, they are trying to gather information that may help prevent future problems, such as unintended pregnancy or sexually transmitted disease. Many adolescents worry about the confidentiality of their responses. If the doctor has not clarified whether parents will be informed, the teenager has every right to ask the doctor about confidentiality before answering the questions.

The overriding goal of this part of the history is to evaluate how well the teenager is progressing with the developmental tasks of adolescence (Chapter 1). By asking broad, open-ended questions, the doctor can gather health-related information and can give the teenager a chance to discuss issues that are troubling or confusing. The types of questions a doctor may ask include:

"How are you getting along with your parents? Your brothers and sisters?"

"How is school going? What extracurricular activities are you doing? What are your special interests, hobbies?"

"Do you have a job? How many hours a week are you working? Are you feeling tired during the day?"

"How are you getting along with your friends? Do you have a best friend?"

"How do you handle the situation when your friends are drinking? Do any of them drink and drive? What would you do if a friend was drinking and tried to drive? Do your friends use drugs?"

"Have you ever smoked a cigarette? How much do you smoke? Have you tried alcohol? Where do you drink?"

"Have you tried marijuana? What about other drugs?"

"Do you go to parties? Have you begun to date? Do you have a boyfriend? a girlfriend? Have you had a sexual relationship with anyone? Have these relationships been with males? females? both? What do you do to prevent pregnancy? Do you use condoms? How often?"

"Do you wear a seat belt every time you ride in a car? Do you skateboard? Ride a bike or motorcycle? Do you wear a helmet?"

Some teenagers may wonder why a doctor would ask such questions. They give the physician a chance to mention that adolescence may be a time of trying new and sometimes risky things that can result in injury or illness. The doctor is not prying or lecturing, but offering information and opening the door to treatment or counseling if the teenager needs it.

Similarly, when the physician asks about a teenager's mood or relationships with friends and family, the intent is to assess and guide. Some of the emotional illnesses of adulthood begin to emerge during adolescence, and depression is more common during adolescence than during childhood. The doctor asks these questions to determine whether the teenager needs help now. The same holds true for questions about sexual activity. Early discussion and counseling are essential parts of the visit because most individuals have sexual intercourse before they leave their teen years.

The Physical Examination

Once the physician and the adolescent have completed the history, the physical examination begins. The teenager will be asked to undress and to put on a cloth or paper robe. On a first visit, a complete physical examination is done. On follow-up visits, the examination may be limited to those parts of the body where a problem was detected or a symptom occurred. A complete physical examination includes the following:

> Height and weight
> Tanner staging (sexual maturation ratings)
> Blood pressure, heart rate, respiratory (breathing) rate
> Visual acuity (using an eye chart)
> Hearing check
> Hair, skin, nails
> Head, eyes, ears, nose, mouth, teeth, gums, and throat
> Neck and thyroid gland
> Lymph nodes
> Breasts
> Chest and lungs
> Heart, pulses in the arms and legs
> Abdomen
> Back
> Extremities (arms and legs)
> Nervous system
> External genitalia (males and females)
> Pelvic examination (for females, if indicated)

Some parts of the teenager's physical examination differ from those for children or adults. For example, Tanner staging is done to evaluate the adolescent's progression through puberty. Height and weight change very rapidly in adolescence, coincident with the growth spurt. Blood pressure may begin to climb, especially in boys, and pulse rate decreases. Acne peaks in mid- to late adolescence and affects 85 percent of teenagers. The child with 20/20 vision may become an adolescent who needs glasses to see the blackboard because of a change in the shape of the lens during puberty. The lymph nodes grow rapidly in late childhood and early adolescence and often are easily felt in the neck, under the arms, or in the groin.

Gynecomastia, or breast enlargement in boys, occurs frequently during adolescence. Up to 40 percent of adolescents have heart murmurs discovered on routine examinations, the majority of which do *not* indicate underlying heart disease. Examination of the back and spine is extremely important because scoliosis, or curvature of the spine (Chapter 31), is present in about 5 percent of teenagers. If scoliosis is suspected from this examination, the doctor may refer the teenager for an X-ray of the spine or to an orthopedist (a doctor specializing in bone conditions).

The breast examination may cause anxiety in adolescent girls, especially if there is a family history of breast cancer. Breast cancer is exceedingly rare during adolescence. Benign breast lumps, called fibroadenomas, are common during adolescence and often disappear after one or two menstrual cycles. Girls should be shown how to examine their breasts monthly, after their menstrual periods. Any breast lump that persists beyond two menstrual periods should be reported to the doctor (Chapter 26).

THE PELVIC EXAMINATION

An internal examination of the vagina, cervix, uterus, and ovaries is indicated for adolescent females who have a history of sexual intercourse, vaginal discharge, pelvic pain, severe menstrual pain, or heavy menstrual bleeding. If none of these indications exist, the first pelvic examination usually is done between ages sixteen and twenty-one.

During the pelvic examination, the adolescent is asked to lie on her back with her knees apart. If the physician is a male, a female attendant will be present throughout the examination. The doctor will wear surgical gloves and will first examine the outside of the vagina. A plastic or metal instrument called a speculum then will be placed gently in the vagina. The speculum can be opened slightly, like a duck's bill, to allow the doctor to see the inside walls of the vagina and the cervix, which is the opening to the uterus.

The doctor then takes some samples of the vaginal fluid or may swab the cervix with a cotton-tip applicator for cultures or for the Papanicolaou ("Pap") smear. The cultures are sent to the laboratory to be checked for bacteria that cause disease. The Pap smear is sent to the laboratory to be examined for signs of cervical cancer and for abnormalities that increase the future risk of cervical cancer. After the speculum is removed from the vagina, the doctor will place one or two gloved fingers in the vagina and will place the other hand on the lower abdomen. This allows the uterus and ovaries to be examined for abnormalities in size and shape. The last part of the examination is a rectal examination (one finger in the rectum), which allows the doctor to feel the back of the uterus.

Many adolescents—and adults—are embarrassed by the pelvic examination or are afraid that it will be painful. Usually the expectation is much worse than the examination. Although the position is awkward, the examination is not painful. Some adolescents are more comfortable if they can see what the doctor is doing. This can be accomplished by propping up the head of the examination table and by giving the adolescent a small mirror to hold.

If the first pelvic examination is done for a problem that subsequently clears, the examination need not be repeated until age eighteen to twenty-one. Once an adolescent has had sexual intercourse—even if only once—a pelvic examination should be done at least yearly because of the risk of sexually transmitted diseases. Many physicians recommend that sexually active adolescents have pelvic examinations every six months, with cervical cultures for sexually transmitted diseases every six months and Pap smears every year.

EXAMINATION OF THE MALE GENITALIA

During this part of the routine physical examination, the doctor will feel the scrotum and groin for signs of a hernia (Chapter 18). Many physicians will teach adolescents to examine themselves regularly for testicular masses, or lumps, because testicular cancer is the most common solid tumor that occurs in young men. It should be remembered, however, that testicular tumors occur very infrequently—in less than one of every 10,000 males (Chapter 18). Males who have had sexual intercourse should have yearly swabs taken from the urethra (which ends at the tip of the penis). These swabs are sent to the laboratory to culture for bacteria that cause sexually transmitted disease.

Laboratory Tests

Healthy adolescents with no symptoms require few laboratory tests. Your doctor may suggest the following:

HEMOGLOBIN/HEMATOCRIT

Anemia due to iron deficiency is common during adolescence because of rapid growth, inadequate iron in the diet, or menstrual blood loss in girls (Chapter 35). A hemoglobin or hematocrit test, therefore, is usually done on the first visit and again when puberty is completed. The test is simple, inexpensive, and requires only a finger prick for a drop of blood.

URINALYSIS

This test is also a simple, inexpensive screen that requires only a sample of urine. A dipstick test is done to look for blood, protein, or sugar—none of which should be present in the urine. A drop of urine is also examined under the microscope for cells or crystals. An abnormal urinalysis can be an early indicator of a urinary tract infection, diabetes, kidney stones, or other irregularities of the kidneys, bladder, or urethra.

SICKLE CELL SCREENING

The prevalence of sickle cell trait and sickle cell anemia (Chapter 35) is highest in individuals of African descent. African-American adolescents who have not been screened in childhood should have the blood test done during the first adolescent visit.

LABORATORY TESTS FOR SEXUALLY ACTIVE ADOLESCENTS

The importance of once or twice yearly examinations of all adolescents who have had sexual intercourse is discussed earlier in this chapter (see The Physical Examination). The specific laboratory tests that should be done for sexually active adolescent girls include the annual Pap smear for cervical cancer or other abnormalities of cervical cells, a blood test for syphilis, and annual or twice yearly cervical samples for gonorrhea and chlamydia (Chapter 21).

Heterosexual males should have an annual blood test for syphilis and annual urethral samples for gonorrhea and chlamydia. Homosexual and bisexual males are at high risk for sexually transmitted diseases, including syphilis, gonorrhea, chlamydia, hepatitis B, and HIV infection. They should be screened for these infections at least yearly, should receive the hepatitis B vaccine if the blood test does not indicate past infection, and should be urged always to use condoms.

Bisexual females are at the same risk as heterosexual females. Homosexual females are at some risk, although less than homosexual males or heterosexual females. The medical issues of homosexual and bisexual youth are discussed in detail in Chapter 16.

Assessment and Plan

The final portion of the adolescent's health screening offers an opportunity for the doctor to discuss the teenager's overall state of health as well as any particular problems, additional tests, treatment plans, referrals, or need for future visits. This discussion is usually held after the physical examination, once the teenager has dressed. The parent is invited in to hear and discuss the doctor's findings, but as mentioned earlier, any concerns expressed by the teenager in confidence are not discussed unless they are life-threatening or unless the teenager wishes to have the doctor mention them to the parent.

This final segment of the health screening should be a time for the teenager, parent, and doctor to discuss any lingering concerns or unanswered questions. Teenagers should ask for clarification of anything that they do not fully understand, and they should be encouraged to contact the physician whenever they have questions or problems in the future.

II

SPECIAL HEALTH ISSUES

4

Exercise and Sports

The President's Council on Physical Fitness, founded in 1956, provided the impetus for new sports programs and encouraged a positive public attitude toward exercise. In just one generation, athletic opportunities for adolescents have changed dramatically. The variety of sports and fitness programs has expanded and more adolescents—especially girls—are participating than ever before. Mothers of today's teenagers rarely joined Little League or soccer teams. Their athletic role models were older women. Many of today's outstanding athletes become role models when they are teenagers themselves.

Teenagers see sports and exercise continue throughout adult life. Grandparents are swimming laps, skiing downhill races, and running marathons. As the age range has widened, resources have increased to meet the growing demand for athletic opportunities. Today's teenagers are surrounded by fitness centers, health clubs, community teams, and school sports programs.

Regular exercise means healthier bodies, improved vigor, stronger hearts, better muscle tone. It also offers pure pleasure—the joy of sinking a jump shot, of walking eighteen rolling fairways, of smashing a lob deep to the backcourt corner. For teenagers, athletic involvement enhances self-confidence and promotes the development of skills that can last a lifetime.

Sports also teach some of life's more difficult lessons—losing or winning with grace, working as a team, handling pressure. A teenager who wants desperately to make a shot, but sees a teammate in an open position, must make an instant decision between shooting or passing, between self or team. Opportunities like this provide lessons quite different from those of textbooks or term papers.

For the vast majority of adolescents, athletic participation should be encouraged. For teenagers who have medical conditions that limit their activity, less strenuous sports can be suggested. Regardless of skill or ability, all teenagers who participate in sports face some small, but real, risk. This may be the physical risk of an injury or the psychological risk of a disappointing performance.

This chapter deals with preventing and treating the problems that may arise when a teenager participates in sports. It begins with the sports physical examination and discusses some of the reasons for limiting an adolescent's athletic participation. It then reviews conditioning, nutrition, and preparing for an important athletic event. The last few sections discuss the prevention and management of sports-related injuries, illnesses, and psychological stress.

The benefits of athletic activity far outweigh the risks when several precautions are taken. The primary goal of health professionals, coaches, and parents should be to minimize risks by providing appropriate preparticipation screening, safe equipment, injury prevention counseling, and guidance about healthy competition.

The Sports Physical Examination

The first precaution is a physical examination geared especially for the young athlete and the sport in which he or she will participate. This is a more targeted examination than the general examination described in Chapter 3. In a sports physical examination, the physician will look closely at muscles, ligaments, joints, and bones. The teenager's musculoskeletal system is still growing, and the examination can assess the adolescent's physical readiness to participate in a given sport. The early detection of musculoskeletal problems may help protect against injury.

During the sport-specific examination, the physician will consider such questions as: Is there a "swimmer's shoulder"? Has the soccer goalie had sufficient rehabilitation of his sprained ankle? Does the running back have weak ligaments? Does the field hockey link have scoliosis, or curvature of the spine (Chapter 31)? For female athletes, the physician will also ask for a menstrual history. Has the first period occurred? Is it delayed? Are the periods regular (page 189–92)?

The physician will closely examine the athlete's cardiovascular system. Has the teenage athlete experienced shortness of breath, light-headedness, fainting, or chest pain during exercise? Is there a family history of early heart disease or unexplained sudden death (page 354–56)?

Many coaches and school districts ask that physicians make recommendations about adolescent participation in specific sports. The American Academy of Pediatrics divides sports into five categories depending on the amount of contact, the chance of collision, and the strenuousness of the sport (Table 4.1).

TABLE 4.1

CATAGORIES OF CONTACT AND COLLISION BY SPORT

Contact/ Collision	Limited Contact/Impact	Noncontact		
		Strenuous	*Moderately Strenuous*	*Nonstrenuous*
Boxing	Baseball	Aerobic	Badminton	Archery
Field	Basketball	dancing	Curling	Golf
hockey	Bicycling	Crew	Table tennis	Riflery
Football	Diving	Fencing		
Ice hockey	Field	Field		
Lacrosse	High jump	Discus		
Martial arts	Pole vault	Javelin		
Rodeo	Gymnastics	Shot put		
Soccer	Horseback riding	Running		
Wrestling	Skating	Swimming		
	Ice	Tennis		
	Roller	Track		
	Skiing	Weight lifting		
	Cross-country			
	Downhill			
	Water			
	Softball			
	Squash, handball			
	Volleyball			

(Reprinted by permission of the American Academy of Pediatrics. "Recommendations for Participation in Competitive Sports," *Pediatrics*, 1988; 81:605–607.)

The physician may use these categories when deciding if a given sport is appropriate for the adolescent. For example, a contact/collision sport may pose an unacceptable risk for an adolescent with a single kidney because a blow to the torso could damage the kidney. An adolescent with high blood pressure may be advised to avoid weight lifting or rowing until the blood pressure is lowered by appropriate treatment (page 363-64). In other situations, all sports may be acceptable but exertion from any cause may exacerbate an adolescent's problem. For instance, exercise can trigger wheezing in some teenagers with asthma. The physician can adjust the type or timing of the asthma medications to avoid or decrease the likelihood of an asthma attack (page 343-45).

These problems are just a few examples of the many that can occur. The physician, teenager, and parent ultimately must decide together what is a safe form of exercise.

Conditioning

"Conditioning" is not the same as "training." Conditioning helps athletes in all sports by improving energy efficiency, speed, endurance, muscle strength, and flexibility. Training is sport-specific and is designed to develop particular skills, such as fielding for baseball or vaulting for gymnastics.

Good physical conditioning requires exercises to build endurance, speed, and strength. Aerobic exercises, such as swimming, cycling, and walking, involve the sustained activity of large muscle groups and efficient work by the heart and lungs. Anaerobic exercises, such as sprinting or diving, involve short, intense bursts of movement. Resistance exercises, using free weights or weight machines, build and help balance the muscles so that they protect the bones and joints from injury.

There is some controversy about whether resistance training is appropriate for children and younger teenagers. Research indicates that working with weights is safe for youngsters when the program is short-term and supervised by well-trained adults. High school programs increasingly utilize weights as a part of overall conditioning. The program must be adjusted to the adolescent's level of physical maturity and must be closely monitored. Injuries do occur with weight training and include stress fractures of bone, muscle strain, and damage to the disks that cushion the bones of the back (Chapter 31).

The United States Weight and Power Lifting Federations recommend that teenage athletes should not be allowed to lift maximal weights until age fourteen. The American Academy of Pediatrics recommends that weight lifting and body building should be delayed until puberty is completed (Tanner stage five) and bone growth is complete. A bone tends to grow at its ends. If this area is damaged during puberty, further growth of that bone may be hampered.

Another component of conditioning is warming up and cooling down to promote flexibility. Slow, prolonged stretches lengthen the muscles and make the body more supple and less vulnerable to injury. Stretching should be done for several minutes both before and after exercising.

Nutrition and the Adolescent Athlete

The dietary patterns of athletes a generation ago were very different than they are today. Then it was common to eat high-protein foods on nonplaying days, to eat less food for a few days before competing, to skip breakfast on the day of the game, to drink little during the game, and to eat lightly afterward.

Today, nutritionists believe that athletes can increase their endurance by eating a high-carbohydrate meal the night before a game. In addition to protein and fat from meat and milk, such a meal would include carbohydrates from pasta, breads, or fruit. On the day of the game, the athlete might eat a low-fat, easily digestible meal three to five hours before competing.

Teenage athletes do not need nutritional supplements if they are eating healthy, well-balanced meals. All of the ingredients in nutritional supplements can be found in the everyday foods that most American teenagers consume. For these youth, supplemental proteins, amino acids, vitamins, and minerals will not enhance performance.

During sports participation, it is very important that athletes drink liquids *before* they feel thirsty. An athlete can lose up to 2 liters of fluid before the brain registers "thirst." (A liter is slightly more than a quart.) During a one-hour workout, a swimmer may lose 1.5 liters of fluid. In hot weather, a runner may perspire as much as 2.5 liters per hour. This fluid loss can limit performance and can cause painful muscle cramping. Once the fluid is lost, it is impossible to replace it all during the exercise.

A cup of cool water is suggested just before a game on warm

days, with another every fifteen minutes during the event. Athletes who compete in several events spaced throughout the day (such as swimming, track and field, gymnastics) should also drink fluids right after each event.

Steroids and Other Drugs

Anabolic steroids should not be used in an attempt to increase muscle size and strength. Steroids have very serious side effects, including liver damage, decreased testicular size, acne, masculinization in women, aggressiveness, and hostility. In teenagers who have not completed puberty, anabolic steroids can cause the bones to stop growing too early, resulting in short stature. The International Olympic Committee has banned the use of steroids. The American College of Sports Medicine has condemned their use. And most importantly, it is a violation of federal law for anyone to dispense anabolic steroids to athletes for the purpose of improved athletic performance.

The International Olympic Committee also has banned the use of stimulants such as amphetamines and cocaine to fight muscular and psychological fatigue. These drugs produce serious—and sometimes deadly—side effects, including high blood pressure, rapid or irregular heart rate, increased body temperature, heart attack, anxiety, and depression. Blood or urine tests can be done to screen for the use of both anabolic steroids and stimulants.

Anti-inflammatory drugs often are used to reduce inflammation and relieve pain. They are effective but should be used cautiously because they can mask the pain that signals serious injury. Any persistent discomfort should be evaluated rather than simply controlled with medication.

Preventing Sports Injuries

Athletics are safer and more enjoyable when teenagers, parents, and coaches take the following precautions:

- Teach proper skills and techniques;
- Enforce safety rules;
- Match teams or players by weight and stage of maturation rather than age or grade alone;
- Condition year-round, with warm-up and cool-down;

- Avoid excessive training, especially if there is pain and over-use of muscles and joints;
- Rehabilitate old injuries thoroughly before returning to play;
- Provide good supervision and appropriate safety equipment.

SPORT-SPECIFIC INJURIES

In spite of these precautions, sports injuries do occur. Up to 40 percent of boys and 20 percent of girls who play interscholastic sports are injured each year. One-quarter to one-third of these high school injuries are significant. The injury risk and type depends on the sport. Consider the following:

Football has the highest rate of injury. Among the one million high school boys who play interscholastic football each year, approximately 28 percent sustain mild injuries, 6 percent moderate injuries, and 3 percent major injuries. One survey found that 81 percent of high school football players are on the bench for up to four days each season because of injuries. In another study, one player per team required hospitalization and another required surgery each year because of injury. The knee and ankle are the most commonly injured sites in football. Up to 25 percent of players with knee injuries continue to restrict their activity a decade later.

Catastrophic head and neck injuries put football at the high-risk end of adolescent athletics. Spinal cord damage resulting in paralysis has been significantly reduced since "spearing" (using the head as a battering ram to block or tackle) was outlawed in 1976. But up to 20 percent of high school football players continue to suffer concussions each year from head injury.

Wrestling injury rates approach those of football. Sprained knees, strained backs, and sprained shoulders are the most common injuries. (Sprains are injured ligaments and strains are pulled muscles.) Wrestlers also are prone to some unique problems. For example, skin infections, spread between wrestlers on the mat, are common. Parents should also be aware that some teenage wrestlers will deprive themselves of food or fluid to "make weight," that is, to fall within a desired weight class. Food restriction can impair the adolescent's growth during wrestling season, and dehydration increases the risk of overheating during the match. The American College of Sports Medicine has condemned these behaviors and has issued guidelines for wrestling coaches.

Ice hockey players must wear helmets and face guards. Common injuries on the ice include concussions, dental trauma, fractures, contusions (blows to a muscle), lacerations (cuts), sprains, strains, and dislocated or separated joints. Similar injuries can occur in field hockey, as well.

Gymnastics carries a significant risk of injury, especially as the level of competition increases. One study found that 39 percent of high school gymnasts become injured, with 16 percent of them on the sidelines for more than four days. Over half of all gymnastic injuries are to the legs, especially the knees and ankles. The most devastating injuries in gymnastics have occurred on the trampoline. Cervical spine injuries resulting in death or paralysis happen even among experienced gymnasts who are well supervised. Gymnasts, like wrestlers, dancers, and runners, may attempt to restrict their weight gain. This may result in delayed puberty or irregular menstrual cycles.

Baseball, the all-American sport, is rarely considered dangerous. Yet, one study found an injury rate of 18 percent among high school players. Shoulder and elbow injuries are common, particularly among pitchers whose muscle strength is not fully developed. Serious eye injuries also are more common in baseball than in other junior and senior high school sports. Protective eyewear is recommended by the American Academy of Pediatrics, particularly if the player has uncorrectable poor vision in one eye. Baseball and softball players should be instructed in correct sliding techniques to avoid ankle and knee sprains and lower leg and ankle fractures.

Soccer has become an increasingly popular sport in the United States. Although it is a relatively safe sport, up to 30 percent of interscholastic soccer players are injured each year. Most soccer injuries are contusions, followed by sprains and strains. Concussion, despite heading of the ball, is uncommon.

Swimming is also a relatively safe sport when the swimmer is in good condition. Shoulder pain is common, affecting over 80 percent of competitors in the butterfly and freestyle. Breaststroke swimmers may suffer low back pain from muscle strain, or knee pain caused by ligament sprain.

Basketball players incur most of their injuries from sprains and strains in their legs, particularly their ankles. Like baseball, basketball carries a significant risk of eye injury, and eye protection is essential for players with uncorrectable poor vision in one eye.

Tennis players commonly experience low back strain, ankle sprains, and tendonitis of the hand, wrist, and knee. Elbow and shoulder pain tend to affect older players, although adolescents may develop these problems from overuse. Eye protection is recommended for tennis as well as for squash and racquetball.

Track and distance running injuries appear to cost young athletes more missed participation time than most other sports-related injuries. The most common track and field injuries include muscle and tendon injuries to the lower leg, and knee inflammation. Boys are more commonly injured during hurdling, while girls are more likely to be injured during short-distance sprints.

There is some concern that children and young adolescents who compete in long-distance runs may be at risk for injuries to growing bones. Long-distance runners also tend to maintain low body weights, which can interfere with pubertal development or menstrual function.

Treating Athletic Injuries

As stated earlier, this book is not a substitute for professional medical care. When adolescents are injured during conditioning or on the playing field, medical attention should be sought. Even if the injury appears mild, examination and counseling can help to prevent reinjury or overuse. Common injuries, such as ankle sprains, should be evaluated and treated immediately, before swelling obscures the damage. In many cases, X-rays are required to distinguish between a sprain and a fracture.

An acronym for the treatment of injuries to muscles and ligaments is RICE—Rest, Ice, Compression, Elevation.

• *Rest* of the injured area for twenty-four to seventy-two hours reduces the chances of further injury and of bleeding into the surrounding tissue.

• *Ice* has been used since Hippocrates' day to numb pain and reduce swelling. Ice diminishes muscle spasm, reduces bleeding into the injured tissues, and shortens the period of disability. A plastic bag full of ice chips or an insulated, disposable cup filled with frozen water should be applied to the injured area for ten to twenty minutes, but never for more than thirty minutes.

• *Compression* controls edema, or swelling of the tissues at the injury site. An elastic bandage can be used for several days, with removal every so often for ice treatments. The bandage should not be wrapped too tightly.

• *Elevation* of an injured arm or leg also helps to reduce edema. Elevation will lower the pressure that forces fluid from the blood vessels into the tissues. It also helps the lymph system drain fluids away from the injured tissues.

Teenagers often are anxious to get back into play and may resist taking time out to rehabilitate an injury. A period of rehabilitation is as important as the immediate care. Beginning two or three days after the injury, rehabilitation may involve a ten-minute application of ice followed by range-of-motion exercises. Weight-bearing exercises should not begin until the teenager is free of pain. Knees and ankles may require support for months until fully healed. A doctor or trainer may also suggest muscle-strengthening exercises. Recovery and rehabilitation time will depend on the degree of injury, but teenage athletes should never be pushed back into play until the injury is fully rehabilitated.

Special Problems

Specific medical conditions and problems are detailed in Part V. Several specific problems relating to adolescent athletes are discussed here:

Menstrual disorders, such as delayed menarche, amenorrhea (the cessation of menstruation), and irregular menstrual periods, have become more apparent as the number of young female athletes has increased. In many female athletes, a low proportion of body fat contributes to these problems. It remains unclear why some female athletes with normal body fat have menstrual disorders. Young women who participate in sports should have evaluations of menstruation, body fat, nutrition, and diet before they begin training and should be monitored as long as they participate. Adolescents with menstrual irregularities should be fully evaluated. In some cases, the reason may be unrelated to exercise (Chapter 17).

Exercise-induced asthma has received more attention in recent years because the incidence of asthma has increased and because more children and adolescents are participating in sports. Approximately 10 percent of individuals without asthma and 80 percent with asthma will experience wheezing during exercise. Sometimes the adolescent with exercise-induced asthma will describe symptoms other than wheezing, such as difficulty breathing, chest pain, or fatigue. In most cases, the correct diagnosis can be made by history and physical examination, without other tests.

Adolescents with asthma need not be excluded from athletic participation. The key is to work with a physician who can design a treatment regimen that prevents asthma attacks during exercise. The type and timing of the medication, usually in the form of inhalers, can do much to maximize the teenager's comfort and function (Chapter 27).

High blood pressure, or hypertension, is defined by at least three separate blood pressure readings that are above the ninety-fifth percentile for age (Chapter 28). The diagnosis should not be made on the basis of one or two measurements because blood pressure can vary widely, depending on the adolescent's anxiety or level of stress. Decisions about athletic participation also should be reviewed regularly because nearly half of adolescents with high blood pressure may have normal blood pressure on subsequent testing.

Blood pressure normally increases during exercise, especially if the exercise involves weight lifting. Exercise poses little risk for most teenagers with mild hypertension when it is controlled by diet or medication. In fact, exercise may help lower the resting blood pressure in many hypertensive adolescents. When the blood pressure is markedly elevated, however, the physician usually will recommend limiting exercise until good blood pressure control is achieved. Once the pressure is controlled, exercise should be encouraged and restrictions should be kept to a minimum.

Heart disease includes a wide array of problems and must be evaluated by a physician before a decision about sports participation can be made. The risk for most teenagers with heart disease is different than the risk for most adults with heart disease. The most common problem in adults is coronary artery disease, which reduces blood flow to the heart muscle and can cause myocardial infarction, or heart attack. In adolescents, significant coronary artery disease is rare. The more common problems in teenagers include congenital heart disease, inflammation of the heart muscle (myocarditis), and irregular heart rhythm (arrhythmia).

All adolescents with heart disease should be evaluated before sports participation. Some may require exercise stress testing to assess the heart's rhythm and function during exercise. Others may require twenty-four-hour monitoring of the heart's rate and rhythm both at rest and during exercise. In other instances, a thorough history and physical examination may be sufficient.

Sudden cardiac death among athletes is a rare but tragic occurrence. The enormous grief following a young person's unexpected death often leads to feelings of guilt and anxiety that a correctable problem was overlooked. In over 75 percent of these sudden deaths, there were no warning signs or symptoms that even the most thorough physical examination would have revealed.

A very common finding in teenagers that is *not* associated with sudden death is mitral valve prolapse, a benign condition that affects over 5 percent of the population. The diagnosis is made on physical examination by hearing a clicking sound often associated with a murmur. It can be confirmed by an echocardiogram, a test that uses sound waves to outline the structure of the heart. The majority of adolescents with mitral valve prolapse should be allowed to participate in all sports (Chapter 28).

Stress and the Teenage Athlete

Athletic competition naturally brings pressure—pressure to win, to do one's best, to be a strong team member. Some degree of stress is beneficial. If it comes in small, manageable doses, it can help the teenager learn to handle pressures both on the field and in other life situations. If stress becomes excessive or chronic, it can impair health and can increase the risk of injury during sports participation.

When stress becomes a problem, teenagers and their parents should try to understand its source: Does it come from a motivation to please coaches or parents? Does it come from a fear of failing? Does it come from comparison with, or pressure from, peers? Has the sport become a way of measuring self-worth?

Stress associated with athletics should receive as much attention and care as a physical injury on the playing field. An impartial adult—a physician, school counselor, teacher, or relative—can help the teenager understand the reasons for the stress and can support a healthier perspective toward the sport. Many schools and athletic organizations have begun to assist adolescents by providing relaxation and stress management programs. Teenagers should be encouraged to learn and use such techniques to cope with pressure. Ultimately, they will become healthier athletes and happier young people.

5

Nutrition

Many teenagers are knowledgeable and concerned about nutrition. They exercise, watch their weight, and avoid foods that are high in saturated fat, salt, and refined sugar.

Healthy eating can be difficult, though, for even the best-informed and well-intentioned adolescents. Consider the demons:

• French fries, double cheeseburgers, or pepperoni pizza after the game or movie. *"Oh, why not? I know I shouldn't but everybody else is."*

• Tempting desserts in the cafeteria line or snack foods in vending machines. *"The pot roast and mashed potatoes look sick! I'll just have a bag of chips and a piece of pie."*

• Time. Or lack of it. Grab the bookbag, gulp some orange juice, and run for the bus . . . *"I can't sit down for dinner, Mom. I've got to write a paper tonight."*

Teenage eating habits are riddled with problems. Hectic schedules encourage eating-on-the-run, snacking, unbalanced meals, and fast foods, which are usually low in nutritional value and high in calories, fats, and salt. The teenager's normal quest for autonomy often means breaking away from family meals and adult notions of what constitutes proper nutrition. Identifying with peers and eating with the crowd is more likely to mean burgers and fries than fish and brown rice. Even for adolescents who have most of their meals at home, time demands on working parents may limit nutritional planning. There may be little supervision of breakfast or after-school snacks. Parents and teenagers may know what constitutes healthy eating but face the competing responsibilities of job, school, homework, and extracurricular activities.

The nutritional needs of puberty, along with the pace and pressure of modern American life, may contribute to the prevalence of eating disorders among adolescents. The three major eating disorders—obesity, anorexia nervosa, and bulimia—are discussed in Chapters 6 and 7. This chapter addresses the nutritional needs of the average, healthy American teenager.

The Importance of a Balanced Diet

A healthy teenage diet should meet two goals. It should provide the nutrients needed for optimal growth and well-being during adolescence, and it should minimize the risk of disease during adulthood. The first goal is fairly obvious, but the second is often overlooked.

Problems associated with diet are the leading causes of death and illness in the United States. Diet has been implicated in heart disease, stroke, and some forms of cancer, such as cancer of the colon, breast, and prostate. Excessive calories and salt increase the risk of high blood pressure. Excessive calories and carbohydrates increase the risk of diabetes mellitus in adulthood. Inadequate dietary calcium may increase the risk of osteoporosis and hip fracture, especially in older women. Diets low in fiber are associated with constipation and diseases of the large intestine. Dental cavities, associated with concentrated carbohydrates and inadequate fluoride, occur in most children before puberty. By age seventeen, the average adolescent has had eight cavities.

Increasing evidence suggests that eating habits can have an important effect on the development and severity of disease. These habits begin during childhood, under parental supervision, and become well established by adolescence or young adulthood. The current-day emphasis on weight and exercise has influenced a generation of adolescents who, for the most part, have some understanding of calories and weight control. They may be far less aware, though, of other important aspects of nutrition, such as their intake of protein, fat, carbohydrates, cholesterol, fiber, minerals, and vitamins.

Many dietary guidelines have been published for the general American population. The Food and Nutrition Board of the National Research Council has compiled a table of recommended dietary allowances (RDAs) for adolescents (Table 5.1). The labels on most packaged foods estimate the amount of each nutrient and give the percentages of the RDAs contained in the food. Diets to decrease the risk of cancer have been developed by the National Research Council, the American Cancer Society, and the National Cancer Institute. The National Cholesterol Education Program has published dietary guidelines for cholesterol and fat intake that are designed specifically for children and adolescents.

TABLE 5.1

RECOMMENDED DIETARY ALLOWANCES

	Males			Females		
	11–14 Yr	*15–18 Yr*	*19–24 Yr*	*11–14 Yr*	*15–18 Yr*	*19–24 Yr*
Total calories	2,500	3,000	2,900	2,200	2,200	2,200
Protein (g)*	45	59	58	46	44	46
Vitamin A (mcg)	1,000	1,000	1,000	800	800	800
Vitamin D (mcg)	10	10	10	10	10	10
Vitamin E (mg)	10	10	10	8	8	8
Vitamin K (mcg)	45	65	70	45	55	60
Vitamin C (mg)	50	60	60	50	60	60
Thiamine (mg)	1.3	1.5	1.5	1.1	1.1	1.1
Riboflavin (mg)	1.5	1.8	1.7	1.3	1.3	1.3
Niacin (mg)	17	20	19	15	15	15
Vitamin B_6 (mg)	1.7	2.0	2.0	1.4	1.5	1.6
Folate (mcg)	150	200	200	150	180	180
Vitamin B_{12} (mcg)	2.0	2.0	2.0	2.0	2.0	2.0
Calcium (mg)	1,200	1,200	1,200	1,200	1,200	1,200
Phosphorus (mg)	1,200	1,200	1,200	1,200	1,200	1,200
Magnesium (mg)	270	400	350	280	300	280
Iron (mg)	12	12	10	15	15	15
Zinc (mg)	15	15	15	12	12	12
Iodine (mcg)	150	150	150	150	150	150
Selenium (mcg)	40	50	70	45	50	55

*g = grams, mg = milligrams, mcg = micrograms

Adapted with permission from *Recommended Dietary Allowances: 10th Edition.* Copyright 1989 by the National Academy of Sciences. Courtesy of the National Academy Press, Washington, D.C.

These guidelines should be used as flexible recommendations rather than rigid limit-setters. Whether in full meals or snacks, food provides more than physical sustenance. Eating together is an important part of social interaction and offers an opportunity for independent decision making. Adolescents must be allowed the room to make choices, decide preferences, and achieve ultimate balance. The goal of these, or any, guidelines is to provide a framework for the development of healthy eating habits.

The body depends on energy to maintain itself, to grow, and to exercise. This energy, measured in kilocalories, comes from protein, fat, and carbohydrates. A gram of fat has over twice as much energy, or kilocalories, as a gram of protein or carbohydrates. That is why high-fat snacks and most fast foods are considered more "fattening" than vegetables, fruits, and high-protein foods such as fish, poultry, or lean meats.

Most of the energy that the body requires is used to maintain the status quo. The rest is divided between growth and activity. A growing adolescent needs more calories in the daily diet than does an adult who is the same height and weight and is just as active. Extra calories in the teenager result in further growth in height, while extra calories in the adult result in weight gain. If calories are withheld from a normal-weight adolescent and the exercise level does not decrease, the rate of growth may be delayed or slowed. In the adult, weight will be lost.

Teenagers of the same age may have very different caloric needs, depending on gender, pubertal stage, metabolism, and physical activity. Boys' caloric requirements tend to increase from about 2,500 calories at ages eleven to fourteen to 3,000 at ages fifteen to eighteen. Girls' caloric requirements tend to stay the same throughout adolescence at about 2,200 calories. For some girls, the caloric requirement may even begin to decrease by age fifteen to eighteen. It is important to realize that an intake of 2,200 calories by a fourteen-year-old girl who is on a swim team and in the midst of her growth spurt may mean weight loss, while another fourteen-year-old girl who is physically mature, less active, and on the same diet may gain weight.

Fat and cholesterol. A balanced diet must include some fat to provide essential fatty acids and fat-soluble vitamins. The problem with fats is that they generally take up a greater proportion of the typical diet than they should. At least 40 percent of the daily calories in the average American diet comes from fat. Ideally, this proportion should be no more than 30 percent. More importantly, no more than 10 percent of the total daily calories should be *saturated* fat, which comes primarily from animal sources such as meat, butter, and cheese. The remaining dietary fat (20 percent of total calories) should be polyunsaturated fat, which comes from plant sources, such as vegetable oils or liquid margarines.

Strong evidence indicates that reducing dietary fat, especially saturated fat, decreases the risk of adult heart disease. Limiting dietary cholesterol to 300 milligrams (mg) a day also is recommended but may be less important than the amount of saturated fat. Cholesterol and fat are *not* the same thing. Foods containing no cholesterol may still contain significant amounts of fat.

Food labels usually give—in fine print—cholesterol and fat content. The large-print words like "light" and "cholesterol free" may be misleading. A beef hot dog package, for example, boasts "25 percent less fat," but 82 percent of the calories in each hot dog still comes from fat. A peanut butter label says "no cholesterol," which is true, yet 70 percent of the calories in a two-tablespoon serving comes from fat. That is not to say that a teenager should never eat a peanut butter sandwich. Just balance the lunch by choosing an apple instead of ice cream for dessert.

The National Cholesterol Education Program has defined normal total blood cholesterol levels as below 170 for children and adolescents. The indications for testing an adolescent's blood cholesterol level and the treatment approaches for high cholesterol levels are discussed fully in Chapter 28.

The best way to keep dietary cholesterol at a minimum is to eat less fat overall. Foods from animal sources tend to be high in both cholesterol and saturated fat; they include red meats, egg yolks, organ products such as liver, and high-fat dairy products such as butter, cream, and whole milk.

How does a teenager translate a concern for lower dietary fat and less cholesterol into realistic eating habits? A fast-food double cheeseburger, for example, has between 560 and 935 calories, depending on whether it has been fried or broiled, the type of cheese, the bun, and the condiments. Fat makes up 52 to 60 percent of those calories. In contrast, a grilled chicken sandwich without mayonnaise has 252 to 400 calories, and only 14 to 16 percent is fat. Table 5.2 lists foods to choose and foods to decrease for a diet that is low in saturated fats and cholesterol. Remember, the goal is balance, *not* an absolute exclusion of fat-containing foods.

TABLE 5.2
FOODS TO CHOOSE AND DECREASE

Food Group	Choose	Decrease
Meat, poultry, and fish	Beef, pork, lamb—lean cuts well trimmed before cooking	Beef, pork, lamb—regular ground beef, fatty cuts, spare ribs, organ meats, sausage, regular luncheon meats, hot dogs, bacon
	Poultry without skin	Poultry with skin, fried chicken
	Fish, shellfish	Fried fish, fried shellfish
Egg	Egg whites (two whites equal one whole egg in recipes), cholesterol-free egg substitute	Egg yolks
Dairy products	Milk—skim or 1% fat (fluid, powdered, evaporated), buttermilk	Whole milk (fluid, evaporated, condensed), 2% low-fat milk, imitation milk
	Yogurt—nonfat or low-fat yogurt or yogurt beverages	Whole-milk yogurt, whole-milk yogurt beverages
	Cheese—low-fat natural or processed cheese (part-skim mozzarella, ricotta)	Regular cheeses (American, blue, Brie, cheddar, Colby, Edam, Monterey, whole-milk mozzarella, Parmesan, Swiss), cream cheese, Neufchâtel cheese
	Cottage cheese—low-fat, nonfat, or dry curd (0–2% fat)	Cottage cheese (4% fat)
	Frozen dairy dessert—ice milk, frozen yogurt (low-fat or nonfat)	Ice cream Cream, half & half, whipping cream, nondairy creamer, whipped topping, sour cream
Fats and oils	Unsaturated oils—safflower, sunflower, corn, soybean, cottonseed, canola, olive, peanut	Coconut oil, palm kernel oil, palm oil
	Margarine—made from unsaturated oils listed above, light or diet margarine	Butter, lard, shortening, bacon fat

Food Group	Choose	Decrease
Fats and oils	Salad dressings—made with unsaturated oils listed above, low-fat or oil-free	Dressings made with egg yolk, cheese, sour cream, whole milk
	Seeds and nuts—peanut butter, other nut butters	Coconut
	Cocoa powder	Chocolate
Breads and cereals	Breads—whole grain bread, hamburger and hot dog bun, corn tortilla	Bread in which eggs are a major ingredient, croissants
	Cereals—oat, wheat, corn, multigrain	Granola made with coconut
	Pasta	Egg noodles and pasta containing egg yolk
	Rice	
	Dry beans and peas	
	Crackers, low-fat—animal-type, graham, saltine-type	High-fat crackers
	Homemade baked goods using unsaturated oil, skim or 1% milk, and egg substitute—quick breads, biscuits, cornbread muffins, bran muffins, pancakes, waffles	Commercial baked pastries, muffins, biscuits
	Soup—chicken or beef noodle, minestrone, tomato, vegetarian, potato	Soup containing whole milk, cream, meat fat, poultry fat, or poultry skin
Vegetables	Fresh, frozen, or canned	Vegetables prepared with butter, cheese, or cream sauce
Fruits	Fruit—fresh, frozen, canned, or dried	Fried fruit or fruit served with butter or cream sauce
	Fruit juice—fresh, frozen, or canned	
Sweets and modified fat desserts	Beverages—fruit-flavored drinks, lemonade, fruit punch	
	Sweets—sugar, syrup, honey, jam, preserves, candy made without fat (candy corn, gumdrops, hard	Candy made with chocolate, coconut oil, palm kernel oil, palm oil

Food Group	Choose	Decrease
Sweets and modified fat desserts	candy), fruit-flavored gelatin	
	Frozen desserts—sherbet, sorbet, fruit ice, Popsicles	Ice cream and frozen treats made with ice cream
	Cookies, cake, pie, pudding—prepared with egg whites, egg substitute, skim milk or 1% milk, and unsaturated oil or margarine; gingersnaps; fig bar cookies; angel food cake	Commercial baked pies, cakes, doughnuts, high-fat cookies, cream pies

Adapted with permission of *Pediatrics,* Vol. 89, page 557, 1992.

Carbohydrates and fiber. One way to lower dietary fat is to eat foods that are high in complex carbohydrates, such as cereals, whole grain breads, pasta, fresh fruits, and vegetables. These foods are also a good source of dietary fiber.

Carbohydrates have a lower caloric density than fats and provide a faster-burning fuel for the body as it expends energy. Complex carbohydrates are preferable to simple carbohydrates, such as table sugar or honey, because they are less damaging to teeth. Complex carbohydrates should supply 50 to 60 percent of an adolescent's daily calories. Unfortunately, more than half of the carbohydrates consumed by the average American is in the form of simple carbohydrates. Decreasing soda and candy, while increasing grains and vegetables, should be the goal.

Protein. Between 10 and 15 percent of an adolescent's total daily calories should come from protein. High-protein foods, which provide all essential amino acids, include lean meats, poultry, fish, eggs, milk, and other dairy products. Amino acids are the building blocks of protein. Some amino acids are made by the body. The "essential" amino acids are those that must come from food because the body cannot produce them. Vegetarian diets that eliminate all animal foods, including milk, tend to be low in essential amino acids. Specific vegetables must be added in these diets to assure that protein intake is adequate.

Vitamins. The rapid growth of adolescence requires energy, and vitamins are needed to convert carbohydrates into energy. Teenagers need more vitamins, such as dietary thiamine, riboflavin, and niacin, than younger children for their accelerated growth. Folate and vitamin B_{12} are needed to support the production of new body tissues that translate into height and increasing muscle mass. Growing bones require more dietary vitamin D. Vitamins A, C, and E are necessary for new cells to maintain their structure and function. Good sources of folate and vitamins A, B-complex, and C include fresh fruits, yellow vegetables, green leafy vegetables, and whole grains.

Most American teenagers do not need to supplement their diets with vitamin tablets. In fact, high doses of vitamins may be detrimental to health. A single multivitamin tablet daily usually is neither harmful nor necessary.

Minerals. The most important minerals to pay attention to during adolescence are iron, calcium, and zinc. The requirements for these minerals increase, and the adolescent diet may not keep pace.

Iron deficiency anemia is one of the most common disorders in adolescent girls and boys. Iron is needed for the production of muscle and red blood cells. The RDA for elemental iron up to age eighteen is the same (18 mg) for males and females because both have increased needs due to growth. After age eighteen, however, the RDA drops to 10 mg for males but remains at 18 mg for females because they tend to lose iron with menstruation. Adolescents with iron deficiency anemia usually require about one month of supplemental iron therapy (Chapter 35).

The RDA for calcium is 1,200 mg per day for both teenage males and females through age eighteen. The body's ability to absorb calcium and incorporate it into bone is affected by other dietary factors, such as vitamin D and phosphorus. Foods high in both calcium and vitamin D include milk products, tofu, and sardines.

Calcium is often short-changed in the typical teenager's diet. Many young people—especially girls—are not consuming enough calcium to protect against osteoporosis, or weakening of the bone, as they grow older. Osteoporosis can result in many problems in older adults, such as hip fracture, other broken bones, loss of height because of compression of the bones in the spinal column, and bent posture. Bone mass and strength increase steadily during adolescence and young adulthood. About 45 percent of the adult skeleton is built during the adolescent years alone. By age thirty-five, the bone mass reaches a peak and then begins to decline. A goal, therefore, is to maximize bone development during the teens and twenties.

Unfortunately, research reveals that calcium intake is often considerably below the 1,200-mg requirement for teenagers. One study showed that only 16 percent of eleven- to eighteen-year-old girls met the recommended 1,200-mg calcium requirement. In place of a can of soda, teenagers should consider an eight-ounce glass of milk, which has 349 mg of calcium, or a six-ounce glass of calcium-enriched orange juice, which has 225 mg. Other good sources of calcium include yogurt, cheese, broccoli, spinach, and salmon.

Zinc is another important mineral during adolescence. The growth spurt of puberty requires an increase from 10 mg to 15 mg of zinc a day. Good sources of zinc include fish, poultry, meat, unrefined cereals, peas, beans, and peanuts.

The most important consideration in any adolescent's diet is not the precise milligrams of a vitamin or mineral, or the exact percentage of protein in any one meal, but *balance*. A balanced diet is rich in variety and harmony of proteins, fats, fiber, carbohydrates, vitamins, and minerals. Narrow, rigid diets quickly become boring and are far less satisfying than a balanced variety of healthy foods.

Special Nutritional Concerns

VEGETARIAN DIETS

As adolescents become more aware of the world economy, the animal rights movement, the environment, religious customs, and philosophical issues, many decide to abandon animal and dairy foods for vegetarianism. Parents may worry about whether a vegetarian diet can meet the nutritional needs of a growing teenager. Vegetarian diets vary widely. Some include fish and milk but exclude meat. Others include milk but exclude eggs, poultry, fish, and meat. Some include eggs but exclude milk, meat, poultry, and fish. The most restrictive vegetarian diets exclude all foods derived from animals and include only vegetable foods.

Some vegetarian diets may require vitamin or protein supplements to avoid deficiencies of essential nutrients. For example, diets that exclude milk products and all other animal foods tend to be low in zinc, iron, calcium, riboflavin, and vitamins B_6 and B_{12}.

Adolescents who follow vegetarian diets must educate themselves about the nutrient value of allowable foods. Careful attention must be given to the protein and amino acid content of their meals. Extreme vegetarianism places the growing adolescent at risk for significant malnutrition and should be discouraged. Adolescents who want to eliminate animal and dairy foods from their diets should consult a nutritionist and the many books that offer guidelines for well-balanced vegetarian meals.

WEIGHT-REDUCING DIETS

Nearly half of all young adolescent girls have experimented with weight-reducing diets. Images of thin celebrities and fashion models have so permeated the popular culture that dieting begins as early as fourth grade for up to 40 percent of girls. Healthy, active, normal-weight girls commonly think they are "overweight" and periodically abstain from certain foods until they shed a few pounds. Although the majority of dieters are girls, teenage boys also diet to look thinner or to remain within lower athletic weight classes.

Dieting is only necessary if the teenager is consistently overweight and inactive. Adolescents are still growing and require increased calories from a healthy variety of food sources. All too often, fad diets catch on among teenagers and become detrimental to their health. If a teenager is overweight (10 to 20 percent above ideal body weight for height, age, and sex) or obese (more than 20 percent above ideal body weight), a weight-loss diet can be planned with the help and supervision of a health professional who understands adolescent nutrition. The best weight reduction plans rely on both decreased calories and increased exercise.

Body contour has a great impact on how adolescents feel about themselves. Nevertheless, eating and weight should not become the central focus of life. Weight issues or eating patterns that interfere with overall physical and emotional health require professional intervention (Chapters 6 and 7).

NUTRITION FOR THE ADOLESCENT ATHLETE

As mentioned in Chapter 4, athletic, growing teenagers have high nutritional needs. It is not unusual, for instance, for an active, still-growing teenager to consume 3,000 calories a day. If those calories are obtained from foods that are nutritionally balanced, most adolescent athletes do not need supplemental proteins, vitamins, or minerals.

Adolescent athletes often do need to increase their sodium, potassium, and fluids during periods of increased training or competition. For a teenage athlete who exercises heavily for two hours a day, about 800 to 1,700 extra calories a day are needed, beyond those recommended for their age, sex, height, and weight. Caloric restrictions and rapid weight fluctuations should be avoided during the growth spurt.

Assessing Nutritional Status

If teenagers or their parents are concerned about dietary adequacy, there are ways to assess nutritional status. The first step is a standard history and physical examination, as discussed in Chapter 3. If the history suggests poor eating habits overall, the physician may refer the adolescent to a nutritionist or dietitian. If a specific nutritional deficiency is found, further evaluation to identify its cause may be necessary.

Nutritional deficiencies can produce many distinctive physical signs. For example, inadequate niacin or riboflavin can produce cracking at the corners of the eyes or mouth. Vitamin B_{12} deficiency can cause redness and smoothing out of the tongue. Severe deficiency of vitamin C causes bleeding and swelling of the gums (scurvy). Long-standing vitamin D and calcium deficiency causes thinning of the bones and easy fracturing. Iron deficiency causes weakness, paleness, and anemia. These are only a few of the many clinical signs of nutritional deficiency. In most cases, the deficiencies must be quite severe before the physical signs appear. If these or other findings on physical examination suggest nutritional problems, the physician may recommend further laboratory measurements.

Anthropometric measurements assess height, weight, and body fat in relationship to each other. For example, a weight of 100 pounds may be appropriate for a teenage girl who is five feet tall but too low for a girl who is five feet five inches tall. Skin-fold measurements taken at the triceps, chest, abdomen, or thigh give an indication of the proportion of the body that is fat. The mid-arm muscle circumference tells something about the body's overall muscle composition. These measurements, when considered together, provide helpful information about the adequacy of weight for height and the relationship of fat to lean muscle mass.

Generalized malnutrition and specific dietary deficiencies also can be detected by blood and urine tests. Many of these tests are routine and inexpensive. For example, individuals with malnutrition may have low protein or albumin levels in the blood. Teenagers with anemia often have low iron measurements. Cholesterol, triglyceride, glucose, sodium, and potassium can all be readily measured from a single, small sample of blood. Many other specific measurements of trace minerals and vitamins are available and can be obtained if the physician feels they are indicated.

Physicians and nutritionists may ask the teenager to keep a written record—a food diary—over several days to a week. Such records should include not only mealtime foods, but also snacks, beverages, diet foods, non-nutritive foods, and any unusual foods or eating patterns. Attempts to gain or lose weight and the methods used should be included in the food diary. The goal of the food diary is twofold. First, it may help identify important gaps in the teenager's diet. Second, the food diary may increase the adolescent's awareness of his or her eating patterns. For many teenagers, increased awareness provides the motivation to correct imbalances and to select more nutritious foods.

Encouraging Nutritious Eating Habits

Healthy eating patterns and adolescence may sometimes seem incompatible. Lecturing teenagers about the risks of cancer, diabetes, or heart disease is often futile. The side order of french fries is immediate; long-range health risks seem centuries away. Most adolescents are concerned about their appearance and their health. If they understand that their eating habits can affect the way they look and feel, they are more likely to eat a balanced diet. Teenagers want to maintain an attractive body weight, appear healthy and well-nourished, and feel energized. If the diet promotes current and future health, it does not matter whether the motivation is a trim body, glowing skin, shiny hair, or the prevention of adult cardiovascular disease. The result is the same: eating well during adolescence supports optimal growth and good health today and also improves the chances of well-being later in life.

6

Obesity

O*h, my God! I'm so obese!"* exclaims a five-foot-five, 120-pound sixteen-year-old struggling to button her jeans. She is not obese. She is not even overweight.

Teenagers are familiar with obesity, but many do not know its real meaning and implications. For a problem that is both common and increasing, obesity is widely misunderstood. Consider a few questions:

What causes obesity? What is the difference between "obese" and "overweight"? Why does obesity seem to run in families? Why do dieters have such trouble keeping off lost pounds? What are the psychological ramifications of obesity? What are its medical consequences? When and how should a teenager diet?

Obesity has been studied extensively, but many questions remain unanswered. Obesity is an undisputed problem for many Americans, including children and adolescents. Two facts stand out starkly:

- One in five American children and adolescents is obese.
- The prevalence of obesity has increased dramatically in the last few decades. From 1963 to 1980, the obesity rate among children aged six to eleven increased 54 percent and the rate for adolescents aged twelve to seventeen increased 39 percent.

Several factors contributed to this recent trend. American teenagers are eating faster and on the run. They are skipping breakfast

73

and lunch and are eating heavily at night, particularly in front of the television. They are eating when they are upset or depressed. They consume readily available, non-nutritious foods that are high in fat and low in fiber, protein, vitamins, and minerals. During the twentieth century, Americans of all ages radically changed their eating and exercise patterns. The shift from farm to city and improved transportation meant a decline in physical activity as part of the work day. Compared to our ancestors at the turn of the century, Americans in the 1990s consume 31 percent more fat and are 75 percent less physically active.

If the rising rate of obesity is to be halted or reversed, a better understanding of its definition, causes, consequences, and treatment is necessary. This is particularly important for young people who are establishing eating and exercise patterns that may last a lifetime.

What Is Obesity?

A diagnosis of obesity should not be made by the bathroom scale alone. The definition of obesity is complex and carries with it important health and social implications.

For years, *obesity* was defined as being at least 20 percent above ideal body weight and *overweight* as being 10 to 20 percent above ideal body weight. The concept of ideal body weight comes from weight charts based on age, gender, height, and frame size. Charts for adults were first developed by the Metropolitan Life Insurance Company to provide "desirable" weight guidelines, which were derived from actuarial data about the body weights of adults with the longest life spans. The World Health Organization created similar charts for children, based on age, gender, and height. These charts have important limitations, however, because they do not take into account frame size, pubertal stage, or percentages of fat and lean tissue. Weight tables for any age group—but especially for teenagers—should never be interpreted rigidly. Rather, they should be used as estimates of desirable weight ranges.

Definitions pertaining to weight should consider the proportions of lean and fat body tissue. An adolescent who is overweight is not necessarily obese. For example, an athlete who has increased lean body mass (or muscle) may exceed the standard weight for age, sex, and height, yet may not have excessive adipose tissue (fat). On the other hand, a sedentary adolescent of normal weight may have a high proportion of body fat. In males of ideal weight, approximately 10 to 15 percent of the body weight is fat. In females at menarche at least 17 percent is fat, and in most adult women at least 22 percent of body weight is fat. One definition of obesity requires that adipose tissue makes up over 25 percent of the male body weight and over 30 percent of the female body weight. The percentage of body fat can be estimated by calipers, which assess the thickness of skin folds in the back of the upper arm (triceps area), abdomen, or hips.

Consider three boys of the same height and age who weigh 130, 148, and 160 pounds. The 130-pound boy's weight is normal according to standardized charts. The 148-pound boy is overweight according to the charts, but when his proportion of body fat is calculated, it is low—10 percent. He is an active, fit athlete whose body has a healthy proportion of lean muscle tissue. The 160-pound boy is obese, not only because he is 20 percent above his ideal body weight, but also because his percentage of body weight as fat is high—30 percent.

The distribution of fat throughout the body may be important in determining the risks associated with obesity. The distribution pattern is determined by measuring the waist and hip circumferences. A high waist/hip ratio, exceeding 1.0 in adult males and 0.8 in adult females, may be associated with adult heart disease and stroke.

Causes of Obesity

Only 5 percent of obese adolescents have specific medical problems that cause their excess body weight. For the remaining 95 percent, obesity may be associated with contributing factors but the cause remains unclear.

Family predisposition plays an important role in obesity. Eighty percent of the offspring of two obese parents become obese, compared to less than 15 percent of the offspring of two normal-weight parents. When one parent is obese, the offspring face a 40 percent chance of becoming obese. Is this family tendency toward obesity the result of heredity, environment, or both?

Studies of twins and adult adoptees suggest that obesity is inherited. Identical twins, whose genes are exactly the same, are twice as likely to weigh the same as are fraternal twins, whose genes differ. The weights (corrected for height) of adults who were adopted in childhood correlate closely with the weights of their biologic parents but not with the weights of their adoptive parents.

Heredity does not tell the whole story. Several studies indicate that although genetics may determine a person's metabolic vulnerability to weight gain, it is the environment that determines whether that vulnerability is shielded or nurtured. A child with a genetic vulnerability to obesity who grows up in an environment where a moderate diet and exercise are encouraged may be at lower risk for obesity than a child with the same vulnerability whose life-style is sedentary and whose diet is high in calories. At the present time, the genes for obesity cannot be changed, but the environment— through diet and activity—can be adjusted to prevent and to treat obesity.

Why do different people seem to have different rates of metabolism or different tendencies to gain weight? One theory involves the concept of a "set point" in which the body regulates its weight just as a thermostat regulates a building's heat. When weight drops below an individual's set point, the body resists and pulls the weight back up to that threshold. The set point hypothesis is that this thermostat is located in a part of the brain called the hypothalamus. In obese people, the energy-regulating system may operate at a higher set point, so that eating and metabolism result in higher body weight and fat.

Some research using time-lapse photography suggests that obese people move less and expend fewer calories in daily activities than normal-weight people. Other studies suggest that, even at rest, obese people burn fewer calories than nonobese people. Still others indicate that the signals that control hunger and satiety (the sense of fullness) are abnormal in obesity. Until the cause of obesity is better understood, treatment options depend on two basic approaches: decreased caloric intake (diet) and increased energy expenditure (exercise). At no time are diet and exercise more important than during adolescence, when the foundations of self-image and adult habits are established.

Puberty and Weight Gain

As discussed in Chapter 2, puberty brings about major changes in body shape and size. Lean body tissue increases in both boys and girls, but more so in boys because their higher testosterone levels promote muscle development. This increase in muscle usually coincides with the height spurt. The increase in body fat experienced by girls typically begins about two years before the height spurt and continues throughout puberty.

Teenagers who have been of normal weight throughout childhood may become concerned about body size and shape in early puberty. In girls, the accumulation of fat in the regions of the hips, thighs, and buttocks may precede the rapid increase in height that accompanies the growth spurt. They should be reassured that with growth in height will come further adjustment of the body's contours. There are three times during life when the body's fat cells develop rapidly in preparation for important milestones. The first increase in fat occurs just before birth. The second occurs in infancy, when the baby is ready to crawl and walk. The third is early puberty, when the adolescent is about to grow taller, stronger, and become reproductively mature.

Obesity appears to affect puberty in several ways. Obese teenagers experience earlier sexual maturation and earlier growth spurts than normal-weight teenagers. Obese girls (who make up 60 to 70 percent of obese adolescents) usually menstruate at a younger age than normal-weight girls and have more menstrual disorders, such as irregular cycles and heavy menstrual flow.

Medical Consequences of Obesity

Many obese teenagers have been overweight since childhood. Because the excess weight has been gained gradually over the years, many take their weight for granted. And, because they usually feel well, most do not think about the eventual medical consequences. While obesity usually does not pose an immediate threat to teenagers, childhood and adolescent obesity is strongly associated with adult obesity, and adult obesity is a definite risk factor for serious medical problems.

The longer a child remains obese, the greater the likelihood of adult obesity. Consider the odds: 10 percent of obese infants, 25 percent of obese preschoolers, 40 percent of obese seven-year-olds, and *75 percent* of obese teenagers become obese adults. And adult obesity is associated with coronary heart disease, high blood pressure, some types of cancer, high cholesterol, diabetes, stroke, and musculoskeletal problems.

Even during adolescence, obesity can cause physical problems. During growth, the spine and the long limb bones may not develop properly. Knock knees and flat feet may result. In obese boys, gynecomastia, or excess breast tissue, is common. In girls, menstrual periods may be irregular. Respiratory problems and difficulty exercising may occur. These physical symptoms can exacerbate the emotional and social distress experienced by many obese teenagers.

Psychological Effects of Obesity

Obese adolescents are usually more concerned with the social and emotional aspects of obesity than with its medical ramifications. They worry more about how they look and what others think of them than about the health effects of obesity. Their weight adds to the emotional baggage carried by all adolescents as they strive to establish a positive self-image and find their place in the world.

Many obese teenagers have been teased, scorned, or shunned by their peers since childhood. Society is not kind to overweight people. Contemporary culture, through television, movies, magazines, and billboards, offers a slender ideal. A $33-billion weight-loss industry tells the American public that thin is in.

A cultural bias exists that obese people lack willpower or are lazy and self-indulgent. Children are sometimes cruel in voicing that bias. Adults may be more subtle, but the bias is still present. Overweight adolescents, for example, have lower college admission rates than normal-weight students. Some evidence suggests that guidance counselors and teachers tend to write less enthusiastic letters of recommendation about overweight than normal-weight students. Studies of hiring and promotion in the workplace also reveal a bias against overweight and obese employees.

By the time obese children reach adolescence, many have what psychologists call a "fat body image." They have envisioned themselves as overweight for so long that they have grown accustomed to that image, making weight loss all the more difficult. This does not mean that obese youth are happy about their weight. Rather, they cannot imagine themselves at normal weight. For some adolescents, the problem is further complicated by low self-esteem. Food can become both a culprit and a comfort. Some teenagers turn to food to decrease anxiety, stress, depression, or boredom. Obese teenagers may avoid sports, dances, and other peer activities outside the classroom because they see themselves as awkward. The result can be a sedentary life-style, social isolation, and loneliness.

Treatment of Obesity

Losing weight is not easy at any age. Successful dieting requires motivation and maturity, which many teenagers have not yet achieved. All dieters, but especially children and adolescents, should be cautious about how they proceed with weight loss. Increasing evidence indicates that children and teenagers who are in programs that involve their parents are more successful at losing weight than adolescents who attempt to manage their dieting alone. The family helps the teenager not only with the initial weight loss, but also with the all-important maintenance phase in which the lost weight remains off.

Before a diet begins, the adolescent and the family history of weight and diet attempts should be considered. Has the adolescent lost weight before? Why was the weight regained? What are the current eating habits? What foods are kept in the home? Does the adolescent *want* to follow a diet in order to lose weight? No diet will work if only the parent is motivated. Successful dieting requires desire to reduce on the part of the adolescent and support on the part of the family.

The ideal weight-reducing diet is nutritionally balanced and adequate in all respects except calories. The diet must be adapted to meet the adolescent's tastes and life-style. A successful diet plan is not a quick fix but rather one that induces a slow weight loss (one to two pounds per week) and can be followed for a long time. For adolescents who have completed puberty, diets of 1,200 to 1,500 calories per day usually are safe and well tolerated. All teenagers who require lower-calorie diets to lose weight and all teenagers who are still growing should be supervised by a physician.

Some obese teenagers require diets that are more restricted in calories in order to lose weight. These diets cannot be followed for more than a few months at a time because of their effects on metabolism. In most individuals who are on very low calorie diets, an adaptation occurs in which the resting metabolic rate falls, calories are burned more slowly, and the rate of weight loss decreases.

Protein-supplemented liquid diets tend to be the most extreme in caloric restriction. These diets can be both effective and safe in teenagers but *must* be monitored very closely by a physician. Side effects do occur, including low blood pressure, light-headedness, halitosis (bad breath), diarrhea, changes in hair or skin, fatigue, edema (fluid retention with swelling of the hands or feet), and loss of essential minerals.

Very low calorie diets can result in impressive weight loss, but they are short-term interventions. The adolescent is likely to regain the lost pounds unless the program includes behavior modification to change eating habits, exercise to burn calories and tone muscles, and a maintenance phase to reintroduce normal, balanced eating.

When a teenager is ready to commit to a weight-loss plan, several factors should be considered and discussed with a doctor and/ or nutritionist:

Goals. For weight to be lost and remain off, realistic goals must be set. A teenager may hope that a magic diet will make twenty pounds disappear by next week's prom, but short-term efforts lead to disappointing results. Slow, steady weight loss is both more effective and more easily achieved. A moderately obese teenager usually can cut calories by 30 percent without harming normal growth. Weight can be lost and good health maintained if portions are diminished and high-fat, high-calorie foods are reduced, but meals must be balanced to provide adequate nutrition.

Exercise. Most diets will fail if exercise is not included in the overall weight-loss plan. Dieting and exercise are partners in successful weight reduction and maintenance. Regular exercise increases the body's metabolic rate so that calories are burned more efficiently. It helps to decrease adipose tissue (fat), increase lean muscle tissue, and promote a sense of well-being and energy. Research indicates that exercise can actually decrease appetite and unnecessary eating.

Regular exercise should not be daunting. A dieter need not begin by jogging three miles a day. Brisk walking or dancing to fast music are realistic ways to begin an exercise program. The level and duration of the physical activity then can be increased as endurance and muscle tone improve. Even small changes in daily living can help burn calories—take the stairs instead of the escalator; ride a bike instead of the bus; put away the remote control; run for the wall phone instead of keeping a portable phone by your side. These suggestions may seem trivial, but modern society has lulled us with so much step-saving gadgetry that we forget how sedentary we can become.

Behavior modification. One of the most helpful ways to reduce weight and keep it off is to change one's eating behaviors. This goes hand in hand with eating less and exercising more. Behavior modification involves looking at the role food plays for the adolescent and for the family. It means taking a hard look at *how and why* people eat, not just *what* they eat.

For example: Do we eat when we aren't hungry? Why? Are there emotional issues that trigger eating? Do we eat rapidly? On the run? Do we sit down and have a conversation during mealtimes? Do we eat for recreation, while we watch television? Do we eat candy bars, cookies, or ice cream as rewards? When families consider these questions, they may find it easier to change the family's eating environment and thereby help the overweight adolescent lose weight.

Behavior modification also entails nonfood rewards for avoiding certain foods, for exercising, and for losing weight. Rewards can be simple and inexpensive, such as spending time with someone special or planning a day's outing. The point is not the value of the reward, but the moral support and pat on the back for the successful effort. Weight loss occurs more easily and is better maintained when the dieter and the family focus more on the improvements in exercise and eating than on calories and pounds.

Drug therapies. Some teenagers or their families may become so frustrated by low-calorie diets that they may consider appetite-suppressing drugs ("diet pills") to help them lose weight. Research indicates that these drugs can produce an additional pound of weight loss per week for a short time. But their effect is not long-lasting and, when they are stopped, weight gain always occurs. Hormones, such as thyroid hormone, should never be used for the sole purpose of weight loss. Diuretics cause weight to drop because of fluid loss but commonly cause dehydration and electrolyte imbalance. All drugs are potentially life-threatening and must not be used without qualified medical supervision. No drug has demonstrated long-term effectiveness in the treatment of obesity.

Surgery. Intestinal and gastric bypass procedures to decrease the stomach size and surgical removal of fat are therapies of last resort. They are used only for morbidly obese adolescents (at least 100 percent above ideal body weight) who have major medical complications related to their obesity and who have failed to lose weight by other methods. Surgery is rarely performed for those younger than age sixteen because of the many resulting complications and side effects.

Psychological Support for Weight Reduction

Reducing calories, increasing exercise, and changing eating behaviors all contribute to weight reduction. The key ingredient to successful weight loss is *motivation*. If the adolescent sees no particular benefit in losing weight or is apathetic about a diet plan, attempts by parents and others will fail.

Families can support a teenager's effort to diet by taking the spotlight off the teenager's weight. Nagging, criticizing, or shaming an adolescent into dieting is ineffective and counterproductive. So is focusing on every pound lost or gained. Because adolescence is a time of increasing independence, parental control of the diet plan is likely to impede both weight loss and the adolescent's sense of autonomy.

Family members can be more supportive by taking a low-key approach and by changing overall eating patterns at home. Specifically: Eat at regular times, encourage slower and more leisurely mealtimes with conversation, do more physical activities together, snack less between meals, keep the shelves and refrigerator stocked with fruits and vegetables rather than chips, cookies, ice cream, and candy.

Dieting adolescents also can benefit by support from outside the family. Peer groups of other dieting teenagers offer emotional support and socialization. Overweight adolescents often withdraw from social activities, and these groups help them recognize that they are not alone. The school nurse, family doctor, or nutritionist can help a teenager find a local peer support group.

Teenagers who have been obese for many years may face new or ongoing problems as they lose weight. They may continue to envision themselves as obese. They may still "feel fat," lack self-confidence, or have low self-esteem. Psychological counseling can help them adjust to their changing bodies and deal with the many issues that have been overshadowed by their obesity.

7

Anorexia Nervosa and Bulimia

Eating disorders commonly emerge during adolescence. Anorexia nervosa begins at an average age of 13.7 years, while bulimia usually occurs in late adolescence or young adulthood. Over 90 percent of people with eating disorders are female, but the prevalence appears to be growing among males.

Anorexia and bulimia have serious medical and psychological consequences that can become debilitating and even life-threatening if untreated. Neither disorder is ever purely medical or purely psychological. The treatment of both anorexia nervosa and bulimia requires the integration of medical management and psychotherapy. The earlier a diagnosis is made and therapy is begun, the better the prospects for a successful outcome.

In both disorders, food and weight constitute the central, obsessive focus of a young person's life. Yet neither eating disorder is solely about food or weight. Both have complex emotional roots and ramifications. By focusing on food and weight, a young person with anorexia or bulimia is attempting to control, survive, and cope with psychological dilemmas and conflicts.

Whether a young person takes the anorectic or bulimic route depends on varying personality and family characteristics. Anorexia and bulimia emerge from similar backdrops. Contemporary society broadcasts a powerful message: "Be thin if you want to be happy." Through advertisements, movies, television, videos, and magazines, the mass media project images of smiling, glamorous, THIN models and celebrities. Teenagers—who quite naturally want to be accepted, liked, and attractive—absorb the thin-is-in message and conclude: "I could be happier (that is, more popular and attractive) if I were as slender as those models and stars." This prevailing cultural environment, which fosters an obsession with weight loss, is one of the contributing factors to the rising incidence of eating disorders in the last half of the twentieth century.

Anorexia Nervosa

Anorexia has received much medical and media attention in recent years, but it remains a baffling problem with no single cause and no simple remedy.

SIGNS AND SYMPTOMS

Anorexia typically begins in a young adolescent girl who thinks that she is overweight. In reality, her weight is normal or only slightly above. She decides to diet by restricting her food intake, both in portion size and in type (no more meats or potatoes, for example). She may begin to exercise strenuously, to induce vomiting, or to use laxatives in an attempt to rid her body of food quickly, before it can be absorbed. Even as she loses weight, however, she still thinks she is "too fat." She stops menstruating as her body fat decreases. She continues to diet until her weight falls dangerously low. She often feels cold, so she wears layers of clothes both to keep warm and to conceal her skin-and-bones frame from her family and friends.

She becomes very secretive. She may sit at the dinner table with her family and pretend to eat, but she sneaks most of her food into her napkin and throws it away later. She may skip meals with the excuse, "I'm just not hungry," or "I'm just trying to lose a few pounds." While she shuns meals, she may display an unusual interest in food by preparing elaborate dishes for the rest of the family, but refusing to eat any herself. Her eating patterns become bizarre. She may cut her food into tiny slices, arrange food in precise patterns on her plate, or eat only very low calorie foods, such as salads without dressing.

A young person with anorexia nervosa also withdraws from friends and social activities. She continues to do well in school and even seems to work too hard. She vehemently denies any problems when asked why she's losing weight or not seeing her friends.

Her behaviors may seem contradictory. Her secrecy about her dieting and weight suggests that she is aware that her behavior is inappropriate. She truly believes, though, that she looks "too fat," even when she appears painfully thin. She has a "distorted body image," as psychologists describe it. When she looks in the mirror, she does not see the emaciated girl she has become, but one who still needs to lose a few pounds.

INDIVIDUAL AND FAMILY CHARACTERISTICS

Each young person and each family is unique. But experts who have studied and treated anorexia nervosa describe some common characteristics among young people with the disorder, their families, and their sociocultural environments.

The young adolescent with anorexia is usually female, has low self-esteem, and strives for perfection and achievement. She feels unsure about her personal identity and evolving independence from her parents. She tends to be obsessive or rigid in her behavior. She wants to feel "in control" of her thoughts, habits, and appearance. She is unusually—and abnormally—preoccupied with her body shape and size.

Some might argue that these characteristics apply to many teenagers who never develop anorexia nervosa. Are there other, more objective, biochemical, hormonal, or genetic traits that predispose an adolescent to anorexia? Hormonal changes do occur, but probably as a result, rather than a cause, of the starvation that typifies anorexia nervosa. There is no evidence of a genetic basis for the disease, although there may be familial or environmental patterns of abnormal eating. At the present time, research supports a complex basis for anorexia nervosa, rather than a purely biologic, psychologic, or social cause.

Several factors characterize the family environment of adolescents with anorexia nervosa. Parents tend to be overprotective. Family members are described as *enmeshed;* that is, their lives are tightly interwoven. In place of clear role definitions about who is parent and who is child, the parent may behave more like a peer or the adolescent may function as the parent's confidante. In an enmeshed family, a parent often speaks for the child, answering questions that are addressed to the child. The parent is overly involved in the details of the child's daily life. In other words, the parent may live through the child, rather than exemplifying a model for separate, adult autonomy.

One or both parents may be highly successful or achievement oriented. The children may assume that the same is expected of them. Adolescents with anorexia often are described as having been model children who caused their parents no distress or turmoil. Their families are regarded as solid citizens of the community, yet often are somewhat removed from friends or colleagues. Families of adolescents with anorexia also tend to be rigid and uncomfortable with change. In their attempt to avoid conflict, they minimize open discussion of problems. The children often become entangled in simmering, unspoken tensions between parents.

Parents or older siblings may also be highly concerned with food, diet, and their own body weight, shape, appearance, or physical condition. Occasionally someone else in the family has had an eating disorder or a mood disorder, such as anxiety or depression.

Anorexia affects families with many age, size, ethnic, and socioeconomic characteristics. It no longer is considered a disease solely of the white, upper-middle-class adolescent girl.

MEDICAL CONSEQUENCES

A young person who has anorexia *starves* herself. She refuses to maintain a minimum acceptable weight for her height and age because she is intensely afraid of gaining weight and becoming obese. Even as she becomes emaciated, her body image is so disturbed that she sees herself as fat. When her weight drops to 85 percent of what is expected for her height and age, she is considered to have anorexia nervosa and is at medical risk.

The physical consequences of anorexia nervosa are similar to those of malnutrition and starvation from any cause. For a still-growing adolescent, anorexia presents particular problems. They include the following:

Delayed growth and sexual maturation. A certain percentage of body fat is necessary for ovulation and menstruation. When the body fat falls below this critical value, whether from anorexia nervosa or another cause, menstruation will cease (amenorrhea). This is because the female sex hormones, estrogen and progesterone, are produced in abnormally low levels. Over time, estrogen deficiency contributes to osteoporosis, a weakening of the bones. This places a young person at risk for easy fractures. If she has not yet finished her growth spurt, anorexia may limit her full height potential and increase the risk of bone deformities. Anorexia also affects a young adolescent's sexual maturation. A ten-to-fourteen-year-old girl with anorexia will not have adequate body fat for puberty to advance. She will continue to appear childlike, with little or no breast development or secondary sexual characteristics.

Cardiac problems. An individual with anorexia may have an irregular or low heart rate, low blood pressure, thinning of the heart muscle, decreased size of the heart chambers, and electrolyte imbalance. Her body temperature drops because her heart pumps less blood and she has lost insulating body fat.

Gastrointestinal problems. She may have abdominal pain or constipation from delayed emptying of the stomach and intestines. When she feels bloated, she may overuse laxatives both for relief of symptoms and to promote weight loss. The resulting diarrhea can cause dehydration and serious electrolyte imbalance. Vomiting to rid herself of food can cause inflammation of the esophagus or pancreas, tears of the esophagus, dental cavities, and swelling of the parotid glands in the cheeks resulting in a chipmunk-like appearance.

Endocrine and metabolic problems. She may experience low blood sugar (hypoglycemia) with episodes of light-headedness, sweating, tremors, or confusion because she has lost normal sugar and fat stores. Weakness, fatigue, muscle cramps, and restlessness may result from malnutrition and electrolyte imbalance. Self-induced vomiting can cause life-threatening falls in the potassium level. Hormonal and kidney abnormalities can cause excessive loss of water and dehydration. The metabolism of fats can be affected, causing high cholesterol levels despite virtually no cholesterol or fat in the diet.

Skin and hair. Anorexia nervosa commonly causes the growth of fine, downy hair called lanugo on the shoulders, back, arms, and face. Scalp hair becomes brittle and dull. Pubic and underarm hair may thin. The palms may appear yellow- or orange-tinged from high carotene intake if the teenager has been eating primarily yellow vegetables. The skin usually is dry and often mottled. Very low protein levels from malnutrition can cause swelling of the feet, or edema, from leakage of fluid into the skin.

PSYCHOLOGICAL CONSEQUENCES

An adolescent's psychological makeup—her feelings about herself, her relationships with family and friends, and her future outlook—contribute to the development of anorexia nervosa. But once the disorder is established, it takes on a psychology of its own. Starvation and malnutrition cause biological changes that affect mood and behavior. The teenager may be cranky, stubborn, or apathetic because of her diminished energy reserve. This contributes to her denial of the problem and her resistance to treatment. She may misinterpret or ignore common physical sensations such as cold, hunger, or fatigue. She tries very hard to control everything in her life—from her diet, to her relationships, to the physical symptoms she experiences. Adolescents with anorexia nervosa may be obsessed with order; they may keep elaborate diaries of the food they have eaten, the pounds they have lost, or the hours they have exercised.

Depression is a common effect of starvation. As her weight falls and she struggles to maintain order with diminishing energy reserves, the anorectic adolescent suffers increasing anxiety and a sense of hopelessness and despair. The fear that she will lose control intensifies and she responds by tightening the reins on everything—but especially on her eating. Emaciated and exhausted, she continues to fight for control even as she loses it in a downward spiral of falling weight and deteriorating health.

TREATMENT

When parents suspect anorectic behavior in a teenager, it is *imperative* that they seek immediate professional help. Anorexia nervosa is not just another fad diet or a passing phase. It is a very serious disease with both medical and psychological consequences. The first step is to consult a physician. The teenager should be given time to talk with the physician alone, but the parents also must be permitted to give their side of the story. The parents' suspicions must be shared with both the adolescent and the physician together. When the history and physical examination support a diagnosis of anorexia nervosa, little laboratory testing is necessary. If the diagnosis is suspected but questionable, diagnostic testing and psychological evaluation should proceed simultaneously.

Anorexia will not be cured simply by urging the teenager to eat. A physician can begin by explaining the medical complications and insisting that sufficient weight must be regained to keep her medically safe. The doctor will reassure her that the goal is not to make her fat or to make her gain all of the lost weight in a week. The goal is to establish healthy eating and exercise habits that allow her to reach a weight that is appropriate for her age and height. The doctor will also make it clear that if the adolescent continues to lose weight or fails to maintain a minimum acceptable weight, hospitalization will be necessary.

The physician should refer the teenager and her family to a psychotherapist who is experienced in treating patients with eating disorders. The most successful treatment plans for adolescents incorporate medical monitoring, nutritional counseling, individual therapy, and family therapy. Because most adolescents still live with their families, the adolescent's eating disorder both affects and reflects the underlying family function. The likelihood that the teenager will overcome the problem is increased when the family understands its roots and works constructively toward a solution.

PROGNOSIS

Long-term follow-up studies indicate that up to 20 percent of adults with a history of anorexia nervosa remain underweight. Many continue to induce vomiting or abuse laxatives as adults. Up to half continue to have amenorrhea or infrequent menstrual periods. Most do well in school or work, but over a quarter continue to experience depression or anxiety as adults. The mortality associated with anorexia nervosa is one of the highest of all psychiatric disorders. Some of the deaths are due to the medical complications of starvation, but most are the result of suicide.

Certain factors seem to be associated with a good prognosis. These include younger age at onset and treatment, good educational achievement, improvement in self-image after gaining weight, and a supportive family. The fear associated with anorexia nervosa can result in a postponement of diagnosis and treatment. Teenagers and parents should recognize that there is effective treatment and that an immediate, unified approach provides the best chance for success.

BULIMIA

Like anorexia nervosa, bulimia is a disorder in which food and weight become an obsessive focus. The hallmark of bulimia is binge eating, counterbalanced with one or more behaviors to control weight. These behaviors include self-induced vomiting, periods of fasting, laxative abuse, and excessive exercise. Unlike anorexia nervosa, bulimia is not associated with profound weight loss. In fact, the bulimic adolescent typically is of normal weight and development. Her normal appearance camouflages her markedly abnormal eating and often delays recognition of the disease.

An individual with bulimia consumes large quantities of easily digestible food in a short time span, usually less than two hours. During the binge, she feels both driven to continue eating and afraid that she will be unable to stop eating. After the binge, she fears that the food will turn to fat and she tries to rid herself of the calories. This may mean self-induced vomiting or the use of escalating doses of laxatives. For some adolescents, the counterpoint becomes days of severe fasting or rigorous physical exercise. The binge-purge or binge-fast pattern of bulimia becomes a vicious cycle. It is much more than a once or twice experience of overeating. It may begin that way, but in full-fledged bulimia the episodes assume a regular, recurrent pattern, occurring at least twice weekly for at least three months. Like any habit, the longer the pattern goes on, the harder it is to break and the more it controls the individual.

SIGNS AND SYMPTOMS

The binge-and-purge episodes are almost always covert, or hidden, from family and friends. Family members may begin to notice that food is disappearing from the kitchen. Last night, five or six brownies were left in the baking pan. By morning, only a few crumbs remain. The carton of ice cream was nearly full. Now it is in the wastebasket, empty. As brother takes out the trash, he notices numerous potato chip and pretzel bags. Strange, he thinks, because Mom never buys junk food. Dad is sure he had three ten-dollar bills in his wallet. Why are there only two now? Mom is doing the laundry when she notices laxatives in the pockets of her daughter's jeans.

Not long after these minor mysteries, the parents begin to notice that their daughter excuses herself from the dinner table rather abruptly and heads for the bathroom. Sometimes they hear retching sounds and the toilet flushing. When they ask her if anything is wrong, she simply says, "Oh, no. I'm fine." A few nights later, at about 2:00 A.M., her father hears noises in the kitchen. On cat's feet, he walks downstairs and discovers his daughter, sitting on the floor in front of the open refrigerator. She is ravenously stuffing herself with last night's leftovers.

Family and friends may witness odd, secretive behaviors from time to time, but they may not realize the full extent of the young person's bulimia because her body size does not change noticeably. Over the long term, her weight is relatively stable. Over a matter of days, though, it may swing up and down by as much as ten pounds.

By the time the bulimic episodes become regular, several physical signs and symptoms may develop. Scratches, scars, or calluses appear on her hands because she uses her fingers to induce vomiting. Her face may appear round because the parotid gland between the jaw and ear enlarges from the repeated vomiting. She may complain of a burning sensation in her chest or a sour taste in her mouth from the chronic vomiting. Electrolyte imbalance and dehydration from vomiting, laxatives, or diuretics can cause muscle cramping, fatigue, light-headedness, or palpitations.

During a routing check up, the dentist may notice damaged tooth enamel on the inner side of the teeth, caused by the acid content of the vomitus. Numerous cavities and gum disease alert the dentist that vomiting has become frequent.

Family and friends may notice behavioral as well as physical signs of bulimia. The adolescent's moods may swing widely from euphoria to depression. Or she may be more irritable or anxious than usual. Her sleep pattern may be erratic because of nocturnal bingeing, diarrhea from laxatives, or insomnia from diet pills. She may be caught stealing food in a market or money from a parent or sibling. The overall picture is one of enormous conflict, anxiety, and out-of-control behavior.

FAMILY CHARACTERISTICS

The family portrait in bulimia differs somewhat from that of anorexia nervosa. Common characteristics found in families of bulimic youth include anger, emotional chaos and conflict, parental discord, impulsive behaviors, and indirect, unpredictable, or contradictory styles of communication between family members.

Families of bulimic youth often are disengaged and less trusting and nurturing than other families. Stress within the family is common, including alcoholism, drug abuse, gambling, depression, and abusiveness. An increasing number of adults now in treatment for bulimia are revealing that they were sexually abused during childhood and adolescence. Some experts believe that bulimia, in some cases, may be a delayed manifestation of these earlier assaults.

MEDICAL CONSEQUENCES

While body weight does not impose a health risk in bulimia, the binge–purge cycles do take a physical toll. The symptoms noted earlier can progress to life-threatening situations. Repeated vomiting causes loss of hydrochloric acid and fluid from the stomach. When the body attempts to make up for this dehydration, normal kidney function is disturbed and electrolyte imbalances occur. The results are weakness, muscle fatigue or spasms, temporary paralysis, numbness, and seizures. In the worst cases, there can be fatal irregularities of the heart's rhythm (arrhythmias).

The adolescent who uses syrup of ipecac to vomit runs a deadly risk. Many families stock ipecac in the medicine cabinet in case a young child swallows a harmful substance. If parents suspect that a teenager is using ipecac, they should remove it from the house immediately. Ipecac can be absorbed and stored in the heart muscle, eventually poisoning and killing this vital tissue.

The dehydration resulting from repeated purging can cause serious kidney problems. As the urine becomes more concentrated from the dehydration, crystals can precipitate and form stones within the kidneys, ureters, or bladder. Severe potassium deficiency, caused by vomiting, diuretics, or laxatives, can result in progressive kidney failure.

During bulimic binges, the favorite foods are often sweet. The pancreas responds to high-sugar foods by releasing extra insulin. This, in turn, drives sugar into the body's cells, causing blood sugar levels to drop quickly and creating an even greater craving for more sweets. The signs and symptoms of hypoglycemia (low blood sugar) are readily apparent: sweating, pallor, tremulousness, changes in mental alertness, fainting, or even seizures.

Gastrointestinal problems are the most common medical problems seen in bulimia. Ingesting handfuls of laxatives to purge calories is both dangerous and futile. Laxatives work on the large intestine after the stomach and small intestine have begun to digest food and absorb calories. Laxatives are therefore ineffective in reducing most of the caloric load. The body also develops a tolerance to laxatives, so that what begins as one or two tablets to induce diarrhea soon becomes a boxful. Eventually the result is chronic abdominal pain and severe constipation.

Other gastrointestinal complications of bingeing and vomiting include inflammation of the esophagus, stomach, and pancreas; ulcers of the stomach and small intestine; tears of the esophagus; and rupture of the stomach. Another consequence of frequent, prolonged vomiting is painful, uncontrollable, spontaneous regurgitation. The bulimic patient who has reached this state has trouble keeping down any food for more than a few minutes. Hospitalization, with intravenous feeding, is required.

PSYCHOLOGICAL CONSEQUENCES

As in anorexia nervosa, a young person with bulimia has low self-esteem and unresolved family conflicts. But unlike anorexia, a bulimic individual recognizes that she has an eating disorder. She may binge and purge in secret, but she does not deny the problem to herself. Once confronted, she is typically less stubborn and less resistant to the idea of treatment than is an adolescent with anorexia.

Bulimia has other psychological consequences distinct from anorexia nervosa. In focusing on food as a means to cope with problems, a bulimic adolescent experiences a wide range of emotions and demonstrates fluctuating moods and behaviors. She is impulsive before the binge, depressed and angry after it, and relieved when her weight is down and the bingeing quiescent. She constantly feels "controlled" by food. The next binge–purge episode is always on her mind. Some individuals describe a feeling of ecstasy or abandoned control at the onset of the binge, followed by a trancelike sensation during the binge. For most, however, this progresses to an intense fear that they will be unable to stop eating and halt the cycle.

Bulimia can seem contradictory because food is both friend and foe. A bulimic adolescent wants to know that food is readily available, as a comfort, when she next needs it. Yet she dreads that next binge. She also is very lonely. She views the binge–purge behavior as bizarre and may believe that she is the only one in the world who engages in it. She harbors her secret because she fears repulsion, should others discover it. To the outside world, she may seem fine, but inside she is terribly alone.

Young people with bulimia seem to be at increased risk for abuse of substances other than food. Their use of alcohol, sedatives, amphetamines, and cocaine surpasses that of people without bulimia.

One study of adults with bulimia indicated that 50 percent had substance abuse problems.

TREATMENT

The greatest impediment to effective treatment is the length of time a young person engages in bulimia before it is recognized. Because the behavior is so secretive and because the young person is of normal weight, parents may not realize that their daughter has struggled for months or years. The typical young woman with bulimia has binged and purged for two to five years before she begins treatment.

Treatment with a psychotherapist who understands the disease should begin as soon as the bulimia is recognized. If medical problems are present, a physician must become involved. A nutritionist may also be part of the treatment team to help the adolescent reestablish healthy food habits. For example, nutritional counseling can help her avoid foods that trigger a binge (such as concentrated sweets or baked goods) and can encourage her to eat three regular meals a day with fewer between-meal snacks. If she can begin to reduce her binges, the purges will decrease as well. Exercise should be encouraged—in moderation—as a healthier weight control method than purging.

Some physicians prescribe antidepressant medication for bulimia. This is not a cure for bulimia but may help decrease the use of bingeing to regulate mood. Before beginning any medication, the teenager and parents should discuss the benefits, risks, and side effects with a physician.

Medical and nutritional intervention is only part of a good treatment plan. Long-term treatment requires psychotherapy to help the young person understand the roots of her disorder and to support her search for better ways to cope with conflict or stress. Family and individual therapy is recommended for most adolescents, particularly in the beginning of treatment. As therapy progresses, as she leaves home for college or moves out on her own, individual therapy without family may become more appropriate. Many support groups exist for young people with eating disorders, as well as for their families. These groups provide important moral support, encouragement, and information. But they are not a substitute for skilled psychotherapy. Groups are best used as a supplement to, rather than a replacement for, therapy.

PROGNOSIS

Reliable statistics about the prognosis for young people with bulimia do not exist. Some studies indicate that one-quarter recover with treatment; that is, they stop bingeing and purging. For most individuals with bulimia, relapses occur both with and without treatment. These relapses are most likely to emerge during times of change or stress, such as leaving home for a job or for college. With good counseling, the young person with bulimia can begin to identify the precipitating factors. Sometimes these factors can be avoided or minimized. At other times, she can develop healthy coping strategies that break the binge–purge cycle and allow her to lead a more balanced, happier life.

8

Sleep, Energy, and Fatigue

An alarm clock is ineffective. A loud knock on the door brings a groggy response: "Okay, I'm awake." Ten minutes later, the teenager is sound asleep.

Parents often worry about the amount of sleep that adolescents do—or do not—get. How much is enough? How much is too much? Is something wrong if he sleeps thirteen hours straight on a weekend? Why does she insist on staying up so late when she must awaken at dawn to catch the school bus?

To put these questions in some perspective, consider the transition in sleep that occurs from birth through adulthood. Most infants sleep fifteen to twenty hours a day during their first six months. By a year of age, babies usually sleep through the night and are awake up to eight hours at a stretch. Toddlers average twelve to fourteen hours of sleep a day. Preschoolers require ten hours at night, plus a midday nap. The need for sleep decreases during childhood but does not usually fall below ten hours a night. Most adults require six to eight hours of sleep each night to feel rested.

Between childhood and adulthood, teenagers approach the diminished sleep requirements of adulthood with the same conflict that characterizes many other aspects of development. Their rapidly growing bodies demand sleep even as their life-styles expand to fill every waking hour. After school, there are sports, homework, chores, television, and phone calls. Parents who are asleep by midnight may not realize that their teenager is on the phone until 1:00

A.M. When she must arise five hours later, it is no wonder that she is tired throughout the day.

Most teenagers need at least eight hours of sleep each night. Rapid growth requires energy, and energy requires periods of rest for refueling. Hormone secretion, which is responsible for growth and development, also depends on predictable patterns of sleep. The release of growth hormone occurs in bursts that reach a peak within an hour of falling asleep. More than two-thirds of the total growth hormone in the bloodstream is secreted at night, during sleep. The beginning of puberty is heralded by nighttime increases in the release of a hormone called luteinizing hormone (LH). The LH travels through the bloodstream and stimulates the ovaries to produce estrogen and the testes to produce testosterone. As puberty and sexual maturation proceed, the nocturnal secretion of LH gradually changes to the adult pattern of intermittent secretion throughout the twenty-four-hour period.

When adolescents hear that they need at least eight hours of sleep each night, the common response is, "No problem. I'll sleep late on the weekend." But this catch-up phenomenon rarely works. Weekends are busy with friends and activities out of school. Nights are late and days are full. The sleep that occurs at noontime is interrupted by daylight, household noise, and the normal physiologic drive to be awake. Teenagers should set a goal of eight hours sleep *each* night, throughout the week and weekend. While difficult to achieve at times, this pattern promotes a sense of restfulness and well-being.

Many teenagers find it a challenge to organize their time efficiently. It often seems impossible to cram everything, including sleep, into a twenty-four-hour day. Juggling many demands may mean studying past midnight for tomorrow's history test. But a maturing (and tired) teenager will realize the next morning that had the telephone hour after dinner been spent studying, there could have been an extra hour of sleep. Parents may warn adolescents of this in advance, but their suggestions and urging are usually less successful than the teenager's own experience.

Adolescents vary widely in their individual sleep patterns. Just as some adults are morning larks and others are night owls, teenagers also develop different styles. Some are light sleepers; others sleep deeply. Some nap; others never do. The exact number of hours of sleep will differ from one adolescent to the next. But all adolescents need a consistent pattern of uninterrupted nighttime sleep to support their growth, their active life-styles, and their over-all health.

Sleep Disorders

Adolescents usually fall asleep easily and quickly. They may lie in bed for a short while to replay the day's events, think about friends, or decide what they will do tomorrow. But as those thoughts fade, sleep comes readily for most teenagers. And sleep offers a healthy respite from the worries and pressures of adolescence.

In the 1989 National Adolescent Student Health Survey, only 6 percent of teenagers described themselves as "often sleepless." Fifty percent reported "never" experiencing sleeplessness and 44 percent said they "sometimes" do.

When sleep disorders occur during adolescence, they most commonly appear as daytime drowsiness or fatigue. The cause may become clearer if the adolescent keeps a written record of sleep patterns for a few weeks. The record should note the total amount and times of nighttime sleep and daytime naps. It also should note any sleep-related problems, such as:

- trouble falling asleep at night,
- trouble staying asleep at night,
- trouble waking up in the morning,
- trouble staying awake during the day,
- nightmares, sleepwalking,
- bed-wetting,
- snoring or trouble breathing during sleep,
- unusual movement or restlessness during sleep.

Sometimes the record will help the adolescent understand and correct the reason for the sleep problem. If it persists, a doctor should be consulted. Share the sleep record with the physician. The evaluation will include a review of the sleep record, a thorough medical history, and a physical examination.

Drowsiness may be caused by something other than lack of sleep. Stress, anxiety, depression, other psychological problems, and drug or alcohol use can all cause fatigue. Or there may be an underlying medical problem, such as iron deficiency anemia, which is common during adolescence (Chapter 35). Extreme obesity and enlarged tonsils occasionally cause blocked airways during sleep, resulting in loud snoring and difficulty breathing. Teenagers with this problem often complain of nightmares, restlessness during sleep, trouble waking up in the morning, and trouble staying awake during the day. Adolescents with asthma may have nighttime wheezing, coughing, or other respiratory problems that disrupt sleep. Nighttime snacking, resulting in a full stomach or full urinary bladder, may interrupt sleep.

Insomnia, the most frequent sleep disorder, includes trouble falling asleep, trouble staying asleep, or waking up earlier than desired. Physical illness, pain, or substance abuse can cause insomnia. But it is more often attributable to stress, anxiety, depression, and irregular bedtime routines. A teenager with insomnia should consider the following:

- Make bedtime and awakening times more routine; try to arise at the same time each day and avoid daytime naps and long stretches of sleep on weekends.
- Try to think about problems during the day, before getting into bed at night; set aside twenty minutes to listen to quiet music; learn and practice relaxation techniques; if the feelings of stress or worry persist, seek counseling early.
- Change the bedroom environment; keep it dark and quiet; remove the television or phone from the bedroom.
- Avoid caffeine-containing soda, coffee, tea, and chocolate.
- Get more exercise, but do it early in the day.

Enuresis (bed-wetting) rarely begins in adolescence but it persists from childhood in up to 5 percent of teenagers. All adolescents with enuresis should be evaluated by a physician. If the enuresis is new, it is more likely that the cause is medical rather than psychological (Chapter 30).

Narcolepsy is a rare condition characterized by an uncontrollable urge to fall asleep, resulting in "sleep attacks" lasting from a minute to an hour or longer. These sleep attacks are not just sleepy feelings or dozing during boring lectures. They happen at any time or place—even in the middle of a dance or a horror movie—and the individual cannot resist sleep. The attacks occur most frequently after meals, late in the day, and after slow-paced, quiet periods. When narcolepsy occurs, the muscles may be temporarily limp; immediately before falling asleep or on awakening, the individual may be unable to move. Narcolepsy typically appears between the ages of ten and twenty-five and probably has an inherited component; 10 to 50 percent of people with narcolepsy have close relatives with the disorder.

If narcolepsy is suspected, a physician should be consulted immediately. The disease can be treated by stimulant medication, which is taken in the morning or midday. Brief daytime naps also may help prevent the sleep attacks. Teenagers with narcolepsy should avoid driving cars or engaging in any other activities during which a sleep attack could place them or others in danger.

Sleep apnea, or hypersomnia, may be confused with narcolepsy. The drive to sleep is less powerful than in narcolepsy, but the sleep episodes are more prolonged. A teenager who suffers sleep apnea has disturbed nighttime sleep and feels tired all day long. Schoolwork and behavior are seriously disrupted by constant daytime drowsiness.

Sleep apnea is a manifestation of an underlying physical problem. Obstructive sleep apnea occurs when the airway is blocked during sleep. The most common cause of this during adolescence is markedly enlarged tonsils and adenoids. Central sleep apnea occurs when the respiratory center in the brain fails to regulate breathing normally. The resulting retention of carbon dioxide by the lungs results in fatigue, sleep, or even coma. The diagnosis of sleep apnea, whether obstructive or central, usually requires an overnight sleep study in a facility that is prepared to monitor respiration, heart rate, and brain wave activity. Sleep apnea is a potentially life-threatening problem that demands evaluation and treatment.

Sleepwalking, nightmares, and night terrors, occur infrequently during adolescence. Sleepwalking (or somnambulism) is more common during childhood and usually disappears spontaneously before adolescence. It is relatively harmless, but precautions should be taken to move objects out of the way and to lock doors.

Night terrors and nightmares also are more common during childhood than during adolescence. Night terrors affect boys more than girls and are far more disturbing to both the child and parent than are nightmares. Night terrors are accompanied by intense fear and anxiety, as well as screaming, moaning, or restless behavior. It is difficult to awaken someone who is having a night terror. After awakening, there is little memory of the terror. Medication may be prescribed for a brief period to suppress night terrors.

A young person having a nightmare, on the other hand, usually does not cry or scream, is awakened easily, and has clear recall of the dream. Nightmares tend to have a psychological rather than a physical cause but can be associated with problems such as sleep apnea or drug abuse.

Fatigue

Most healthy teenagers complain of fatigue from time to time. But fatigue is nebulous, both as a term and as a symptom. When a teenager says, "I'm exhausted," or "I don't have any energy," or "I feel weak," it is difficult to determine the seriousness of the complaint and its cause. "I feel weak" may mean "My muscles have no strength" or "I feel tired . . . or achy . . . or faint . . . or light-headed." And even if the teenager describes the symptoms clearly, the cause often remains unclear: Is the teenager generally over-exerting—staying up too late, partying too much, working too long at a part-time job? Is there an underlying physical problem, such as an infection or anemia? Or is the fatigue a manifestation of a psychological problem, such as depression, anxiety, or stress?

When an adolescent complains of fatigue, begin by considering recent activities. If there has been considerable physical or mental exertion recently—increased athletic training or cramming for exams—the fatigue probably is a normal response to the metabolic effects of overwork. This common, everyday fatigue is transient; it will pass once the body is rested and re-energized.

If overexertion has not occurred, review the teenager's daily pattern of sleep and nutrition. Look also at the teenager's moods: Have there been recent or abrupt mood swings? unusual signs of passivity or indifference? a drop in motivation? change in school performance or activities? change in friends? These problems suggest a psychological basis for the fatigue. The best approach to the evaluation of this adolescent's fatigue is to explore the psychological and physical avenues simultaneously.

Fatigue is a common symptom of underlying physical disease but it usually is not the only symptom. Chronic infections, such as hepatitis or mononucleosis, cause fatigue but also cause fever, or rash, or swollen glands, or abdominal discomfort. Anemia is one disorder that can appear as only weakness or fatigue; it is readily detected by a red blood cell count. Other causes of fatigue that a physician will consider include metabolic, hormonal, nutritional, muscle, or nerve problems. Whenever fatigue persists, whether alone or with other symptoms, a physician should be consulted.

Chronic Fatigue Syndrome

Chronic fatigue syndrome (CFS) has received widespread attention in recent years. Despite much research, its cause is elusive and no treatment has been proven effective. CFS is not the normal fatigue that follows overexertion or accompanies periods of emotional distress. CFS is persistent and debilitating. It comes on suddenly, often coincident with a viral infection, but the fatigue persists long beyond the other viral-type symptoms. CFS often is called chronic postinfectious fatigue syndrome or postviral fatigue syndrome, even though a viral cause remains unproven.

Diagnosing CFS is a process of elimination. There is no laboratory test that confirms CFS. When doctors exclude other causes of fatigue—such as anemia, underactive thyroid, malnutrition, infection, pregnancy, sleep disorder, emotional problems—CFS becomes suspect. The fatigue usually is accompanied by other symptoms in varying degrees: fever, headache, sore throat, swollen glands, achy muscles, joint pain, depression, forgetfulness, confusion, or difficulty concentrating.

The fatigue and flulike symptoms of CFS may be constant or may wax and wane. The diagnosis depends on symptoms that have occurred so persistently over a six-month period that the individual's overall functioning is impaired. People with CFS commonly report that their fatigue is precipitated by exercise but is out of proportion to the amount of exertion. Some experience drenching night sweats, morning stiffness, light-headedness, sleep problems, irritability, and distractibility. Before the onset of the syndrome, most were active, healthy, young people.

CFS typically appears in late adolescence or early adulthood, although it has been diagnosed in children. It occurs twice as often in females as in males. Megavitamins, special diets, and numerous medications have been tried for CFS, but with little success. In most instances, the symptoms abate spontaneously, over a course of months or years. Until then, many patients, especially adolescents, benefit from psychological counseling to help them deal with the debilitating symptoms of their illness.

CFS is not a common problem. The vast majority of adolescents who complain of fatigue will improve after some adjustments of their busy schedules. Remember that fatigue is a common symptom that often is a healthy reminder that it is time for rest and refueling.

9

Dealing with Chronic Conditions

• Donald has diabetes. He gives himself insulin injections and must have snacks to balance his blood sugar. Donald feels self-conscious about eating in class. The stares and teasing remarks of his classmates are hard to ignore.

• Rob survived a childhood brain tumor. He has beaten the malignancy, but the surgery and radiation therapy impaired his growth. He is shorter than his classmates and hates the thought of once again standing in the front row for the class picture.

• Cara lobbies her parents for a driver's license. Afterall, she is eighteen, and her sixteen-year-old brother has started driver education classes. "Is it because I have Down syndrome that I can't drive?" she asks.

• Laura is paralyzed below the waist from a childhood infection of the spinal cord. She spent months in the hospital and was well known to the pediatric staff. At age nineteen, she was admitted to the hospital's adult floor. No one knew her. There were no familiar faces. Laura felt suddenly, abruptly alone.

Donald, Rob, Cara, and Laura are four of the approximately two million American children and teenagers who have chronic illnesses or disabilities. Some will not survive to adulthood. Others will remain physically or cognitively limited throughout their lives. Still others can expect cures or treatments that will improve the quality of their lives far beyond the predictions of a few years earlier.

Whatever their present or future medical conditions, they are first and foremost teenagers. They share the concerns of all adolescents—body image, sexual maturity, independence, school performance, peer relationships. But adolescents with chronic illness or disability face additional challenges. The process of maturation is complicated by health-related issues and by constraints imposed by parents, physicians, schools, and environment. A chronic condition during adolescence can be even more upsetting or frightening than an acute or sudden condition. An acute illness generally brings with it an expectation or hope of full recovery. Years of living with a chronic illness or disability bring the frustrating reality that a complete recovery or cure is unlikely. As teenagers work toward autonomy and an independent adulthood, this reality may become increasingly difficult to accept.

Adolescent tasks, such as developing a strong personal identity, assuming greater responsibility, and planning for the future, cannot be separated from the illness or disability. They are part of the adolescent's overall health and well-being. The rapid physical and emotional changes of puberty can complicate the management of an underlying medical problem. One teenager's story illustrates many of the challenges confronting young people with chronic illnesses or disabilities:

Sarah is sixteen and has cystic fibrosis, a chronic disease of the lungs (Chapter 27). Her identity has been colored by her illness since early childhood. She needed oxygen for a bout of the flu. She was in the hospital for her junior prom. She coughed her way through the school play. Sarah says, "I feel like I'm always wearing a sandwich board that says **cystic fibrosis.**"

Sarah had been a compliant child, willing to follow instructions and take her medications. As a teenager she began to bristle at the decisions made by her doctors and parents. She missed several clinic appointments. She often refused the daily physical therapy that helped relieve congestion in her lungs. Sarah knew she should take responsibility for her care, but she resented the pull away from the "normal" life of her peers.

At the time of her diagnosis, Sarah's parents were told that the average life expectancy for children with cystic fibrosis was nineteen years of age. Believing that she would not reach adulthood, her parents gave her everything she wanted. As Sarah grew older, more effective ways to treat cystic fibrosis were discovered. Life expectancy improved dramatically. Her parents began to wonder if, in their love and concern for Sarah, their overprotection had shielded her from important opportunities to make her own decisions, try new things, prepare for adulthood.

Like Sarah, many teenagers with chronic problems have improved health prospects. Medical advances now help 84 percent of children with chronic illness and disability reach adulthood. The survival rate of children with congenital heart disease, for example, has increased 300 percent since 1965. The survival rates for leukemia and spina bifida (an incomplete formation or fusion of the spinal canal) have increased 200 percent. Premature infants who, twenty years ago, would not have survived the first month of life, now are approaching their teens thanks to new medical technology. Such advances give families great hope, but they do not erase the many complexities of chronic disease or disability as a young person progresses through adolescence.

Effects of Chronic Conditions on Teenagers

A major task of adolescence is moving from childhood dependence toward adult independence. When a teenager has a chronic condition, medical restrictions may prolong dependency on parents, physicians, and other adults. This takes a heavy toll on the teenager who strives to be more autonomous but recognizes that adults must continue to make important medical and social decisions that interfere with the normal life of a typical teenager. Frustrated by these conflicts and limitations, an adolescent may be a "good," compliant child one day, and a rebellious, obstreperous teenager the next. The reasons for these fluctuations in behavior stem from the struggle to adjust to increasing personal competence, an evolving peer network, and rapidly changing bodies.

Body image is a concern of all teenagers, but for the young person with a visible condition, it assumes even greater importance. Adolescents are highly aware of their appearance. They compare their changing bodies with those of their friends. Most want to blend into the crowd and to feel reassured that what is happening to them is happening to their friends in similar ways. For a teenager in a wheelchair or one with thinning hair from chemotherapy, the outward sign becomes a conspicuous red flag of "difference."

For some teenagers, the underlying condition or its treatment may affect the onset or progression of puberty. Radiation therapy or chemotherapy for childhood cancer, for instance, may result in shorter physical stature or delayed sexual maturation. Many chronic diseases, such as chronic kidney failure, Crohn disease (a type of inflammatory bowel disease), and cystic fibrosis, are associated with pubertal delay. Early or precocious puberty can result from other conditions, such as spina bifida or hormone-producing tumors. All of these conditions are discussed in more detail in Part V. The objective here is not to describe the specific effects of each, but to emphasize that a chronic condition can influence physical maturation and that this effect may be most pronounced and apparent during puberty.

For an adolescent whose body cannot approach the ideal portrayed in magazines and television advertisements, puberty can be a time of social isolation and self-doubt. Unsure about how to cope with stares, unwanted attention, and unkind or intrusive remarks, teenagers with visible conditions may prefer to avoid social situations, including school. As the adolescent experiences increasing anxiety about appearance, friendships, and sexual relationships, there may be a growing reluctance to discuss these issues.

It is more than visible signs, however, that contribute to a feeling of difference for adolescents with chronic conditions. In fact, studies show that teenagers with nonvisible conditions, such as congenital heart disease, experience more emotional distress than those with more apparent conditions. The reasons for this are unclear, but may be related to the tension of trying to keep the illness hidden, to appear and function normally despite the ever-present physical limitations. Other people may add to this burden because they do not understand the limitations of a condition that they cannot see.

Adolescents with chronic illness and disability may experience more conflict and challenge than their able-bodied peers, but there is no evidence that they are more likely to develop serious psychiatric problems. Youth with chronic conditions demonstrate a flexibility that often carries them through their teenage years with grace and fortitude. It is this extraordinary strength that the adolescent, family, and health professionals must hold on to during the times of greatest turmoil.

As adulthood approaches, the questions and concerns begin to shift from present to future. Will I be able to move away from home? Will I always be dependent on my parents? What kind of job can I get? Will I be able to support myself? Will anybody find me attractive? Will I be able to have normal sexual relations? Can I have children? Will they have the same medical problems that I have? These are just a few concerns that require sensitive, honest discussion with knowledgeable adults. Parents usually cannot provide all the answers. Access to physicians, nurses, social workers, and adults with similar conditions becomes very important as these questions arise.

Many teenagers benefit from getting to know adults with the same conditions. These adults have a level of understanding and a perspective that comes from personal experience. Having coped with the disability and adolescence, adults with chronic conditions offer teenagers a window on the future.

Expectations about the future can affect behavior today. A teenager who expects to die before adulthood may seek instant gratification whenever possible. At some level, parents understand—and may agree—with the adolescent's motivation. At a deeper level, they rightfully worry about the risks involved. The risks may take many forms, from skipping medication doses, to dropping out of school, to more overtly dangerous behaviors. These negative actions may reflect the only control that the adolescent can exert over an unfair and seemingly hopeless situation. Understanding why the behaviors occur cannot remove the underlying illness, but it can help reduce the conflict that arises between frustrated, frightened adolescents and their parents.

How Teenagers Cope with Disease and Disability

Involved, loving families can help adolescents with chronic conditions cope with challenges successfully. But even in the most supportive families, difficulties can arise as the inevitable behavioral, emotional, and cognitive changes of adolescence occur. Mood and behavior can seesaw—almost overnight—from regression and dependence to maturity and autonomy. These are normal coping mechanisms, reflecting the teenager's attempt to adjust to the underlying condition while simultaneously negotiating the tasks of adolescence. It is helpful for families to understand and anticipate the strategies that teenagers may use to cope with their illness or disability:[7]

• *Denial* is a common reaction, particularly in early and mid-adolescence, which can lead to defiance or noncompliance—skipping medications, therapies, and doctors' appointments. Denial is usually the initial defense mechanism, occurring soon after a new diagnosis or medical setback.

• *Acceptance* of the condition and its limitations is uncommon in early and mid-adolescence. As the older adolescent matures and gains greater cognitive insight, acceptance begins to develop. Calm, intellectual interest in the condition does not necessarily imply acceptance. People of all ages, when faced with a debilitating illness, may avoid their feelings by intellectualizing; that is, they demonstrate great interest in the medical details in an attempt to avoid dealing with their anxiety, fear, frustration, or anger. Intellectualizing usually occurs in mid- to late adolescence, once the young person has developed the cognitive capability for abstract, complex reasoning. This is also the stage at which the persistence of the condition into adulthood begins to force a confrontation with feelings.

• *Projection* is a method of transferring emotions to others; snapping at a nurse or yelling at a parent, for example.

• *Displacement* is another way to shift unpleasant feelings elsewhere—complaining about lengthy delays in the waiting room, when the teenager is actually frightened about the impending bone marrow biopsy. With increased stress, the teenager may escalate from displacement to aggressive behavior, such as throwing a bedpan.

• *Compensation* is a positive way of coping with the constraints of disease or disability. A teenager who must forego certain sports because of physical limitations, for example, may develop artistic or musical abilities.

• *Identification with the aggressor* is a way of turning a negative experience into something positive; a teenager with leukemia may talk about going to medical school to become an oncologist, a doctor who treats cancer.

• *Regression* is a common reaction to a stressful situation or a medical crisis. When apprehensive about a new development, teenagers may regress to a childlike dependency on adults—parents, doctors, nurses. Adolescents who have been ill or disabled since childhood often have strong ties with their pediatricians and, during stressful periods, may try to recapture those comfortable, dependent relationships. Sometimes this is an appropriate and effective mechanism for the adolescent. At other times, especially for the young adult, reinforcing such dependency impedes the transition to adult care. Returning to the pediatric setting in these instances can convey the incorrect message that it is allowed because the prognosis for adult survival is poor.

Depending on their medical status and their social, emotional, and cognitive development at a given moment, teenagers may use any of these behaviors to help them cope with their emerging identities within the context of their chronic conditions.

Families and health professionals can smooth the way by maximizing teenagers' participation in medical decision-making and management. Ideally, the process of enlisting children as active players begins early, before adolescence. Older children with diabetes, for example, can give themselves insulin injections and can be responsible for monitoring their diets. Today, youth with cancer usually are told the diagnosis and are involved in the decisions regarding surgery, chemotherapy, or radiation therapy.

Increasingly, health professionals are urging adolescents to take responsibility for making and keeping doctors' appointments, taking their medications, and avoiding certain foods or activities. Teenagers who take an active role tend to comply better with medical regimens and manage their conditions more successfully than those who are not encouraged to do so. Giving responsibility to a teenager can breed responsibility. As adults demonstrate their trust, adolescents begin to trust their own competence as young adults.

The Family Circle

Families pay enormous costs in emotion, time, energy, and money whenever a child has a chronic medical problem. For many families, these costs have been mounting since the child's birth. Over the years, many families develop coping strategies which, they hope, will carry them through their child's adolescence. Mom or Dad may have taken an extra job to pay for expenses not covered by medical insurance. Friends and neighbors may have formed a supportive network to assist with the child's physical therapy. No matter how well a family has accepted the condition and made plans to manage it, adolescence usually brings new, unexpected twists. The child who happily cooperated with volunteers, for instance, becomes a teenager who demands privacy. She now sees their assistance as an unwanted invasion.

One of the most common struggles between parents and teenagers is about protectiveness. Parents naturally want to safeguard their child from danger. The teenager may see their limits as overly restrictive. A rule that was accepted throughout childhood may suddenly be met with an angry "Stop babying me!" As the teenager lashes out, parents may feel hurt and confused.

Parents walk a tightrope as they try to balance protection and letting go, safety and freedom. On the one hand, they must set some firm limits. On the other hand, they need to allow the teenager to branch out, to take safe risks, to develop a healthy, full social life. Some of these challenges are independent of the adolescent's disease or disability. Most, though, are affected by it in some way— either through the potential risk to the adolescent or through the anxiety and concern experienced by the parents. Adolescents and parents agree that it is often difficult to maintain the balance between health and illness, safety and risk, reliance and independence.

Siblings and spouse may be overlooked as a parent attends to the many needs of an adolescent with a chronic condition. No parent deliberately neglects the other parent or the healthy siblings, but it is difficult to apportion attention equally to each member of the family. During childhood, siblings may not voice their feelings. They may feel guilty about complaining when a parent makes a hospital visit instead of attending their ball game. They may fear that something bad will happen to their brother or sister if they misbehave. They may worry about their own health, focusing on minor aches and pains.

Parents sometimes hope that growing up with a chronically ill or disabled sibling will promote sensitivity or compassion. When siblings reach adolescence, they usually grasp the details of their brother or sister's condition, but their emotional understanding may lag behind their medical understanding. They may begin to voice frustration or anger: "You give her more attention," "You care more about her," "You never have time for me." Healthy teenagers often are torn by the love and resentment they feel toward both their parents and their disabled sibling. Parents can help by recognizing these conflicts and by encouraging siblings to vent their feelings in constructive discussions.

Managing Chronic Conditions

Medical management is best handled by a team of health professionals who know the adolescent well and are knowledgeable about the specific disease or disability. Several general suggestions can help teenagers and their families integrate the medical, psychological, social, and financial aspects of care.

The overall goal during adolescence is to promote a smooth transition from the pediatric or childhood health care environment to an adult health care setting. During this transition, the adolescent assumes increasing responsibility for the management of the condition and for general health and well-being. Parents, siblings, physicians, nurses, therapists, school personnel, social workers—everyone involved with the teenager—can ease this transition in several ways:

• Discuss the condition openly, from its limits to its reasonable expectations. Don't condescend or withhold information, especially when the teenager asks direct questions.

• Encourage the teenager to talk with health professionals directly and to ask for clarification when confused. Give the adolescent time alone with the doctor or nurse. Avoid answering questions that are directed to the teenager. Encourage the teenager to provide the medical history. Parents are often surprised about how accurate and thorough that history can be.

• Include the adolescent in planning the transition from pediatric to adult care. Do not push a move away from a well-loved pediatrician until the teenager is ready. Many children with chronic conditions have grown up with a team of specialists rather than a single primary care physician. It may help to identify one team member who will be an advocate and an anchor during the transition to adult care.

• Do not overlook nonmedical issues. Other problems (such as athletics or school) may be causing the teenager as much—or more—concern than the underlying disability.

• Encourage the adolescent to discuss emotions, to voice anger or frustration. Psychological counseling can be very helpful during adolescence, when privacy and confidentiality begin to alter the parent–child relationship. Support groups of other teenagers or adults with chronic medical problems also offer a network for socialization and role-modeling.

• Discuss the teenager's social, educational, and vocational skills with the health care team. A social worker who is knowledgeable about community resources can help the adolescent focus goals and plan for the future.

• Prepare for health insurance coverage when the adolescent reaches adulthood. Payment is the most important barrier to health care for people with chronic conditions. Hospital-based social workers usually are well versed about available options and can help the family plan for adult coverage.

• Address the teenager's sexual questions and concerns. Encourage the adolescent to ask health professionals for information and counseling about sexual development, sexual function, menstruation, contraception, and fertility.

When an illness or disability has been present since childhood, there is a tendency to consider the condition first and the teenager second. After months or years of medical procedures, medications, therapies, doctors' appointments, and hospitalizations, the teenager may disappear into the role of "patient." Adolescents with chronic conditions may have trouble seeing themselves outside the "sick" or "disabled" role. Most young people are able to correct the image and view themselves as emerging adults, mature and competent. All adolescents—healthy or ill, able-bodied or disabled—yearn for a sense of independence and responsibility. Families must also remember that most people, regardless of age, want to feel safe and protected, especially at times of crisis or ill health. The adolescent with repeated medical setbacks will mature but may do so more slowly, with more frequent periods of regression or childlike behavior. The difficult task before families and health professionals alike is to instill a sense of hope and forward momentum while maintaining an aura of trust, calm, and constancy.

Labeling can be especially hurtful to an adolescent's evolving identity. No teenager wants to be described as "the diabetic," "the cancer patient," or "the Down syndrome kid." It is more respectful and accurate to refer to the adolescent by name first. When descriptions are needed, the condition should be a noun rather than an adjective labeling the person—"Donald, the boy who has diabetes," or "Amy, the patient with cancer," or "Tom, the teenager who has Down syndrome."

It may be difficult for others to see beyond the illness or disability, particularly when it is visible. Gently remind them that the adolescent with a chronic condition shares the same joys, hopes, fears, and worries of all teenagers. This adolescent does not want pity, sympathy, overprotection, or overinvolvement from adults. This adolescent wants to live a full, productive life.

Special Concerns About Mental Retardation

Teenagers with mental retardation are like most teenagers. They love music and junk food. Their bodies mature. They feel sexual attractions. They may take risks. They also face many of the same challenges—restrictions, looking or feeling "different"—as teenagers with the chronic physical problems previously described. What sets them apart, however, is a limited intellectual capacity. This affects behavior and health and requires extra teaching and patience from families. First, the behaviors:

BEHAVIORAL ISSUES

Teenagers with mental retardation tend to have fewer chances to socialize than teenagers with normal intelligence. They may be lonely and isolated because they do not drive, do not go on unchaperoned dates, and do not take part in many of the independent activities of other teenagers. Their limited intelligence hinders their ability to understand and accept frustrations. At the same time, they are experiencing the hormonal changes of adolescence. The combination of frustration and hormones can lead to unexpected, and sometimes undesirable, behaviors.

Parents are baffled when their sweet-tempered child exhibits new behaviors: emotional outbursts, defiance, moody withdrawal. Individual situations should be discussed with an experienced doctor or counselor, but don't panic; much of this is an expected part of development. Adolescents with mental retardation have a wide range of emotions like other teenagers. They may require some special attention, however, because they have more difficulty expressing their emotions and understanding the causes. They need to be taught alternate ways to vent their feelings before they lead to unacceptable behaviors.

When the teenager was a child, parents probably used some behavior modification techniques to reward good performance and discourage negative behaviors. These methods can be updated and made age-appropriate for teenagers. If they are insufficient, it may be necessary to seek counseling. Teenagers with mental retardation need to understand that certain behaviors are acceptable and others are not. Words or actions that were okay at age six are no longer appropriate at age sixteen.

Families can reinforce social skills by taking advantage of "teachable moments" when a behavior has just occurred or is about to occur. It is unrealistic to expect that, once taught, these skills will last without frequent repetition, review, and reinforcement.

Occasionally, behaviors spin out of control and the question of medication arises. Psychiatric drugs have been used in institutional settings far more often than in individual family settings. Regardless of where the young person lives, medication should be used only after careful evaluation of many factors. The behavior needs to be examined within the broadest context: Is it a new behavior? How often does it occur? What triggers it? Can circumstances be altered to prevent the behavior? The best way to answer these questions is a joint consultation between the people who are most familiar with the teenager's daily behavior and a psychiatrist who is experienced in treating young people with mental retardation.

Medications can play a role, but they should not be given simply to sedate. Individuals with mental retardation can have depression and other psychiatric disorders that—when properly diagnosed—can be helped by medication. A clear treatment goal should be established, and the adolescent taking medicine should be monitored closely.

MEDICAL ISSUES

One pediatrician may have cared for the teenager since infancy, or several specialists may have been consulted along the way. Adolescence is the time to make a smooth transition to adult health care and a doctor who is familiar with the particular type of retardation and its medical aspects. If the doctor is unfamiliar with the condition, parents can share information about family support networks, advocacy groups, or other sources. Doctors usually appreciate the information because most see few patients with mental retardation.

This chapter cannot address each medical concern associated with every form of mental retardation, but three general guidelines can be offered: (1) These teenagers should have the same health examination described in Chapter 3 for all adolescents. (2) Special attention should be paid to growth, skin, vision, hearing, and skeletal and dental conditions. (3) Education about sexuality and reproduction is essential.

Several medical issues deserve special attention during adolescence:

• Physical inactivity—sitting and snacking in front of the television for hours—is unhealthy for *all* teenagers. It is very important to establish lifelong exercise and nutrition habits (Chapters 4 and 5). Many opportunities exist to promote fitness: Special Olympics, community recreation programs, exercise videotapes, etc. Physical activity on a regular basis promotes health and keeps boredom at bay. As they prepare for more independent living as adults, teenagers with mental retardation also should be taught the basics of good nutrition and the health risks of smoking cigarettes, drinking alcohol, and using drugs.

• Certain medical problems are associated with particular types of retardation. Thyroid and orthopedic problems, for example, are common in young people with Down syndrome. Other types of retardation are associated with seizures. Individual problems should be followed through adolescence and into adulthood.

• Teenagers with limited intellectual capabilities deserve to understand the changes taking place in their bodies. Elaborate physiological details and diagrams can be confusing. They should be told, in simple but correct terminology, about menstruation, sexual intercourse, pregnancy, and sexually transmitted diseases. Schools and libraries can provide information for different cognitive levels. The basic points should emphasize safe, appropriate sexual and social behaviors. Many families, for example, are comfortable with the message that masturbation is permissible in one's bedroom but not in public. Teenagers with mental retardation can learn the difference between public and private.

• Their limited intellectual capacity makes them vulnerable to people who will take advantage of them. They must be taught, in very specific ways, how to avoid situations that put them at risk for sexual or physical abuse.

• Adolescents with mental retardation need to learn how to use condoms correctly before they become sexually active. They should know that condoms can fail, and some backup contraceptive method should be used. The information in Chapters 15 through 23 should be explained to teenagers with mental retardation. It should be discussed and reviewed to ensure that they understand it and can apply it in their own lives.

Teenagers with mental retardation have many more educational, vocational, and social opportunities today than ever before. If they are to function successfully in their communities, they must be taught appropriate behaviors and given clear, useful information to ensure their well-being.

10

Consent and Confidentiality

• Will and Erika want advice about birth control. They are afraid to go to a clinic because they think their parents will be informed.

• John thinks he has a sexually transmitted disease. He worries that his family doctor will tell his parents or require their consent for treatment.

• Jerry has a drug problem and wants to enter a treatment program. He assumes that the program will insist on parental consent and payment. But Jerry's parents know nothing of his problem, and he is certain that they will never allow him to return home if they find out.

• Sandy is pregnant. She knows that she should seek care soon, but she is afraid to tell her parents. If she decides to have an abortion, will she need her parents' permission? If she decides to have the baby, who will pay the medical bills?

In a perfect world, all teenagers could share health concerns openly with their parents. They could go to a doctor together, discuss options, and decide upon treatment. There would be no need for secrecy. No fear that confidentiality might be broken. No worry about repercussions. Some families achieve this balance, but many teenagers and parents disagree about health-related behaviors. As a result, many adolescents delay seeing health professionals for fear that parents will be informed, permission required, or payment demanded. The overwhelming feeling may be one of confusion: "Where should I go? Who will be told? How will I pay?"

Adolescents have good reason to be confused about their legal standing in the health care system. Laws pertaining to the care of minors vary from state to state, and their interpretation can be inconsistent and ambiguous. A patchwork quilt prevails—common law, state laws, Supreme Court rulings, lower court decisions, agency regulations. Parents and health care providers often are just as baffled as teenagers about legal rights and responsibilities.

This chapter cannot give the state-by-state status of ever-changing laws related to adolescent health care. It can help clarify the two cornerstones of this complex area: *consent* (permission for care) and *confidentiality* (privacy about care). More detailed legal information can be obtained through local bar associations, county or state medical societies, community health departments, or social service agencies.

Parents can help by discussing legal, ethical, and financial issues of health care with their teenagers before crises arise. The common goal of parents, teens, and health professionals should be to maximize and protect adolescent health and well-being. To achieve this, adolescents must understand where and how to get care. Hopefully, this care will come with their parents' full knowledge and agreement. But when parental involvement endangers health or delays necessary care, adolescents must understand their rights and must be prepared to function as independent health care consumers.

Consent

A paradox exists in adolescent medicine. Health is the top priority, yet teenagers avoid health care when parental consent is the prerequisite. Is this right? Is it legal? Is it ethical? Should parental permission deter necessary care?

In medical emergencies, children of all ages can be treated without parental consent. Emergency need not imply life-threatening. A wound that needs sutures (stitches) should be treated promptly. It is legal to do so, and delay would be considered negligent in most cases. Health professionals must try to contact legal guardians in emergency situations, but they are not expected to delay treatment when immediate attention is indicated.

Non-emergencies pose the more common and controversial situations. In legal history, the concept of parental consent dates back to seventh-century England when a minor (then anyone under age twenty-one) was considered the father's property. A doctor who treated a minor without the father's permission, even if the treatment was necessary, could be sued for interfering with the father's legal right to manage his property.[8] Common law prohibited minors from making contracts on their own. Because medical care was considered a contract between patient and physician, adolescents were not free to seek health care without permission.

This historical concept of parental consent assumed that adolescents lacked the maturity, experience, and judgment to make their own decisions about health care. By the 1700s, Anglo-American courts began to recognize *emancipated minors,* or adolescents who live on their own, support themselves, and are not supervised by parents. In the 1930s, courts expanded this concept, allowing minors who were not emancipated to give *informed consent* for many types of health care. Informed consent means that the individual understands the treatment, its benefits, risks, and alternatives. *Minor* refers to anyone under eighteen in all states except Alaska, Nebraska, and Wyoming, where the legal age of majority is nineteen.

The term "emancipated minor" today includes self-supporting adolescents, those in the military, college students, adolescent mothers, and—in some states—pregnant adolescents. These teenagers are legally adults, and parental permission *never* is required for their health care.

Adolescents aged fourteen and older who are not emancipated can consent to treatment if they understand the treatment and risk, if the treatment does not pose major risk, and if the physician decides that the adolescent can consent as capably as an adult. When this *mature minor* doctrine is applied to non-emergency, elective care, parents usually are not held financially responsible. The minor is considered responsible, though often is unable to meet the full payment.

The problem of payment has led to different applications of the mature minor doctrine for inpatient versus outpatient care. ("Inpatient" refers to admission to a hospital. "Outpatient" refers to a clinic or office visit.) Outpatient care generally entails less serious disease, less risky treatment, and less expense. When the adolescent is unable to pay for a clinic visit, the provider may be willing to forego payment. A hospital admission, on the other hand, is costly and frequently involves more risk. Few adolescents have health insurance independent of their parents. It is unlikely that a hospital will admit an adolescent on a non-emergency basis without first obtaining the parents' health insurance information or willingness to assume financial responsibility. The mature minor doctrine, in theory, protects the adolescent's right to all care but, in practice, is applied far less to inpatient than outpatient treatment.

Even in the outpatient setting, the application and interpretation of the mature minor doctrine vary widely. State guidelines are often vague, and most states do not have specific mature minor laws. The doctrine is supported, though, by a substantial body of law. This support has resulted in more care for adolescents and more legal protection for the physicians who provide that care.

The issue of adolescent consent can arise in any medical situation, but most typically occurs in five areas: family planning services, abortion, treatment of sexually transmitted disease, mental health care, and treatment of adolescents who have been sexually abused. Even within a given state, laws regarding these aspects of care may differ. The following discussion of each of these health areas attempts to give general guidelines that apply in most areas of the country.

FAMILY PLANNING SERVICES

In 1977, the Supreme Court established that minors have a right to privacy with regard to contraception. Half the states now have laws allowing minors to obtain services for the prevention of pregnancy without parental consent. In some of these states, there are restrictions, such as a minimum age. Many states specifically exclude abortion. The right to contraceptive services—separate from abortion—has been an area of much legal debate since the early 1980s when the U.S. Department of Health and Human Services tried to require federally funded family planning clinics to notify parents when minors were given contraceptives. This "squeal rule" was found unconstitutional in 1983. These federal court decisions assure an adolescent's constitutional right to contraceptive services if sought at a federally funded facility. Private physicians and clinics not receiving federal funds, however, may refuse to provide contraceptives to teenagers.

Most states have laws that allow pregnant adolescents to obtain prenatal care without parental consent. Most of these laws also do not require that parents be notified of the care. About one quarter of the states allow for notification if the health professional so decides.

ABORTION

In 1973, the U.S. Supreme Court legalized abortion with the landmark *Roe* v. *Wade* decision. The Court simultaneously stated, though, that individual states could regulate abortions, resulting in considerable variation between states for women of all ages. Laws pertaining specifically to adolescents are even more confusing. The Supreme Court has ruled that parents cannot absolutely veto a minor's decision to have an abortion. If a state requires parental consent for abortion, it must also allow for judicial bypass. Under this procedure, an adolescent can obtain court approval, without parental notification, for abortion if she can demonstrate that she is mature enough to make the decision and that the decision is in her best interest. Judicial bypass also protects the adolescent's right to confidentiality about the abortion.

Since the Supreme Court's 1989 Webster decision, which gave states more leeway in restricting abortion, constitutional law concerning abortion and its availability have been in question for women of all ages. Minors typically constitute the first group to be affected by restrictive rulings pertaining to abortion. This is an area of the law that is in great flux and that varies widely between states. Adolescents and parents who face a decision about abortion must become familiar with their own state's rulings.

SERVICES FOR SEXUALLY TRANSMITTED DISEASES AND AIDS

Lawmakers nationwide recognize that health care for adolescents must be readily accessible to reduce the high rates of sexually transmitted disease. Most states have passed legislation permitting minors to be evaluated and treated for sexually transmitted disease without parental permission. Most of these laws do not stipulate an age limit, but a few specify that a minor must be twelve or fourteen. Some states specifically allow minors to consent to testing for HIV and AIDS. Most states do not have specific legislation, but do have general laws pertaining to infectious disease that could be interpreted to include HIV and AIDS.

Some laws address the issue of parental notification once an infection has been diagnosed or treated in an adolescent. Most states allow the physician to decide if parents should be informed.

The question of parental notification is an issue that the teenager can and should discuss with the physician early in the course of care.

DRUG AND/OR ALCOHOL ABUSE

All states except Alaska, Arkansas, Oregon, Utah, Wyoming, and the District of Columbia allow minors to consent to and receive drug- or alcohol-related care without parental consent.

MENTAL HEALTH SERVICES

Some adolescents with emotional problems are reluctant to discuss their distress with parents. Recognizing that these teenagers will not receive care if parental consent is required, nearly half the states have passed laws permitting outpatient treatment without parental consent.

Inpatient treatment, which requires a minimum of one night's stay at a hospital or mental health facility, presents a more complex problem. Half the states allow minors to apply for inpatient admission to a mental health service without parental consent, usually at a minimum age of sixteen. Some states require that *both* the teenager and parent consent to the inpatient care.

The most difficult scenario occurs when a teenager resists inpatient treatment that is recommended by the physician and agreed upon by parents. In general, "voluntary" commitment of a minor by the legal guardian is allowed, even when the minor resists the hospitalization. In 1979, the Supreme Court decided that when the commitment was done to protect the minor, a formal hearing was not required. The Court did decide, however, that an inquiry by a neutral party, such as a caseworker or court-appointed official, was necessary to assure that criteria for admission were met. Unfortunately, states continue to vary widely in their protection of youth against inappropriate institutionalization. Under most current state laws, minors without mental health problems requiring hospitalization still may be committed to inpatient care at the discretion of parents and physicians.

SEXUAL ABUSE, RAPE, AND INCEST

Many states allow adolescents who have been sexually abused to receive treatment related to pregnancy prevention and sexually transmitted disease without parental consent. At the same time, though, these adolescents are subject to child abuse laws requiring health professionals to report the violation to local child protection authorities. This required notification deters some adolescents from seeking care, especially when the perpetrator is a relative or family friend.

The legislation in the specific health areas described above deals far more commonly with parental consent than with parental notification. In other words, courts seem more concerned with who will give permission for care than who will be informed of that care. But the issue for teenagers is more likely to be one of assured privacy and confidentiality than one of signed permission. The adolescent who does not want parents informed cares little whether the notification comes before or after the care is delivered. The end result is the same: a breach in confidentiality and disruption of the doctor–patient relationship.

Confidentiality

Fortunately, federal and state courts have begun to recognize adolescents' need for confidential health care. Far more prevalent than law, though, are the endorsements of health professional organizations. Many groups of physicians, nurses, social workers, psychologists, and others who care for teenagers have issued ethical standards calling for parental involvement whenever possible, but protection of an adolescent's privacy when such involvement is not in the teenager's best interest.

The doctor–patient relationship has long been grounded in confidentiality and trust. When an adult receives medical treatment, the doctor is expected to protect the patient's privacy and the patient is expected to provide honest, pertinent information. The same relationship should apply for adolescents, particularly when they are able to consent to their own care. Teenagers who fear a breach in confidentiality avoid necessary care. Those who have experienced a loss of privacy are reluctant to reenter the health care system, and they forgo important preventive care. Certainly, health professionals should urge adolescents to involve their parents. There are times, though, when insisting on this involvement endangers the teenager (for example, an irate or abusive parent) or decreases the likelihood that the teenager will proceed with the care.

Legal requirements pertaining to confidentiality—informing a minor's parent about test results, prescriptions, or procedures— vary from state to state. Generally, if an adolescent has demonstrated maturity and understanding in the consent for treatment, a health professional is not expected to inform a parent or legal guardian. For the most part, case and statutory law does not specifically address questions of confidentiality and parental notification. In some situations, courts and legislatures decided that adolescents can consent to their own care, but that their parents must be notified of that care. In those instances, parental notification is viewed as less important to the adolescent and health provider than parental consent. But teenagers do not see it that way. For many adolescents, confidentiality and privacy are the heart and soul of health care. Without them, teenagers will seek neither care nor consent.

Adolescents may see the consent and confidentiality issues more clearly than courts and legislators. These issues are frequently inconsistent in the legal world. For example, many states allow minors to receive treatment for substance abuse without parental consent but vary widely when it comes to parental notification. Some do not mention notification; some leave it up to the discretion of the health professional; some require an "attempt" to inform; some stipulate confidentiality in one situation, notification in another. Because the law is inconsistent and confusing, teenagers, parents, and health providers should seek guidance about personal rights and responsibilities. As noted earlier in the chapter, local information can be obtained from city, county, or state health departments, social service departments, bar associations, district attorney's offices, or country and state medical societies. Many communities have special telephone hotlines for adolescents to help clarify an often confusing legal and health care system.

The most important point in these muddy areas is this: Parental consent and notification should never become a barrier to health care for adolescents. If concerns about payment jeopardize care, teenagers and health care providers can discuss alternatives. There usually are local clinics that provide health care at reduced or sliding scale fees. Most state and federally funded family planning programs offer reproductive health services at little or no cost. School-based health clinics and hospital-based adolescent clinics are other possibilities. If the teenager is seeing a private physician, perhaps a payment schedule can be arranged to allow the teenager to pay in small increments from part-time job wages or allowance.

Adolescents should try to involve their parents in their health care decisions. In the vast majority of cases, parents care deeply for their teenager's health and well-being. But when the gap between parents and adolescents seems insurmountable, consent and confidentiality should not block teenagers from seeking and receiving necessary care. Their health—both now and as society's future adults—must be cherished and protected.

III

PSYCHOLOGICAL AND BEHAVIORAL ISSUES

11

Risk Behaviors

Risk and adolescence go hand in hand. Teenagers try new ventures and adult behaviors to determine their capabilities and limits. Positive risks, such as trying out for the varsity team or the school play, can help an adolescent become more competent and independent. Whether the effort succeeds or fails, it challenges the teenager and promotes responsible, mature behavior.

Other risks carry negative consequences that endanger health, well-being, or even life itself. Consider the following:

• A fourteen-year-old girl cuts class to buy cigarettes from a doughnut shop down the street.

• A sixteen-year-old boy drives his parents' van at eighty-five miles an hour along a country road. He and his passengers are not wearing seat belts.

• A seventeen-year-old couple has sexual intercourse at the girl's home after school, before her parents return from work. They use nothing to protect against pregnancy or sexually transmitted disease.

This chapter discusses risk behaviors that may lead to negative outcomes: injury, suicide, homicide, substance abuse, unintended pregnancy, sexually transmitted disease. The behaviors range from the seemingly innocuous, such as smoking a first cigarette, to the clearly dangerous, such as intravenous drug use. All behaviors fall on a spectrum of risk. Each family must identify its own dividing line between acceptable and unacceptable, safe and dangerous.

Risk behaviors cut across social, economic, educational, ethnic, and religious lines. The specific behavior may depend on the teenager's age, gender, race, or family income, but all teenagers encounter some pressure to take negative risks. Families must understand that adolescent risk taking can escalate quickly and that risk behaviors travel together. A teenager who smokes cigarettes is more likely to drink alcohol. A teenager who drives too fast is less likely to wear a seat belt. A teenager who uses drugs is more likely to have multiple sex partners. A teenager who becomes pregnant is less likely to complete her education. These statements are not intended to frighten or to alarm. They simply represent well-documented trends in adolescent behavior.

The Broad Picture

The leading causes of death among adolescents and young adults aged fifteen to twenty-four are injury, homicide, and suicide. Although injuries are often called accidents, most are *preventable*. This makes their cost all the more tragic.

Risk behavior is the common thread that weaves through these causes of death. Consider the following statistics:

• Over 80 percent of adolescent deaths are the result of injury, homicide, or suicide.

• Motor vehicles are responsible for three-quarters of teenage deaths, more than all other causes combined. The motor vehicle death rate for young people aged fifteen through twenty-four is nearly double that for adults aged twenty-five through seventy-five.

• Between early and late adolescence, the mortality increases by over 300 percent. In the mid-1980s, the numbers of deaths per 100,000 adolescents aged ten to fourteen and fifteen to nineteen were 34.9 and 114.7, respectively.

• Homicide, the second leading cause of death among young people, claims 14.2 lives per 100,000 youths aged fifteen to twenty-four. The homicide rate doubled from 1960 to the mid-1980s. One in five American high school students (and almost one in three boys) carries a weapon for protection or use in a fight.

• Suicide, the third leading cause of death among young people, has tripled since the 1950s. Guns, the leading method used in suicide, account for half of teenage suicides (Chapter 13).

Risk behaviors result in morbitity as well as mortality. Morbidity includes chronic disability, unintended pregnancy, sexually transmitted disease, drug and alcohol abuse, and the complications of smoking. Some examples:

• Approximately one million teenagers become pregnant each year (Chapter 20). In 1989, of every 1,000 girls aged fifteen through seventeen and eighteen through nineteen, thirty-six and eighty-six respectively, gave birth.
• Teenagers who are sexually active are at high risk for sexually transmitted disease (Chapter 21). In 1988, over half of fifteen-to-nineteen-year-olds reported having had sexual intercourse within the past three months. Only 22 percent of sexually active females in that age group reported that their partners used condoms. In 1989, 30 percent of all reported cases of gonorrhea in the United States occurred among ten-to-nineteen-year-olds.
• Eighteen to 22 percent of adolescents have mental disorders ranging from anxiety to depression (Chapter 13) to schizophrenia. Feelings of sadness and hopelessness are associated with many self-destructive behaviors, including substance abuse and suicide attempts.
• Alcohol, tobacco, and illicit drugs place young people at risk for both immediate and long-term health problems (Chapter 12). Alcohol-related motor vehicle crashes are the leading cause of teenage death. In addition, alcohol is linked to injuries involving bicycles, skateboards, drownings, fires, firearms, and falls.

Why Do Teenagers Take Risks?

Adolescence is the natural, normal time to test the limits of parents and society. Teenagers take risks for many reasons: to gain peer acceptance or recognition, to boost self-esteem, to assert independence and autonomy, and to show parents that they are no longer children. Problems occur, though, when risk taking crosses the line from occasional, maturity-enhancing experiments to intense, frequent, life-threatening behaviors.

Adolescent risk behavior is intensified by a universal lack of experience. Teenagers have not had the time or opportunity to clarify their physical and psychological limits. They tend to be more impulsive than adults, so that high-risk activities may occur with little planning and no time to make sure that safety nets are in place. Young adolescents may not really accept the link between today's behavior and tomorrow's outcome. The fact that cigarette smoking causes lung cancer, for example, may be of less concern than the more immediate peer pressure to smoke.

A youthful sense of immortality contributes to risk behaviors. When an adolescent drives a car or motorcycle at eighty miles per hour, an injury or death usually is not intended. It is simply not considered. A teenager in the midst of a risk behavior has a sense of it-can't-happen-to-me: "I won't get pregnant the first time I have sex." "I don't need to use a condom with someone I know so well." "I can have a drink and drive because I've done it before." In many situations, it may seem less risky to take a risk, such as drinking one more beer, than to face the risk of rejection or ridicule from friends.

Which Teenagers Take Risks?

Risk behaviors have been studied extensively by health professionals and social scientists. Their research suggests that several factors may help identify which teenagers take risks and when the behaviors are likely to occur.

Timing and stage of development. The biological, psychological, and social phases of adolescent development usually are not completely synchronized. The timing of these events may affect when teenagers begin to take risks. Adolescents who enter puberty earlier or later than their peers may be more prone to engage in risk behaviors. A girl who attains physical and sexual maturity before other girls her age is more likely to be uncomfortable with her physical appearance and to have lower self-esteem. She often receives more attention from older boys but less from girls her own age. She may travel in an older social circle and, as a result, may face greater pressure to try "older" behaviors, such as smoking or drinking. Girls who develop early may *seem* independent and self-sufficient, but their decision-making skills usually are on par with their same-aged classmates. Consequently, they are not ready to foresee or manage the responsibilities that come with these older, riskier behaviors.

Boys enter puberty one or two years later than girls. While the early-maturing girl is the first in her class to show signs of puberty, the early-maturing boy may be somewhat less conspicuous. The late-maturing boy, in contrast, may be the last in his class—boy or girl—to show signs of puberty. He feels and appears quite different from his peers and tends to have lower self-esteem. His classmates may incorrectly equate his smaller stature or slighter build with cognitive or emotional immaturity. Perhaps in response to this, the late-maturing boy sometimes exhibits more impulsivity and rebellion. As he feels increasingly out of synch with his peers, he may take risks to prove himself. Once puberty begins, however, most late-maturing boys develop very quickly. Because their rate of development often is faster than that of boys who enter puberty earlier, boys who begin later actually complete puberty at about the same age as peers who had an earlier start. The period of risk behavior consequently tends to be limited. This may explain why, despite the turbulence, late-maturing boys do not seem more likely to escalate to more dangerous behaviors than their peers.

Gender and hormones. The role of sex hormones in risk behaviors is not fully understood. Testosterone levels in males have been associated with risk behaviors—both sexual and nonsexual. Males are more likely than females to engage in nearly all risk behaviors, and the death rate for teenage boys exceeds that of girls.

Environment. Major changes in school or at home can trigger risk behaviors. An adolescent who moves to a new neighborhood or school may behave in new, riskier ways in an attempt to boost peer acceptance or to test the limits of the new environment. Parental separation, divorce, and remarriage are associated with significant adolescent stress and may result in increased risk behavior.

Individual characteristics. Risk behaviors tend to cluster. An adolescent engaged in one is more likely to escalate to others. Teenagers who repeatedly place themselves at risk often are at odds with their families, demonstrating a drive for independence and a rebelliousness against parental discipline. They may have low expectations about their school achievement and, as a result, express boredom or frustration with classes and teachers. Their academic performance tends to decline as the risk taking increases. They may drop out of extracurricular activities, lose contact with childhood friends, and spend more time alone or with new friends engaged in similar risk behavior. The result can be a terrible paradox. As the need for adult intervention increases, the high-risk adolescent imposes a growing barrier of hostility and alienation.

Prevention of Risk Behaviors

Parents face a difficult challenge when they attempt to prevent risk behaviors. Adolescents face real temptations in their everyday life, from fast cars to suggestive advertising. At the same time, there are more dangers than ever before: HIV infection, crack cocaine, high rates of homicide. The individual parent cannot alter the social milieu. But parents can influence their teenager's response to social demands, especially if guidance and prevention begin early.

Children who have grown up with firm, consistent limits are less likely as teenagers to push their behavior into the danger zone. Limit-setting remains important during adolescence, although parents can become more flexible as their children mature. Teenagers complain about rules, but most want some guidelines and even some hard and fast limits that must not be surpassed. At some level, the teenager who is angry about a curfew recognizes that the parent's underlying message is "I want you home by midnight because I love you and I care about what happens to you." That is a reassuring message for any adolescent.

Parental limits sometimes provide a social safety valve, a way to save face among friends. Parents can say, "I'll play the heavy. Blame me. I still want you home by midnight." The teenager may tell friends, "My parents will ground me if I don't get home before midnight." By "blaming" parents this way, the adolescent may avoid difficult situations in which risk behaviors can occur.

Whether parents are firm or lenient, all adolescents must make decisions about risk behaviors. Families can prepare for these decisions. It is best to have open discussions *before* teenagers are faced with on-the-spot decisions about whether to engage in risk behaviors. These discussions, during non-crisis times, work much better than lectures. Begin with open-ended, non-accusatory questions, such as, "What is the drug situation like at school?" "Where do teenagers who use drugs get them?"

Once the conversation is underway, many teenagers appreciate the opportunity to air issues that they may have considered taboo within the family context. Talking before the point of decision making gives them a chance to plan their response when confronted with the challenge to drink, do drugs, have sexual intercourse, or engage in any other risk behavior. The discussion can evolve into a type of rehearsal or role-play about "what to do in this situation." Later, perhaps long after the discussion, the teenager may feel better prepared to handle a party, for example, where alcohol is served or drugs are offered. Discussions should also include less-charged subjects, such as the importance of seat belts, bicycle helmets, or fluorescent clothing when jogging at night.

Prevention requires parents to define and state their own limits about which behaviors are acceptable and which are not. If, for example, parents accept that their adolescent will drink alcohol at a Saturday night party, they should be direct in asking, "How are you going to get home after the party? Is there a designated driver who will drink no alcohol that night?" Or, "We know there will be some drinking; we would rather drive you and your friends than have you take the car." If, on the other hand, parents consider it unacceptable for their adolescent to drink at any time, they should state that explicitly. Even if the teenager agrees to no alcohol, it is still safest to be sure that the driver, whether friend or parent, is sober.

The bottom line in parent–teen discussions of risk behaviors is this: All adolescents take some risks, but these risks can be decreased if adolescents understand how to protect themselves. They must find ways to avoid unnecessary danger, such as buckling a seat belt, walking home instead of riding with a drunk driver, refusing a cigarette, using a condom. Teenagers *can* avoid adverse consequences by planning prevention before faced with risk.

It is tempting for parents to turn a discussion into a lecture or to give far more information than an adolescent wants or needs. The key to good communication is listening. Parents must *hear* their children's questions and gauge their responses accordingly. They need to admit "I don't know" when that is the case. They must remember that adult and adolescent perceptions differ. What may seem obvious to a parent, such as choosing a designated driver when others are drinking, may not be so apparent to a teenager at the end of a late party. What comes naturally to a parent, like allowing enough time to get home by midnight, still may be difficult for a young adolescent.

If Prevention Fails, What Next?

When risk behavior becomes apparent—empty beer cans in the trash, marijuana in the basement, a speeding ticket in the glove compartment—parents' reactions vary widely. The first time a risk behavior is recognized, parents need to act immediately, firmly, and appropriately. The should condemn the behavior but not the teenager by taking a tone of "I love you, but not the behavior." At the same time, parents should understand that some testing and experimenting are normal. The first time it happens is less worrisome than the second.

When a risk behavior occurs again, parents should gather information about its extent and should seek help if the problem is beyond their control. It is important not to ask questions behind the teenager's back—that will only foster mistrust and anger. Instead, parents can tell their adolescent that they know of the problem and are going to talk with other adults (parents, teachers, coaches, for example) about how widespread it has become. If other teenagers are involved, including all the teenagers and parents in a joint discussion can be helpful. School-sponsored parent meetings on topics such as contraception or sexually transmitted disease can also help individual families recognize and deal with an issue directly.

Whatever the social context, risk behaviors usually have stronger roots at home than at school or among friends. To understand better the causes of risk behaviors, parents can ask themselves several questions: Is there discord or fighting at home? Do we send inconsistent, mixed messages? Does Mom react with horror when her son comes home drunk, while Dad sees little harm in it? What kind of examples are we setting? Do we smoke, but forbid our children to smoke? Do we wear seat belts? Drive too fast? Drive after we've been drinking?

If dangerous behaviors escalate in frequency and severity, parents can take some concrete steps to decrease the risk of catastrophe. For example, if the teenager has been showing signs of depression or talking of suicide, remove firearms from the home and clear the bathroom shelves of *all* medications. If substance abuse is the problem, do not leave cigarettes, alcohol, or money lying around the home. If teenagers are planning a party, find out if the host's parents will be there and if alcohol or drugs will be available. If teenagers are sexually active, discuss ways to prevent sexually transmitted disease and pregnancy, provide phone numbers of family planning clinics, offer to arrange an appointment or to accompany the teenager for a gynecological visit. When parental involvement is offered and accepted, the relationship between parent and teenager can strengthen and mature. Even when refused, the offer has been heard and the lines of communication may have opened.

Seeking Outside Help

Despite attempts to prevent and deal with adolescent risk behaviors, many parents find that events spiral rapidly out of control. It is time to find help outside the family when parents feel that:

- they no longer know how to cope with the problem;
- they know how to cope, but the behaviors continue;
- the teenager is increasingly withdrawn, distant, or depressed.

Once parents or adolescents recognize a need for help, they may feel confused about where to go, who to call, or how to overcome financial and social barriers to care. Accessible, available first contacts include the following:

- other parents (individual parents of their teenager's friends or parent groups such as a PTA or religious group);
- school personnel (guidance counselor, principal, teacher, school psychologist, or coach);
- clergy (minister, rabbi, priest);
- health professional (physician, psychologist, social worker, nurse);
- an adult whom the teenager likes and trusts (grandparent, uncle, aunt, older cousin, neighbor, or parent of a friend).

Many schools have school-based health clinics with highly trained staff who can help with adolescent risk behaviors. Most communities have hotlines that teenagers and their parents can call for information about where to get help with particular problems. Parents can provide the phone numbers, encourage the adolescent to call, and agree not to cross-examine about the results. Community mental health centers offer counseling for high-risk youth and their families. Private psychotherapy is another, although costly, alternative; some hospitals or clinics offer a sliding scale fee schedule that is adjusted to the family's income.

What is most important is to intervene promptly. Even when the problem seems overwhelming, adolescents and parents should remember that it is surmountable and need not be faced alone. This is the time to talk together, involve others, and work actively to promote change and a secure future.

12

Alcohol, Tobacco, and Drugs

On the television screen an egg sizzles in a frying pan while an announcer proclaims, "This is your brain on drugs . . ." Billboards, magazine ads, radio and television spots warn of the dangers of drinking and driving. From kindergarten to high school graduation, schools teach about the hazards of smoking tobacco, drinking alcohol, and using illegal drugs.

In the late 1980s and early 1990s, educational and media campaigns to combat substance abuse were pervasive and began to work. Drug and alcohol use among adolescents declined. Teenagers took greater responsibility when they drank by choosing designated drivers, exerted more peer pressure against heavy drinking and drug use, and joined groups like SADD (Students Against Drunk Driving).

Yet adolescent substance abuse remains a pressing national problem and challenge to every family. Recent evidence suggests that the rates of use may be on the rise, especially among young adolescents. Thousands of young lives are lost because of drugs and alcohol—8,000 adolescents die in alcohol-related motor vehicle collisions each year and 45,000 more are injured. Each young life that is lost or disabled is all the more tragic because this is preventable.

Adults who worry about teenage substance abuse commonly envision cocaine, crack, amphetamines, or heroin. These drugs certainly do endanger adolescent health, but they are used by far fewer youth than three other harmful drugs—tobacco, alcohol, and mari-

138

juana. Tobacco is responsible for more lost years of life than all other drugs combined. Alcohol is implicated in over half of all motor vehicle fatalities among adolescents. Marijuana impairs memory, learning, and coordination.

Tobacco, alcohol, and illicit drugs all carry risk, and each is considered a substance in this chapter. Differentiating adolescent experimentation from use, use from abuse, and abuse from dependence can be difficult for parents and physicians alike. When making these decisions, parents should consider a few facts. First, the younger a teenager is when the use begins, the greater the chance that the use will progress. Second, adolescents often are less able to limit their behavior than adults. Third, whether parents consider adolescent drinking acceptable or not, it is illegal to serve minors and it is illegal for minors to purchase alcohol. Fourth, the teenage experience with illicit drugs today is different than it was when parents may have experimented as youth of the 1960s or 1970s. Marijuana, for example, then contained less than 0.2 percent THC (delta-9-tetrahydro-cannabinol). Today, it contains an average of 2 to 6 percent and up to 14 percent. Finally, the use of all illicit drugs, no matter where or by whom, is a criminal offense.

The Scope of the Problem

Every year since 1975, thousands of high school students across the country have been surveyed by the University of Michigan's Institute for Social Research. This nationwide survey, sponsored by the National Institute on Drug Abuse, is considered the best source of information about teenage tobacco, alcohol, and drug use. The survey provides important descriptions about adolescents who are in school, but tells nothing about school dropouts (15 to 20 percent of the high school–age population) or about students who are absent on survey day (another 16 to 23 percent). Its results, therefore, may underestimate the rates of substance use among all adolescents. The survey reveals several trends:

• The use of illegal drugs and alcohol by high school students was on the decline in the early 1990s. The last few years suggest that the rates may be increasing among eighth graders.

• Tobacco use has not decreased; cigarette smoking has reached a plateau and the use of smokeless (chewing) tobacco has increased.

• Males use most drugs more than females. Cigarettes, stimulants, and tranquilizers are used more commonly by females.
• College-bound seniors use substances less than classmates who are not headed for college.
• More than half of the seniors who use cigarettes, alcohol, marijuana, or inhalants began before tenth grade. Follow-up surveys indicate that individuals who experiment with substances in childhood and early adolescence are more likely to use drugs or alcohol as adults than are those who delay first experimentation.
• Student perceptions of the dangers associated with substance abuse are decreasing, and disapproval of peer use is decreasing. Research suggests that these trends are the harbingers of increasing drug use among teenagers.

When crack, the cheaper form of cocaine, first appeared in the United States in 1986, there was great concern that its use by adolescents would increase quickly. The school-based surveys do not indicate that this has occurred. The proportion of seniors who have tried crack or cocaine dropped from 15 percent in 1987 to 6 percent in 1993. Marijuana use fell from a peak of 60 percent in 1979 to 32 percent in 1992 but increased in 1993 to 35 percent.

A 1991 survey by the Surgeon General revealed that more than half of 20.7 million junior and senior high school students drink alcohol. Eight million said they drink on a weekly basis; 5.4 million said they occasionally binge-drink (five or more drinks in a row); a half million said they binge-drink weekly. In 1993, 27 percent of seniors reported binge-drinking in the last month.

Adolescents seem to have limited understanding of the risks associated with alcohol use or the alcohol content of various drinks. Almost 80 percent of adolescents do not know that a can of beer contains as much alcohol as a shot of whiskey; one in three does not realize that wine coolers contain alcohol; one in four is uncertain about the legal age to purchase alcohol. (Answer: Age twenty-one in all fifty states.)

Unlike drug and alcohol use, cigarette smoking by teenagers has not diminished. One of eight American teenagers aged twelve to eighteen smoked regularly, according to a 1991 study by the Centers for Disease Control. Although cigarettes may seem less risky than illegal drugs in the short run, they are responsible for more years of lost life than the total of all other drugs. A habit that begins in adolescence may mean death from premature heart or lung disease in mid-adulthood.

Why Do Teenagers Use Substances?

When asked why they smoke cigarettes, teenagers often mention peer pressure, curiosity, imitation, independence, rebellion, or an attempt to appear "cool." Cigarette manufacturers capitalize on the image factor by featuring glamorous models smoking in beautiful or exciting settings.

When asked why they drink alcohol, teenagers give explanations like these:

"It helps me relax."

"Everyone else does."

"I like it. It's fun."

"Because I'm stressed out. To escape."

"Why not? I don't drink that much."

In the 1991 Surgeon General's survey, 25 percent of adolescents said that they drink to get high and 66 percent said because they are stressed or bored. Thirty-one percent reported that they drink when they are alone. When the survey was released, the Surgeon General at the time, Antonia Novello, called the trend in teenage drinking "alarming" and explained, "They drink deliberately to change the way they feel. And we know that the use of alcohol to, in effect, self-medicate is the trap door to full-blown alcoholism."

Why do teenagers use illegal drugs? Adolescents who experiment with drugs, such as crack, cocaine, amphetamines, or hallucinogens, give reasons similar to those described for tobacco, alcohol, and marijuana: family use, peer pressure, low self-esteem, anxiety or depression, stress, boredom, and rebellion. Tobacco, alcohol, and marijuana often are called the gateway drugs because they tend to precede the use of other illegal drugs.

Although adolescents are bombarded with information about the dangers of drugs and alcohol, no teenager is immune to their social influence or their easy availability. This is especially true for teenagers whose parents smoke, drink, or use drugs. A young person, watching others use substances, must decide, "What role will this play in my life?"

Many teenagers answer that question with, "I'll just try it once, to see what it's like." Experimenting with drugs is dangerous. Although a legal drug like nicotine in cigarettes may be perceived as innocent, it can be both physically and psychologically addictive. A couple of drinks can lead to impulsivity, poor judgment, and tragedies such as motor vehicle fatalities.

Who Is at Risk?

The simplistic answer is, "All teenagers." Alcohol and drugs are readily available, and most adolescents experience some pressure to try them. Some adolescents are at higher risk of substance use than others. Three important factors contributing to risk are family history, peer use, and individual characteristics.

Teenagers are at greater risk if parents or siblings smoke, drink, or use drugs. For alcohol, this risk reflects both genetics and environment. For cigarettes and other drugs, the effect is predominantly environmental. Teenagers are also at increased risk for substance use if parents condone the use either through their own use behavior or through inconsistent discipline of their adolescents' use. Teenagers who have been physically or sexually abused and those who have run away from home are at increased risk. Adolescent substance use is more common in families who are socially withdrawn or isolated and in those who have experienced stresses such as separation, divorce, remarriage, frequent moves, unemployment, serious illness, or death.

One of the strongest predictors of adolescent substance use is peer use. A teenager whose close friends use tobacco, alcohol, or drugs is more likely to experiment with them than is a teenager whose friends avoid and disapprove of them. Peer use is especially influential in the preteen and early adolescent years. Postponing the age at which a teenager first experiments with cigarettes, alcohol, and marijuana appears to diminish both use of these substances in adulthood and progression to other substances.

Certain individual personality and behavioral characteristics may be indicators of adolescent substance abuse. Adolescents who use drugs or alcohol are more likely than nonusers to be anxious, depressed, alienated from family, rebellious, truant from school, or delinquent. Because most drugs decrease impulse control, users may engage repeatedly in dangerous or sensation-seeking behaviors. These behaviors, accompanied by the poor muscle coordination and delayed reflex time associated with alcohol and drugs, increase the adolescent's risk of injury and even death.

Children who have particular emotional or behavioral problems (Chapter 14) may be at increased risk of substance use during adolescence. Young people who have experienced years of academic underachievement or difficulty controlling their behavior in social settings may turn to drugs as an escape; they may falsely believe that illegal drugs improve their behavior or make them more socially acceptable. The many new medications and treatment options that are now available offer far better relief and a bright outlook for future achievement.

Recognizing the Problem

Parents, siblings, and friends may notice gradual changes in behavior as a teenager progresses from experimentation to regular alcohol or drug use. Without intervention, the adolescent eventually will experience physical symptoms and signs of deteriorating health.

Four stages of escalating substance use, described by Dr. Donald Ian Macdonald, author of *Drugs, Drinking, and Adolescence,* can help families and friends recognize behavioral changes and determine the frequency of use.

During the first stage, adolescents begin to learn the mood swing that accompanies alcohol and drug use. In this early stage, teenagers experience good feelings and few consequences as they experiment with alcohol, marijuana, or inhalants on weekends among friends. Family and friends may notice little or no change in behavior. If caught, most teenagers in this first stage will deny or lie about their use.

In the second stage, teenagers seek the mood swing brought about by drug or alcohol use. They experience feelings of excitement and some early pangs of guilt. The drugs of choice during the second stage may still include tobacco, marijuana, alcohol, and inhalants, but often expand to include stimulants, tranquilizers, or hallucinogens, such as LSD. The frequency of use in the second stage increases to four or five times a week. The teenagers may begin to use drugs alone, apart from the peer group. Changes in behavior become more noticeable: declining or erratic schoolwork, dropping out of extracurricular activities, different friends, changes in dress style, mood swings, dishonesty.

Teenagers in the third stage of drug use are preoccupied with the mood swing. They use drugs every day and use them alone as much as in the company of friends. Their emotions range from euphoric highs to depressive lows, including thoughts of suicide. They may now use many different types of drugs, including crack, cocaine, heroin, and other narcotics. Teenagers in this stage may depend on selling drugs to finance their own use. Behavioral changes include school failure, truancy, lost jobs, fighting, stealing, a shift away from "straight" friends, and pathologic lying.

By the fourth stage of drug use, teenagers rely on drugs just to make it through the day and to prevent the symptoms of psychological and physical withdrawal. They experience chronic guilt, shame, remorse, depression, and suicidal thoughts. They will use whatever drug is available and will obtain it in any way they can. The frequency of use has now escalated to all day, every day. They overdose frequently. They drop out of school. Their mental and physical health deteriorates. Their drug abuse is life-threatening and undeniable.

The physical signs and symptoms of substance abuse vary with the type of drug and the frequency of use. They may include:

• Recurrent bronchitis, chronic cough, stained teeth, halitosis (bad breath), chronic runny nose, frequent nose bleeds, recurrent sinus infections, red eyes;
• Skin bruising, unexplained skin sores, needle marks;
• High blood pressure, rapid or irregular heartbeat, chest pain;
• Abdominal pain, weight loss, loss of appetite, nausea, vomiting, liver enlargement, stomach or intestinal ulcers;
• Poor muscle tone, weakness, lack of energy, fatigue;
• Memory loss, inattention, irritability, tremor, clumsiness;
• Poor judgment, disorientation, confusion, hallucinations, and delusions.

Recognizing substance abuse and identifying which drug is being used is complicated by the many drugs that are available and their numerous names (Table 12.1).

Facing the Problem

When families suspect substance abuse, they face the question, What do we do about it? It is usually ineffective to confront a teenager at midnight when he or she staggers in drunk. Preaching, screaming, and punishing the moment marijuana is discovered in the sock drawer also tends to have limited effect. If the teenager does not appear to be in acute danger, it is better to discuss the substance use when he or she is not high and when tempers are

TABLE 12.1

COMMON SLANG TERMS FOR ILLICIT DRUGS

A's	amphetamine
Acapulco gold	high-grade marijuana
acid	LSD, D-lysergic acid, diethylamide tartrate
angel dust	DMT or PCP sprinkled over parsley or tobacco
barbs	barbiturates
base	cocaine
Beast	LSD
bennies	Benzedrine, a brand of amphetamine sulfate
black beauty	methamphetamine
blues	amobarbital sodium
brown	heroin
cactus	mescaline
candy	barbiturates
chalk	powder form of methamphetamine hydrochloride
Charlie	cocaine
china white	heroin, fentanyl
coke	cocaine
copilots	amphetamines
crank	methamphetamine hydrochloride
crap	heroin
crystal	methamphetamine hyrochloride in powder or crystal form
cubes	LSD
dexies	Dexedrine, or dextroamphetamine sulfate
downers	depressants
dust	cocaine, PCP
flake	cocaine
footballs	oval-shaped amphetamine tablets
ganja	hashish
gold dust	cocaine
goof balls	barbiturates
grass	marijuana
H	heroin
hash	hashish
hearts	Dexedrine, or dextroamphetamine sulfate
hog	PCP
horse	heroin
ice	crystal form of methamphetamine
joint	marijuana cigarette
juice	PCP

junk	heroin
ludes	methaqualone (Quaalude)
magic mushroom	mushroom containing psilocybin
mesc	mescaline
meth	methamphetamine
Mickey	combination of alcohol and chloral hydrate
MJ	marijuana
pinks	secobarbital sodium
pot	marijuana
primo	marijuana cigarette laced with cocaine
rainbows	barbiturates
reds	secobarbital
roach	butt of marijuana cigarette
rope	hashish
scag	heroin
scat	heroin
smack	heroin
snow	cocaine
speed	methamphetamine
speedball	injected heroin and cocaine
sunshine	LSD
uppers	stimulants
weed	marijuana
whites	amphetamines
yellows	pentobarbital sodium

under control. If there is any question about the teenager's safety, immediate help should be sought from the family doctor or emergency room.

Teenagers sometimes worry about their own use of substances. They may feel confused or uncertain about how much is too much. Remember that *any* use of alcohol by teenagers or illicit drugs by anyone is against the law. Several screening questionnaires have been developed to help teenagers, along with their parents and physicians, decide if there is an alcohol problem (Table 12.2).

Once substance use is suspected or confirmed, it should be confronted quickly and firmly. Parents need to be explicit and consistent in saying that the use must stop. They should emphasize that it is the teenager's *behavior*—not the teenager—that is unacceptable. Anger and denial can be expected initially, but parents are most effective when they remain calm and unwavering in their intolerance of substance use.

TABLE 12.2

THE MICHIGAN ALCOHOL SCREENING TEST

Circle "Yes" or "No," depending on whether the question indicates something true or not true about you. Please answer all questions.

1.	Do you feel you are a normal drinker?	Yes	No
2.	Have you ever awakened the morning after some drinking the night before and found you couldn't remember a part of the evening?	Yes	No
3.	Do your friends or family ever worry or complain about your drinking?	Yes	No
4.	Can you stop drinking without a struggle after one or two drinks?	Yes	No
5.	Do you ever feel bad about your drinking?	Yes	No
6.	Do friends or relatives think you are a normal drinker?	Yes	No
7.	Do you ever try to limit your drinking to certain times of the day or to certain places?	Yes	No
8.	Are you always able to stop drinking when you want to?	Yes	No
9.	Have you ever attended a meeting of Alcoholics Anonymous (AA)?	Yes	No
10.	Have you gotten into fights when drinking?	Yes	No
11.	Has your drinking ever created problems with your friends or family?	Yes	No
12.	Have your friends or any family member ever gone to anyone for help about your drinking?	Yes	No
13.	Have you ever lost friends or spouse because of your drinking?	Yes	No
14.	Have you ever gotten into trouble at work or school because of your drinking?	Yes	No
15.	Have you ever lost a job because of your drinking?	Yes	No
16.	Have you ever neglected your obligations, your family, or your school work for two or more days in a row because you were drinking?	Yes	No
17.	Do you ever drink before noon?	Yes	No
18.	Have you ever been told you have liver trouble?	Yes	No
19.	After heavy drinking, have you ever had delirium tremens (DTs) or severe shaking, heard voices, or seen things that were not there?	Yes	No
20.	Have you ever gone to anyone for help about your drinking?	Yes	No
21.	Have you ever been in a hospital because of your drinking?	Yes	No
22.	Have you ever been a patient in a psychiatric hospital or on		

a psychiatric ward of a general hospital where drinking was
part of the problem? Yes No

23. Have you ever been seen at a psychiatric or mental health
clinic or gone to a doctor, social worker, or clergyman for
help with an emotional problem in which drinking played a
part? Yes No

24. Have you ever been arrested, even for a few hours, because
of drunk behavior? Yes No

25. Have you ever been arrested for drunk driving or driving
after drinking? Yes No

To determine your score, add up the points given for the answers you circled:

Question No.

1. yes = 0, no = 2	9. yes = 5, no = 0	17. yes = 2, no = 0
2. yes = 2, no = 0	10. yes = 1, no = 0	18. yes = 1, no = 0
3. yes = 1, no = 0	11. yes = 2, no = 0	19. yes = 5, no = 0
4. yes = 0, no = 2	12. yes = 2, no = 0	20. yes = 5, no = 0
5. yes = 1, no = 0	13. yes = 2, no = 0	21. yes = 5, no = 0
6. yes = 0, no = 2	14. yes = 2, no = 0	22. yes = 2, no = 0
7. yes = 1, no = 0	15. yes = 2, no = 0	23. yes = 2, no = 0
8. yes = 0, no = 2	16. yes = 2, no = 0	24. yes = 2, no = 0
		25. yes = 2, no = 0

Your score is _____

0–3	Probably not alcoholic
5–10	80 percent risk of alcoholism
10 or more	Definitely alcoholic

Adapted from the *American Journal of Psychiatry* 127:89. Copyright 1971, the American Psychiatric Association. Reprinted by permission.

If experimentation becomes abuse, a health professional should be consulted. A physician who does a thorough health screening will ask every adolescent about tobacco, alcohol, and drug use—not just the adolescent in whom it is suspected. When substance abuse is discovered by a physician, the question of confidentiality arises. A doctor will not always share information about drug use with parents but will inform the teenager of its dangers and methods of curbing it. While respecting confidentiality, however, the doctor will make it clear that parents must be informed if the adolescent does not correct substance use that endangers health or life itself.

Some parents who suspect substance use may ask a doctor to screen for drugs by a blood or urine test without informing the teenager. Cloaking the test as part of a "routine" examination can destroy the teenager's trust in both the doctor and the parents. If the test results turn out to be positive, the doctor and parents will have great difficulty in convincing the teenager to accept treatment.

If the teenager agrees to a drug screen, it is important for parents to recognize that a negative test does not exclude the possibility of drug use. Similarly, a positive test does not confirm beyond doubt that drugs have been used. Results vary, depending on the type of drug, the length of time between use and test, the amount used, and the kind of analysis. In some cases, a second test may be necessary to confirm the first. Some tests, which are easy to perform and inexpensive, carry unacceptably high false-positive rates. The confirming tests are more accurate but often are costly and time-consuming because they require special equipment and trained personnel. It is useful to discuss test procedures, implications, limitations, and cost with the physician before screening. It should also be recognized that test results simply say positive or negative. They say nothing about frequency of use, dependence, or impairment. Drug testing, in other words, is not a final verdict.

Treatment of Substance Abuse

The first step toward effective treatment of substance abuse is the insistence by the parents that all use must stop. If the adolescent does not agree to treatment, the parents and physician must work together to convince the teenager of its importance. If persuasion fails, the adolescent ultimately may need to be forced into treatment. The intensity of the treatment will depend on the severity of the teenager's problem. The site of treatment depends on both the adolescent and the family. Teenagers living in homes where alcohol and drug use is prevalent may need to leave that environment to overcome their own use. For these adolescents, residential treatment programs may be more successful than outpatient programs.

A doctor or other health professional who is skilled in drug and alcohol treatment can manage the care with office visits if the teenager recognizes the need and has not gone far beyond experimental usage. Adolescents, particularly younger ones, who have been using drugs or alcohol more heavily and who have not responded to office-based counseling may be referred to special outpatient programs. This course of treatment also applies to teenage substance abusers who have other psychological or behavioral problems. If substance abuse continues and outpatient care fails, an inpatient program usually is recommended. Inpatient care is essential for teenagers who need detoxification, who are in imminent physical or psychological danger, or who are compulsive substance users.

Many treatment programs are available, but their services and costs vary widely. Families are best served if they consult with a health professional who is well-trained and experienced in substance abuse management or can refer the family to a respected program. The local medical society, Alcoholics Anonymous and Narcotics Anonymous chapters, and the National Clearinghouse for Alcohol and Drug Information in Washington, D.C., can also help families find programs in their communities. (See Resources at the end of this book.)

What makes a treatment program successful? Licensed drug counselors, a requirement of total abstinence, and family involvement are all found in programs that have the highest success rates. A program that offers a quick fix should be avoided because substance abuse has a high relapse rate and requires long-term support.

In searching for effective and appropriate treatment options, families may become baffled by the wide variety of programs available. Before choosing one, parents and teenager should visit several programs and ask questions such as:

• What is the program's philosophy? What are its goals? How does it attempt to reach those goals?
• Does it assess the medical, behavioral, educational, and emotional needs of the teenager and the family?
• Does it have an individualized treatment plan for each teenager? Are both professionally supervised groups and self-help support groups part of the overall program?
• What does it demand of the teenager? Does it require complete and total abstinence? Does it maintain a drug-free environment?
• How long has the program existed? What is its relapse rate? What are the training and experience of its staff? What is the patient–staff ratio? Is there frequent interaction between an assigned counselor and the adolescent? Are there psychiatrists, clinical psychologists, and psychiatric social workers on staff?
• Does the program involve the family in the treatment plan?

Does it work toward the establishment of a functional family unit? Does it help with other living arrangements if the family's home is unsafe for the adolescent?

• Does it include services such as tutoring, educational or vocational assistance, physical exercise, recreational programs, aftercare support and follow-up?

• Does the program help the teenager reduce other dangerous behaviors, such as sexual promiscuity or unprotected sexual intercourse?

• If the program also treats adults, does it separate its teenage patients from the adults?

• What is its cost? How can it be financed?

The answer to the last question depends largely on a family's insurance coverage. In 1990 dollars, the cost of private inpatient treatment programs ranged from $15,000 to $30,000 a month. Even if a family has some health insurance, most policies limit the length of treatment, the kinds of reimbursable services, and the total number of allowable treatments. Prohibitive costs force many people with substance abuse to seek outpatient care even when inpatient programs are indicated. Public, government-financed programs exist but cannot handle all the people who need help. Other treatment options include hospital-based inpatient programs aimed at crisis intervention, short-term residential programs followed by outpatient support, and day programs in which teenagers return home in the evening.

The final decision about treatment for substance abuse depends on many factors, including the severity of the teenager's substance abuse, the family structure and function, and finances. There is no single, ideal form of treatment. The bottom line is to seek and obtain help for an adolescent who is struggling with an overwhelming and debilitating problem. If the treatment options are unclear, talk to physicians, school counselors, social workers, or public health professionals.

13

Anxiety, Depression, and Suicide

The word "teen" has a little known, archaic meaning: "suffering" or "grief." This will not surprise the many adolescents who have experienced emotional pain: a loved one dies . . . a romance breaks up . . . parents fight . . . close friends move away . . . others behave cruelly . . . a classmate is assaulted. . . .

None of these life events is unique to adolescence. Yet all bring a sadness that seems more profound and traumatic during the teen years. Why? Perhaps because many other changes compete for the adolescent's emotional reserve. Or perhaps the teenager's increasing ability to grasp the permanence of some events makes the pain both more acute and long-lasting.

No one sails through adolescence—or life—without some emotional upset. Most teenagers demonstrate remarkable resilience and an impressive capacity to adjust and to cope. This chapter does *not* address the normal ups and downs of adolescence. It concerns those teenagers who are experiencing more extreme and persistent emotional problems. The terms describing these problems vary widely, but they include anxiety, panic, depression, and hopelessness. Signs that these problems exist range from distress felt only by the adolescent, to visible changes in mood or behavior, to physical symptoms related to the emotional upset, to suicidal thoughts or acts. All of these problems demand attention and care. They are every bit as serious and painful as medical problems with well-defined physical causes.

Physical Syptoms of Emotional Distress

Tina's head hurts. Her stomach aches. She is tired and irritable. Her eyes feel blurry. Her ears feel stuffy. Sometimes she feels dizzy. Nothing makes the feelings better or worse, and they have been there, on and off, for several weeks. The exact location of her discomfort changes, and it can occur any time during the day. Tina's parents are concerned but note that she has continued to eat and sleep well, has not lost weight, and looks generally healthy. After a careful examination, Tina's doctor finds nothing abnormal but wonders if Tina's symptoms are related to her grandmother's prolonged illness. Tina is very close to her grandmother and visits her almost daily on her way home from school.

Michael has chest pain that is very vague and difficult to describe. Sometimes it is on his right side, sometimes on his left. Sometimes it is dull and throbbing, sometimes sharp and fleeting. It can last seconds or hours. The pain never prevents him from playing ball, eating, or sleeping. He notices it mostly when he is sitting still and reading or watching television. It began last week, around the time that he learned that his family was going to move to another town.

Tina and Michael have psychosomatic complaints, or symptoms that arise from emotional feelings rather than from identifiable physical abnormalities. That does not mean that the physical feelings are "all in the head," "imagined," or "not really there." The symptoms are very real. They are a powerful message from the brain that something is causing emotional upset or turmoil. The physical symptoms are the brain's method of telling Tina and Michael that something is amiss and needs attention.

How can a teenager or a concerned parent differentiate a psychosomatic complaint from an organic complaint (a physical symptom with a physical cause)? This is one of the most difficult, common, and important distinctions in the entire medical field. Parents and teens often cannot decide without the help of highly trained health professionals. Whenever a symptom persists without a clear cause, help should be found. Even when the cause is known, whether emotional or physical, any persistent symptom warrants some form of treatment. For some problems, the treatment will be a medication. For many, simple reassurance is sufficient. For others, counseling or psychotherapy is indicated.

Psychosomatic complaints do share some common characteristics that help distinguish them from organic complaints. Tina's symptoms are vague aches and pains affecting many different parts of her body. Although bothersome, none of her complaints is severe or disabling. In a teenager who appears well, multisystem complaints (those affecting several body areas) are often psychosomatic in origin when they are unspecified, inconsistent, and hard to describe, and appear only when awake. Adolescents may be more prone to such multisystem feelings because of their rapidly growing and changing bodies. They are experiencing new physical sensations, and it is likely that psychological problems or conflicts will make themselves known through some physical symptoms.

Michael's symptoms are far more localized than Tina's, but they also change from one episode to the next. Michael finds it very difficult to pinpoint any consistency in his pain. Its location, duration, character, and severity all fluctuate. This is very typical of localized psychosomatic pain. Yet Michael is able to identify areas of stress: he has done poorly in school, is upset about the prospect of summer school, and worries about moving to a new town where he will not know anyone.

The management of psychosomatic problems depends on the emotional issues underlying the physical symptoms. When the symptoms reflect overattention to the many physical changes and sensations of puberty, discussion and reassurance by a physician or nurse often are sufficient to reduce concern. Several follow-up visits at intervals of three to six months may ease the process of puberty, making it more understandable and emotionally more comfortable.

Psychosomatic symptoms often are related to stress. This stress may be rather sudden—as when Michael learned of his family's plan to move—or more insidious—as Tina's experience during her grandmother's illness. It may be easier to recognize that the symptoms are related to the stress when the event is sudden. For Tina, the longer period of stress and the outward appearance of good coping camouflaged the association between her sadness about her grandmother and her physical symptoms. A physician can help the teenager recognize the association. Once recognized and understood, the symptoms often begin to abate. Most teenagers who develop psychosomatic symptoms adapt and continue smoothly through adolescence.

There are times, though, when psychosomatic symptoms are

more disabling and persistent. These symptoms may be obscure (such as fatigue) or localized (such as abdominal pain), or may appear as part of a specific medical problem (such as asthma or migraine headaches). Regardless of the symptoms, the common thread is that the teenager no longer functions normally at home or at school, and the symptoms do not fade with time, reassurance, or short-term counseling. Often it is difficult to identify a particular stressful event, though there may be generalized stressors, such as ongoing family discord or school problems.

Confronted with the very real discomfort and disability, adolescents and parents may react angrily when a physician suggests underlying emotional turmoil. The key to evaluation and treatment is to pursue the emotional and physical *simultaneously.* If the family or physician suspects a psychological component to the symptoms, it is generally a mistake to spend weeks or months exploring the physical and ignoring the emotional. The teenager remains in pain, and there may be no identified cause at the end of the process. The more expedient and comprehensive approach is to begin the counseling or psychotherapy while the medical evaluation is in process. This gives the adolescent a chance both to explore possible emotional causes and to develop, with psychological help, a way to cope with the discomfort.

One type of psychosomatic problem that is uncommon but that occurs more during adolescence than at any other age is called *conversion disorder.* This disorder is attributed to an ongoing psychological conflict that may have begun many years earlier. The symptoms can take various forms, but the most common is weakness of an arm or a leg or repetitive movements (called motor tics) that may be as localized as eye blinking or as generalized as seizurelike activity.

The adolescent with a conversion disorder usually is unaware of the psychological turmoil that is producing it. The events that initiated the turmoil may be difficult to identify because they occurred years ago. When a doctor suspects a conversion disorder, psychiatric referral is imperative. The goal of treatment is to help the teenager understand the cause of the symptoms, cope with the conflict, and restore physical function. The earlier this treatment begins, the better the outcome, both physically and psychologically.

Anxiety

Anxiety is very common during adolescence. When it is intermittent and controllable, it can help motivate teenagers to study harder, swim faster, kick the ball farther, or communicate better. When anxiety increases out of control, there is a decline in overall function, often extending beyond the immediate cause of the anxiety. This type of anxiety can take two forms, panic disorder or generalized anxiety disorder.

PANIC DISORDER

This disorder is defined as sudden episodes or attacks of intense fear associated with physical symptoms, such as trouble breathing, a choking sensation, pounding heartbeat, chest pain, light-headedness, trembling, sweating, hot or cold flashes, numbness or tingling sensations, and nausea or abdominal discomfort.

Before the attack occurs, the teenager may experience a sense of impending doom that increases as the physical symptoms mount. During the attack, there is an intense fear of losing control, going crazy, or even dying. At first, panic attacks may be infrequent enough that the adolescent can continue to function normally. The frequency and severity of the attacks eventually can result in marked dysfunction. Some people may experience an overwhelming fear and avoidance of public places (agoraphobia). Others may fear being alone.

Panic disorder is more common in females than males, and in adults in their twenties or thirties than in teenagers. Physical symptoms, rather than the anxiety itself, usually lead to a doctor's visit. The physician will look for an underlying physical problem, such as an overactive thyroid gland, excessive caffeine intake, or drug abuse (especially crack, cocaine, or amphetamines). In most cases, the doctor can make the diagnosis of panic disorder very quickly.

The treatment of panic disorder includes both psychological counseling and, when necessary, medication. Adolescents with this disorder are terrified and need to understand what is causing their symptoms and how to ease them. For some individuals, breathing in and out of a paper (*never* plastic) bag will alleviate the breathlessness, palpitations, and light-headedness. If these simple measures—along with counseling, relaxation techniques, and behavior modification—are insufficient, psychiatric medications can be effective. These medications include antidepressants and antianxiety drugs. They should *never* be used without the full knowledge and supervision of a physician. These medications are helpful when used appropriately but can cause serious side effects and dependence when used inappropriately.

GENERALIZED ANXIETY DISORDER

This condition is a state of persistent, chronic anxiety. When it follows a clearly stressful event (rape, assault, witness to violence, for example) that could produce emotional distress in anyone, it is called posttraumatic stress disorder. When there is no clear precipitating event, it is called generalized anxiety disorder.

The symptoms of generalized anxiety include intense fearfulness, sleep problems, and concentration difficulties. Medication can be helpful for short-term control of the symptoms, but the mainstay of treatment is psychotherapy.

Depression

"I'm depressed" is a familiar adolescent expression: "I'm depressed because we broke up." "Because my parents grounded me." "Because I'm overweight." "Because I failed my math final." In most of these cases, the depressed feelings do not persist and do not endanger the teenager's health and well-being. The word "depression," though, covers a broad spectrum of emotions—from the mild and momentary to the life-threatening.

Depression is a psychiatric and biological disorder that is very treatable. Simple depression will disappear on its own, as quickly as the event that triggered it. Sometimes, though, the depression deepens and persists. It can paralyze an adolescent's social, academic, and emotional life, and it can affect physical health. Depression can lead to self-neglect, self-harm, and suicide. Adolescent depression can be a very serious disease that demands early recognition and treatment.

Depression is defined as a disorder of mood, sometimes called an affective disorder. This umbrella term has several subcategories. For example:

Depressive feelings are responses of sadness to life's disappointing, unpleasant experiences. These feelings do not last longer than a few hours or days.

Reactive depression occurs in response to a specific event. The depressed feelings interfere with normal functioning and can persist for up to six months. The precipitating event usually occurs within three months prior to the depression. The event may be the loss of a friend or relative, parental separation or divorce, change of home or school, or any other stressful life event.

Seasonal affective disorder occurs less often in children and adolescents than in adults. It is a repeated pattern of profound sadness that occurs at a particular season for at least a three-year period. When the season—usually autumn or winter—ends, the depression lifts.

Dysthymia is a frequent sense of unhappiness, depression, or irritability that waxes and wanes for at least one year. Teenagers with dysthymia enjoy little, often feel hopeless, and concentrate poorly. Physical symptoms such as change in appetite, sleep disturbance, and fatigue are common.

Major depression is more severe than dysthymia. It is defined as a marked change in mood, behavior, and function lasting most of every day for at least two weeks. The adolescent feels and appears depressed or irritable and shows no interest or pleasure in activities previously enjoyed. Physical signs and symptoms include significant change in appetite or weight (gain or loss); sleep problems (either too much or too little); an appearance of restlessness or marked slowing; fatigue and loss of energy; low self-esteem and guilt; inability to concentrate and make decisions; recurrent thoughts of death or suicide.

Bipolar disorder is the current term for manic-depressive illness. It involves dramatic mood swings that interfere with personal relationships and school life. During the high (manic) period, the teenager may be extremely expansive, talkative, irritable, overstimulated, and physically "wound up." When the pendulum swings to the opposite pole, there is a low (depressed) period of sadness, withdrawal, and silent moodiness.

STATISTICS

Recent studies indicate that one out of four American children and teenagers has a psychiatric disorder. The likelihood that a child will become depressed increases with age. Less than 10 percent of preschool children show signs of clinical depression, compared to 15 percent of third through ninth graders, and 20 percent of fifteen-year-olds. An estimated 10 percent of adult men and 20 percent of adult women are depressed, making it the most common serious emotional and physical illness in the world.

GENDER DIFFERENCES

Girls are twice as likely as boys to experience depression during adolescence. The rates are equal during childhood, change with puberty, and persist throughout adulthood. During early puberty, self-image among girls seems to decline more commonly than among boys. Several studies of middle school students demonstrate that girls are far more concerned with their appearance than boys and tend to measure their overall self-worth according to their body image. A girl who feels too tall, too short, too fat, or too thin may become highly critical of all aspects of her appearance, personality, and performance. Such preoccupation with a perfect ideal fuels further decline in self-esteem and often results in significant depression.

The basic feelings underlying depression are the same in girls and boys, but the signs and symptoms may differ. Characteristics that are common among girls include distorted body image (seeing oneself differently than one really is), change in appetite and weight (Chapter 7), and a verbalized dissatisfaction with home, school, or social life. Depressed boys more commonly exhibit irritability, anger, hostility, impulsivity, rebelliousness, withdrawal from friends, and decline in school performance.

Girls and boys also seem to cope with depression differently. Girls are more likely to talk about their feelings with friends and sometimes with parents or trusted adults. Boys are more likely to withdraw from friends and family, often delaying both recognition of their depression and much needed care.

DIFFERENCES BETWEEN CHILDHOOD, ADOLESCENT, AND ADULT DEPRESSION

Far less is known about depression in childhood than depression in adulthood, but the signs and symptoms clearly differ. Depression in both children and adolescents commonly is missed because adults assume, and hope, that the signs are part of a transient stage, or normal childish misbehavior, or typical adolescent turmoil. Although depressed teenagers and adults share similar mood changes in terms of sadness and hopelessness, the adolescent often *appears* less depressed than the adult. The teenager's depression is more likely to become apparent through early behavioral changes than is the adult's. Events that begin as irritating but infrequent—a broken curfew, a missed school day—may escalate as the depression deepens.

Childhood depression can appear with persistent low self-esteem, nervousness, boredom, irritability, temper tantrums, and school avoidance. When these signs continue over several months, they are not just passing phases or stages. Depressed children who are impulsive, aggressive, or angry are likely to be noticed on the playground, in the classroom, and at home. Labeled as troublesome, these youngsters may be placed in special classes designed for children with hyperactivity or learning differences (Chapter 14), not for children with depression.

Depressed children who are listless or withdrawn are frequently overlooked. The attention of parents and teachers focuses on the more active, talkative child, while the quiet child is considered well-behaved and, therefore, well-adjusted.

During adolescence, the signs and symptoms of depression tend to be more recognizable. Moodiness, anger, impulsivity, social withdrawal, and changes in sleeping or eating occur more commonly in depressed adolescents than depressed children. Adolescent girls in particular express their low self-esteem more openly and may talk about feeling hopeless. Inattention and difficulty concentrating, common to depression at all ages, may cause a distinct fall in school performance that is detected more readily in adolescence, when academic demands increase, than in childhood. At its most extreme, depression is far more likely to result in life-threatening behaviors, such as substance abuse or suicide attempts, during adolescence than during childhood.

BIOLOGIC FACTORS

The causes of depression are many, and they are interrelated. Environment, biology, and genetics all contribute to its development. An environmental event may trigger depression by producing fluctuations in neurotransmitters, which are chemicals produced in the brain. These chemicals are released into the tiny spaces between nerve cells and transmit a signal from one cell to the next. At least eight different neurotransmitters have been identified. The three that have been linked most directly to depression are serotonin, norepinephrine, and dopamine. When there is an imbalance in the production or breakdown of these neurotransmitters, a mood disorder such as depression may result.

The identification of neurotransmitters has led to a great deal of interest in nutrition and diet as a way to alter mood. At present, there is no proof that any particular group of foods or vitamins alleviates depression. Treatment continues to center on psychotherapy and prescription medications.

MEDICATIONS

The improved understanding of the biologic basis of depression has led to an increased use of medication for its treatment. Antidepressant drugs that have proven effective in the treatment of adult depression are now used increasingly for children and adolescents. The field of pediatric psychopharmacology is relatively new and still somewhat controversial. In adults, antidepressant medications have an 80 percent rate of effectiveness. In children and adolescents, the effectiveness rates also seem high, but the medications have not been used or studied as extensively as in adults. Parents and teenagers should not regard medication as a magic bullet. In virtually all depressed adolescents, medication, when indicated, goes hand in hand with psychotherapy.

Antidepressant medications fall into two major classes: polycyclics and monoamine oxidase (MAO) inhibitors. All of these medications affect special receptors that exist in brain cells. The most commonly used type of polycyclic antidepressant is the tricyclic antidepressant, meaning that it has three rings in its molecular structure. The names of some tricyclics and their trade names are amitriptyline (Elavil), imipramine (Tofranil), nortriptyline (Aventyl or Pamelor), and desipramine (Norpramin). These drugs increase the brain levels of two neurotransmitters, norepinephrine and serotonin. Their major side effects in adolescents include sedation, light-headedness, dry mouth, blurred vision, and rapid heart rate. A rare side effect is cardiac arrhythmia (irregular heartbeat). When appropriate doses are used under a physician's supervision, the risk of an arrhythmia is practically negligible in a teenager without underlying heart disease.

Several newer antidepressant drugs within the polycyclic category do not have the three-ring molecular structure but work similarly to the tricyclics. Some include sertraline (Zoloft), fluoxetine (Prozac), amoxapine (Asendin), maprotiline (Ludiomil), trazodone (Desyrel), and bupropion (Wellbutrin). The side effects of some of these, especially sertraline and fluoxetine, tend to be less in adults than the tricyclics. Because these drugs are newer than the tricyclics, there is less information about their effectiveness in children and adolescents. Close supervision by a doctor who is very familiar with both the adolescent and the medication is essential.

The MAO inhibitors work very differently than the polycyclic antidepressants. MAO (monoamine oxidase) is an enzyme or chemical that breaks down norepinephrine and serotonin. The MAO inhibitors work by blocking this breakdown so that levels of the neurotransmitters in the brain increase. The names of some MAO inhibitors include tranylcypromine (Parnate), phenelzine sulfate (Nardil), and isocarboxazid (Marplan). The most common side effect of the MAO inhibitors is light-headedness when standing. Usually this side effect peaks during the first month of use and then diminishes. Other side effects include sleep disturbance, change in appetite, fluid retention, dry mouth, blurred vision, and rapid heart rate. A rare but dangerous side effect of the MAO inhibitors is sudden high blood pressure after eating certain foods (such as aged cheese, red wine, or pickled herring) or taking stimulating drugs (such as cold/allergy preparations or diet pills). MAO inhibitors usually are used only when the polycyclic antidepressants have proven ineffective.

Medication alone—no matter which type—should *never* be the sole treatment for the depressed adolescent. The vast majority of teenagers who experience depression will *not* require medication if skilled pschotherapy is provided. For those adolescents who do begin medication, virtually all will benefit from some ongoing psychotherapy. The difficult decision confronting adolescents and their parents often is where to go and which of the many types of counseling or therapy is most appropriate.

PSYCHOTHERAPY

Adolescents with short-term depressive feelings or reactive depression usually respond to supportive counseling in which a caring adult listens, reassures, and provides some guidance. For many adolescents, this guidance can come from a parent, teacher, guidance counselor, coach, family physician, or other trusted adult. When the teenager does not respond, however, treatment by a mental health professional always is indicated. Most adolescents respond best to a combination of individual and family therapy. Individual psychotherapy allows the teenager the autonomy to explore his or her own emotions and behaviors. Family therapy helps every member of the family understand the underpinnings of the adolescent's depression and cope with it in a more collaborative way.

A type of therapy that is effective in adults but unproven in adolescents is called cognitive therapy. In this approach, the individual's negative feelings are challenged by the therapist and eventually replaced by more sensible, positive feelings. Another approach, called behavior therapy, attempts to change the teenager's environment by increasing positive events and reinforcing pleasurable behavior. Other types of psychotherapy exist at both the individual and group levels. Regardless of the type, success depends on the skill of the therapist and the rapport with the adolescent.

The most important thing for the depressed teenager to remember is that the depression *will* lift. It *will* get better. In the midst of a depression, it is common to experience overwhelming hopelessness and a sense of permanent unhappiness. Everyone around the teenager must reinforce the temporary nature of the depression. Hope must be instilled. Treatment and support must be immediate, for the adolescent is in the throes of a personal crisis. The cry for help may be silent withdrawal, or psychosomatic complaints, or suicidal behavior. Whatever the signs, the underlying problem is treatable and reversible.

Suicide

Since the late 1960s the rate of teenage suicide has climbed at an alarming pace. Among fifteen-to-nineteen-year-olds, it has doubled. Among ten-to-fourteen-year-olds, it has *tripled.*

Now the third leading cause of mortality among American adolescents, suicide accounts for 10 percent of all deaths of ten-to-nineteen-year-olds. More than 5,000 American youth kill themselves each year. Nearly two million have attempted suicide. Many investigators believe that these estimates are two or three times lower than the actual numbers because suicidal acts are underreported. Up to 10 percent of teenage deaths in single-vehicle crashes may be suicides. Drownings, falls, and drug overdoses may be suicides rather than unintentional injuries. Underreporting probably results from several factors: variations in the definition of suicide and the criteria used to determine cause of death; social pressure to label a young person's death accidental rather than intentional; or practical concerns, such as loss of insurance benefits.

The single most important risk factor for adolescent suicide is a previous attempt. Over 40 percent of teenagers who complete suicide have made previous attempts. Between 3 percent and 10 percent who try to kill themselves succeed within fifteen years. Of adolescents hospitalized for suicide attempts, 10 percent try again within four years.

Another figure paints an even bleaker picture: only 5 percent of teenagers who attempt suicide reach medical attention, despite the fact that up to 50 percent seek medical care shortly before the attempt. Their reasons for seeking care, however, typically do not suggest the underlying emotional turmoil. Rather, their outward complaints are physical symptoms similar to those of the general adolescent population (such as sore throat, abdominal pain, or fatigue). An important goal for physicians and parents is to look beyond minor physical symptoms if there is any suggestion of emotional difficulty. It is always better to ask the teenager directly about suicidal thoughts or behavior than to lose the opportunity to intervene. There is no evidence that asking the question produces the behavior. The problem can be addressed and treated only if it is recognized.

Why does suicide so often come as a shock to family, friends, and school? What signs went unnoticed? Could it have been prevented? Which teenagers are at risk for suicide? How can families, schools, and communities prevent the increasing numbers of adolescent suicides? How should a community respond when confronted with the tragedy of an adolescent suicide? One way to begin searching for answers is to look at the overall data on adolescent suicide:

Demographics. Suicide rates among youth vary widely by age, gender, and race. Ten-to-fourteen-year-olds have far lower rates (1.5 per 100,000 in 1987) than fifteen-to-nineteen-year-olds (10.3 per 100,000 in 1987). The highest rate (which peaked at 27.8 per 100,000 in 1983) exists among white males between twenty and twenty-four. White males are twice as likely to kill themselves as African-American males, four and a half times as likely as white females, and eight times as likely as African-American females. The highest adolescent suicide rates in the United States are reported among Native American youth—two and a half to four times higher than all other ethnic groups.

The ratio of male and female suicides has changed over the twentieth century. In the early 1900s, the female rate exceeded the male rate. By 1983, males were three times as likely as females to kill themselves. The ratio has now reached four to one.

Method. Firearms are the leading cause of suicidal death. In 1985, there were nearly 2,500 deaths from firearms among youth aged fifteen to nineteen, divided evenly between suicides and homicides. With half of all American homes containing guns—some 200 million in all—adolescents have ready access to firearms.

The next most frequent methods of youth suicide are hanging, strangulation, and suffocation. Ingestion of medications and carbon monoxide inhalation (usually from auto exhaust) follow. Among suicide attempts that reach medical attention, drug overdoses account for 38 percent and self-inflicted wounds for 33 percent.

Attempt rates. School-based surveys from 1986 to 1989 revealed that 9 to 14 percent of students in grades seven through twelve reported at least one attempt at some time in their lives. A 1990 national survey of ninth through twelfth graders revealed that 27 percent of students had thought seriously about suicide within the past year, 16 percent had made a suicide plan, 8 percent had attempted suicide, and 2 percent had made an attempt that required medical attention. Although boys had higher rates of completed suicide, girls were more likely to consider, plan, or attempt suicide. Hispanic girls had the highest attempt rates, followed by white girls, and then African-American girls.

Risk factors. As stated earlier, the single most important predictor of suicide is a previous attempt. Yet, important demographic differences exist between the larger population of adolescents who attempt suicide and the smaller group who complete it. Girls are more likely to make attempts; boys are more likely to commit suicide. Adolescents who attempt suicide are somewhat younger than those who commit suicide. Hispanic adolescents have high attempt rates, yet low suicide rates.

Mental health problems are common among both teenagers who attempt suicide and those who complete it. Adolescents with schizophrenia or bipolar depression are at high risk for suicide attempts, and one in twenty-five ultimately commit suicide. An estimated 40 percent of adolescents who commit suicide and 25 percent of those who attempt it have a history of major depression. One study revealed that 35 percent of depressed adolescents attending a clinic for high-risk youth had attempted suicide.

Hopelessness may be even more characteristic of suicidal youth than depression. Nearly all who attempt suicide express a sense of irreversible sadness or believe that their circumstances are irreparable. Some adolescents may reveal all the classic signs of depression. But for other adolescents, warning signs may be very difficult to detect. Teenagers who are troubled, but not necessarily depressed, are far more likely than adults to attempt suicide impulsively, with no advance planning. Young adolescents who have not developed the cognitive maturity to relate current behavior to future outcome may not fully understand that the act may result in death. Swallowing pills may be seen as an immediate relief of current emotional pain rather than as a cause of future death.

Certain family factors increase an adolescent's risk of suicide. The teenager's perception of how the family functions may be as important as the facts of the family's situation. For example, an adolescent from a divorced family who feels loved and supported by both parents probably is at lower risk than an adolescent whose parents live together but who feels isolated and unable to communicate with either parent.

Adolescents who contemplate suicide often believe that their parents do not understand them or do not take their depression or hopelessness seriously. Concerns of great importance to adolescents may seem trivial to parents. If expressions of stress or sadness go unrecognized, teenagers may respond by withdrawing from the family or revealing unhappiness in behavioral rather than verbal ways. Whatever the manifestations, they feel blocked, isolated, and alienated. As the frustration mounts, so too does a sense of futility. They see no options and no ways to take control of their lives. Suicide seems the only escape.

Drugs and/or alcohol use is implicated in 30 to 70 percent of teenage suicides, and probably contributes to its implusivity. A troubled adolescent may turn to drugs or alcohol as a way to alter a depressed mood or to dull the pain of a threatening or stressful situation. The alcohol or drug further impairs the teenager's ability to make decisions or moderate behavior.

Poor school performance is another factor associated with suicidal behavior. Most studies indicate that although adolescents who kill themselves have average to high IQs, their inattention and difficulty concentrating interfere with learning. Just as they have trouble coping with the problems in their lives, they struggle with the problem-solving tasks required in most classrooms.

A recent stressful event, such as parental punishment, a fight with a friend, or a romantic conflict, may be related to the timing of suicidal behavior, but the event never is the sole cause. When a suicide occurs or is attempted, the event becomes a part of a long series of problems or distress. The same or similar events happen to many other teenagers who never consider suicide as the solution. The difference between the nonsuicidal and the suicidal youth is the *response* to the stressful event, not the event itself.

Another risk factor that has received much public attention involves what is called a cluster effect. When one adolescent suicide occurs, other teenagers in the same town or school may consider, attempt, or even commit suicide. It is unclear whether this happens because something in the environment affects each teenager separately, whether there is a copycat effect, or whether media attention inadvertently promotes suicidal behavior. A suicide cluster behaves like an epidemic in that the number of actual adolescent suicides in a given geographic region far exceeds the number that would be expected on the basis of history and population size. The number of adolescents who have died in a single community as part of a cluster phenomenon ranges from two to twenty over a period of several months.

SUICIDE PREVENTION

Parents, friends, educators, and health professionals can work together to prevent adolescent suicide. This begins with early recognition of the signs of depression, hopelessness, reckless behavior, and suicidal behavior. When these signs appear, a prompt response is essential. Sometimes, supportive counseling from a caring friend or adult is enough to prevent a suicidal act. When this is inadequate, professional help must be available—no barriers, no reasons to delay. Adolescents must know that there are confidential mental health services in their communities. They must know how to find them. Telephone hotline numbers should be advertised on billboards and publications that teens read. Crisis intervention services around the country operate twenty-four-hour telephone lines staffed by adult and peer counselors. These services range from referral only to drop-in counseling. Despite their availability, many adolescents remain unaware of the services or fearful that their parents will be informed. These hotlines protect confidentiality and usually do not require name, address, or telephone number before providing help.

What practical steps can parents or friends take when they suspect a teenager is considering suicide? A few specific suggestions:

• Lecturing does not work. Listen and reflect back the adolescent's feelings. Avoid judgmental or critical statements. Take the teenager's problems seriously. Do not minimize, trivialize, or mock.

• Speak honestly about your concerns. Say that you are worried about the teenager. Share your own thoughts about feeling sad and lonely. Let the adolescent know that everyone feels depressed at times and that he or she is not alone.

• Parents or friends of teenagers who appear suicidal sometimes hesitate to bring up the subject for fear that the discussion might promote the idea. Talking about suicide does not precipitate it. Instead, the discussion provides an opportunity to intervene.

• Suicidal teenagers sometimes talk or even joke about suicide. They may become preoccupied with death themes or may give away favorite clothes, tapes, or other prized possessions. Do not ignore these comments and behaviors. Discuss your concern openly with the adolescent and consult a mental health professional immediately.

• Try to discover the roots of the problem and encourage the teenager to consider other solutions or coping strategies. Support the adolescent through the process and make it clear that you are there for the long haul—not just for today's talk.

• Remove potential methods of suicide. If there is a gun in the home, get rid of it permanently. (And, because firearms are the most common method of suicide, support efforts to promote gun control legislation.) Clear the medicine cabinet of all medications, including the seemingly harmless over-the-counter types.

• Adolescents who are unable to control their suicidal tendencies require one-on-one surveillance by adults until they can be placed in a safe, secure environment. Try to buy time by listening and instilling trust until professional help is found and the adolescent is safe.

COMMUNITY RESPONSE TO TEENAGE SUICIDE

In response to the national concern with adolescent suicide clusters, the Centers for Disease Control in 1988 called for community plans to prevent and contain suicide clusters. The CDC recommended that community leaders in education, public health, mental health, and adolescent medicine establish coordinated plans that would go into effect whenever a teenage suicide occurs. Such plans involve adolescents, parents, teachers, coaches, counselors, clergy, and support personnel. At the plan's core is a system of communication. The major goal is to respond to the suicide quickly, to provide honest information without deception or glorification, and to identify other youth who may be at risk for suicide. Support systems should be planned in advance so that help becomes immediately available to all adolescents who need it. After the crisis has passed, the community should review and revise the plan.

Suicide is a tragedy at any age. The death of an adolescent brings immeasurable pain to family and friends and represents an enormous loss to society. Adolescent suicide is a problem that demands attention at all levels—individual, family, community, national. While it is frightening, teenage suicide also is preventable. Most anxious or depressed adolescents will overcome their emotional difficulties and never face suicidal thoughts or acts. Some adolescents continue to suffer and experience increasing hopelessness and despair. These teenagers can benefit from our help. The goals are to recognize, acknowledge, and intervene without delay.

14

Learning and Behavior Problems

When John was in preschool, he fidgeted and wandered while other children sat still for story time. In first grade, he had trouble paying attention in the classroom and squabbled on the playground. By second grade, he was lagging behind his peers in reading and writing skills. John's parents talked with his pediatrician, teachers, and the school psychologist. After careful observation of his behavior, a physical examination, and psychological testing, a diagnosis of attention deficit hyperactivity disorder (ADHD, p. 175–82) was made. John's treatment began with a change in his home and school routine. He was moved to a special class in his public school that had fewer children and was highly structured. At home, his parents tried to set clear limits and to reward John for good behavior rather than just reprimanding him for his frequent misbehavior. These changes helped but did not solve the problem. By third grade, John was well aware that he was often in trouble and out of control. He wanted to comply but could not contain his impulsiveness and daydreaming. His doctor suggested that a medication called methylphenidate (Ritalin) might help John pay attention and curb his overactive behavior.

The medication did help. John did better in school. His relationships with friends and siblings improved as his aggressive behavior diminished. He felt happier about himself and began to hear fewer rebukes from those around him. But the medication was not a panacea. He still had to work hard to concentrate. He had trouble organizing his school responsibilities. And there were some side effects to the medication.

Day-to-day living was a trying experience for John and his family. But when they took the long view, John's parents saw progress. They looked forward to the day when John would no longer need medication. They had read that some children outgrow attention deficit hyperactivity disorder during adolescence. And so they waited . . .

Like John, millions of youngsters have learning or behavior disorders that affect their school performance, their relationships, and their self-esteem. Estimates of the prevalence of learning difficulties among school-age children range from 10 to 30 percent. This range is wide and imprecise because learning problems have many forms and causes, making clear diagnosis somewhat elusive. Within each of the following major categories are many specific diagnoses:

1. Psychological and other causes such as family stress or inadequate teaching;
2. Specific learning problems such as dyslexia and ADHD;
3. Mild or borderline mental retardation;
4. Chronic physical illness or disability;
5. Hearing, vision, and speech impairments;
6. Neurological problems such as frequent seizures that interfere with learning.

A thorough medical evaluation usually will identify causes in the last three categories. Psychological testing, performed by a specially trained psychologist, can help identify adolescents whose learning difficulties are due to mental retardation. Most of these young people are recognized earlier in childhood, but mild deficits (intelligence quotients, or IQs, of 70 to 85) may not become apparent until the increased academic demands of the middle or high school years.

Most teenagers with school problems fall in the first two categories: psychological causes and specific learning problems. Many of the psychosocial causes, such as anxiety and depression (Chapter 13) and substance abuse (Chapter 12), were discussed earlier. The goals of this chapter are to help parents and adolescents recognize when a specific learning problem, such as dyslexia or ADHD exists, to review the treatment options and coping strategies, and to consider the prognosis, or outcome, during adolescence and adulthood.

Learning difficulties usually become apparent before the teenage years. Problems that seemed manageable or stable during childhood can flare as school demands and social distractions increase. The result for many adolescents with learning problems is frustration and diminishing motivation. The challenge is to maintain the teenager's sense of achievement and self-worth. This begins with a careful evaluation of the adolescent's strengths and weaknesses. Parents and teachers can then work together to create an environment that breeds success and optimism about future learning.

Recognizing and Coping with Learning Disabilities

Learning is a highly complex process. Information comes in through the senses of vision, hearing, touch, smell, and taste. The information must then be interpreted through reasoning and stored through concentration and memory. A defect in any of these operations impairs the total learning process and results in a *learning disability*. The specific problem may appear as difficulty in reading, writing, arithmetic, spelling, speaking, listening, or following instructions.

Learning disabilities are often, but not always, diagnosed in elementary school. Some children learn to compensate for the difficulties and make good academic progress. But many children with unrecognized learning disabilities struggle from their earliest school years. By adolescence, they have a track record of repeated failures, conflicts with teachers and other students, and truancy. They dislike school and feel defeated by the process. As the curriculum becomes more difficult, the learning disability takes an even greater toll and they feel hopelessly behind. What began as a specific learning disability becomes a set of complex psychological problems manifesting as frustration, poor self-esteem, misbehavior, and underachievement. These teenagers are in crisis. They need immediate evaluation and help to reverse a downward spiral that began in school and has expanded to all facets of their life.

Learning disabilities that first emerge during adolescence may look more like behavior or mood problems than academic problems. Some of the common signs of a learning disorder in adolescence include:

• Escalating anxiety about schoolwork. The anxiety may become so pervasive that it interferes even more with attention.

• A sense of futility. The teenager may begin to feel that even best efforts are unsuccessful, so "Why try at all?"

• Acting-out behavior. The adolescent's frustration and difficulty meeting adult expectations may lead to defiant behavior toward the adult world.

• Change in friends. Teenagers who meet with repeated failure often seek consolation and support from each other. As childhood friends thrive in school, the learning-disabled adolescent may drift away, toward a new social circle.

• School truancy, absenteeism, dropout. This may begin as frequent absences for minor ailments and progress to missed days without parents' knowledge, and ultimately to an outright refusal to return to school.

• Depression. The sense of failure and hopelessness may extend from the classroom to all aspects of life.

When parents or teachers suspect that an adolescent has a learning disability, they should discuss the issue together to determine if the difficulties observed in school match those observed at home. A school psychologist can evaluate the teenager or suggest a specialist who is skilled in psycho-educational testing and diagnosis. These tests, when considered jointly, may help clarify the specific learning problem and its cause. IQ tests assess overall intelligence. Achievement tests measure levels of knowledge in specific areas such as reading, math, spelling, and writing. Psychological testing can identify behavioral problems related to learning. Hearing and vision tests can discover defects in auditory and visual skills. Neurological tests can identify problems in the central nervous system that affect learning.

Adolescents with learning disorders desperately need encouragement and reassurance about their strengths. They need to identify what they can do well and how to cope with their weaknesses. Many need straightforward information about their intellectual capabilities.

Teenagers with learning disabilities typically have normal IQs. They have the cognitive capability to learn, but tend to approach learning in a way that differs from their peers. Because most schools direct their primary teaching toward the average student, the teenager with a learning disability finds his or her style inefficient. Early recognition of the disability can help teachers structure learning strategies for the adolescent. This may involve breaking tasks down into small steps, using techniques to help the adolescent decode problems, or promoting organizational skills.

Parents can offer support and encouragement on the homefront. During the early years, children with learning disabilities benefit from parental structure and involvement—exact beginning and ending times for homework, sitting with the child during homework time, checking the work. This level of involvement is likely to be met with resistance during adolescence, and parents must begin to relinquish control. Continued overinvolvement may send a painful message that the teenager is such a failure that he or she cannot survive without the parent's help.

Parents of adolescents with learning disabilities can be most supportive if they follow these suggestions:

• Determine your child's learning style. A learning disability is *not* an inability to learn, but rather a different learning style that requires special structure and techniques. The study habits that worked for a parent may be wholly ineffective for the teenager. Similarly, the approach toward school and homework that a parent took with other children in the family simply may not work when applied to an adolescent with a learning disability.

• Be flexible. Working together with the teenager, parents and teachers can experiment with different learning techniques. Gently encourage the adolescent to take academic risks, to try learning something new or challenging.

• Show as much concern for your teenager's feelings as you do for the report card. The teenager's feelings about school are even more important than the performance. Let the adolescent know that you understand the frustration and the struggle. Reward a solid effort, even if the product is less than desired.

• Look for strengths and downplay weaknesses. It is far better to praise and encourage than to criticize.

• Remain open-minded and optimistic about your teenager's future academic and career options. A learning disability that continues into adulthood does not exclude a college education or a professional career. Work with the adolescent and guidance counselor to identify colleges or training programs that meet the needs of students with learning disabilities. Help the teenager make a good match that is challenging yet realistic.

Dyslexia

Dyslexia is a commonly used term that encompasses several different types of reading disorders. Most children with dyslexia are recognized in elementary school, but some manage to compensate or to circumvent the problem until high school when the reading level and volume increase. Some of the signs of dyslexia include:

- reversing letters in words,
- losing the place on a page,
- skipping words or whole lines,
- substituting a new word for the printed one,
- guessing at a word based on its first letter,
- misreading familiar words,
- difficulty decoding unfamiliar words,
- reading haltingly and without expression,
- overlooking punctuation.

When a parent or teacher suspects dyslexia, an evaluation should be done to look for associated problems, such as a vision or hearing deficit, another specific learning disability such as ADHD, or an emotional problem.

The cause of dyslexia is unclear. Some research suggests that it results from delayed development in the brain's ability to interpret written material. This delay probably results from both inborn and external factors. Whatever the cause, the teenager with dyslexia can learn to read and can excel in school. The sooner the reading difficulty is recognized, the more successful and competent the teenager will feel.

Attention Deficit Hyperactivity Disorder (ADHD)

Many adolescents and young adults grew up with the label "hyperactive," "minimal brain dysfunction," or "minimal brain damage." "Hyperactive" was used to describe their impulsive, restless, inattentive behavior. "Minimal" reflected the minor neurological findings, normal or high IQ, and the lack of evidence for brain damage.

Early descriptions of this set of disorders focused on the behavioral component and attempted to separate hyperactivity–attention deficit disorders from learning disorders. Newer evidence indicates that most children with persistent trouble paying attention or concentrating also have learning problems. Some are hyperactive. Some are not. Clearly, there is a wide spectrum of disorders that includes many combinations of attention, learning, and behavior problems. These disorders are now grouped together under the umbrella diagnosis *attention deficit hyperactivity disorder (ADHD)*.

Along with the new term, ADHD, is a shift in our understanding of its outcome during adolescence and adulthood. Before the 1980s, it was commonly believed that children with ADHD outgrew their learning or behavior problems at puberty. Now it is recognized that up to one third of children with ADHD continue to experience some symptoms beyond age eighteen. For many adolescents with ADHD, school and behavior difficulties actually may become worse as the academic demands of secondary school increase.

ADHD is the most common learning–behavior disorder of childhood. Approximately 5 to 10 percent of all school children aged five through twelve have ADHD. Among boys, the rate may be as high as 20 percent. Boys are three to six times more likely than girls to have ADHD. The reasons for this gender difference—and indeed the cause of the disorder—remain unknown. Increasing evidence indicates that ADHD has an inborn, biochemical basis, with low levels of brain neurotransmitters such as norepinephrine and dopamine. (Neurotransmitters are chemicals produced in the brain that transmit signals between nerve cells.)

But biochemistry does not explain all of the difficulties experienced by children and teenagers with ADHD. Psychological makeup and the social environment clearly contribute as well. For example, a student with ADHD who has trouble paying attention is further stymied if the classroom environment is full of distracting noise and movement. The student's fragile ability to concentrate may be shattered by a whispered conversation between classmates or by a wailing fire siren outside. The same student who is given structured tasks in a small, quiet classroom may do very well.

Diagnosing ADHD in teenagers can be more difficult than in younger children. The adolescent with ADHD does not have a new disorder that just developed, but rather a long-standing disorder that was either mild or unrecognized in childhood. Consequently, the difficulties may have compounded over the years so that by adolescence the many minor skill deficits produce major academic problems. The mild misbehaviors of childhood, coupled with years of frustration and criticism, may lead to serious behavioral problems during adolescence.

Consider Greg, a fifteen-year-old with recently diagnosed ADHD. Greg was an overactive, hard to manage child from the time he could walk. He spent much of his childhood in repeated "time outs" for disruptive behavior. His IQ tests indicated superior intelligence, but he never managed more than a C in schoolwork. Greg rarely received the pats on the back for good work that stimulated his classmates to learn and persevere. When he behaved well, teachers stayed out of his way and hoped it would last. When he misbehaved, reprimands were quick as teachers struggled to maintain order in the classroom. Greg increasingly assumed the role of the "bad child," always on the edge of trouble. By early adolescence, his parents felt that they had lost control of his behavior. Greg was cutting school, stealing household money, and lying to his parents. Then he was arrested for driving without a license.

Steven is another fifteen-year-old with newly diagnosed ADHD. As a child, Steven was quiet and withdrawn. His teachers were perplexed by his poor school performance, given his above-average intelligence. They described him as often daydreaming and missing or mis-hearing instructions. At home Steven spent most of his time in front of his computer or television. To his parents, Steven was a quiet boy who never got into real trouble, but they were frustrated by his tendency to forget instructions or dally with homework and other tasks. By adolescence, Steven looked and felt depressed. His parents were worried. He had few friends and participated in no school activities. He communicated little, and they felt increasingly out of touch with him.

Both of these teenagers have attention disorders, yet the manifestations differ. Greg is hyperactive. Steven is not. Greg has developed a conduct disorder, meaning that he violates basic and important rules of society. Steven has become significantly depressed. Underlying these differences is a common thread: inattentiveness. Both boys have a long history of trouble paying attention, following instructions, completing a task. Both Greg and Steven have behavioral features that limit their ability to function normally within the social environment. And both boys have experienced more difficulty over time—not because the underlying cause has changed or become worse, but because the list of frustrations, unlearned skills, underachievement, and criticisms has grown.

PROBLEMS ASSOCIATED WITH ADHD

Greg and Steven have ADHD and other problems commonly associated with ADHD. These associated problems can complicate the teenager's diagnosis and treatment. One of the greatest concerns of parents is that their child with ADHD will, in adolescence, engage in serious behaviors such as lying, stealing, aggression, assault. These types of behavior constitute a serious conduct disorder and are often associated with a personality disorder called antisocial personality. A teenager with an antisocial personality engages in criminal-type behaviors repeatedly and with no sense of remorse or social responsibility. Antisocial behavior is associated with ADHD but tends to occur more frequently in a subgroup of teenage boys who are aggressive in childhood and show ongoing hyperactivity in adolescence. It seems to occur more often when the ADHD was untreated or uncontrolled in childhood and when the adolescent faces significant environmental stress, such as poverty and neighborhood violence.

Alcohol and drug abuse are associated with antisocial or conduct disorders far more than with ADHD. No clear evidence suggests that ADHD alone, especially when treated, predisposes the adolescent to substance abuse. Some investigators believe that teenagers with untreated ADHD who turn to drugs do so in an attempt to self-medicate their out-of-control behavior.

Unintentional injuries and motor vehicle accidents are more common among adolescents with ADHD, probably because of their inattentiveness and distractibility. Among hyperactive youth, the tendency toward risk-taking and impulsive or aggressive behavior also may increase the chance of injury. In about half of children with ADHD, there may be coordination problems such as poor eye–hand coordination, difficulty with gross motor skills (running and jumping, for example), or fine motor skills (such as handwriting). These coordination difficulties can increase the risk of injury and add to the teenager's frustration.

Other movement disorders also may be associated with ADHD. About 20 percent of children with ADHD have tic disorders that range from eye blinking or twitching, to jerking movements, to repeated vocal noises such as grunting or throat clearing. Tic disorders usually appear in mid-childhood, after the symptoms of ADHD appear but before puberty. Tourette syndrome is an uncommon, severe tic disorder involving motor and vocal tics, often with involuntary vocal obscenities. Tourette syndrome is more common in children with ADHD, but also can occur in children without ADHD.

Obsessive–compulsive disorder is related to both ADHD and tic disorders. This disorder usually begins in adolescence as a tremendous preoccupation with a particular behavior such as hand washing. Other psychiatric illnesses that may be related to ADHD include school phobia and avoidant disorder, in which the adolescent avoids social settings and interactions.

The most common problems associated with ADHD are the result of the repeated frustrations and negative feedback experienced over the years. These problems include poor self-image, depression, and lack of motivation or ambition. The most important goal of early diagnosis and treatment is the prevention of these secondary problems.

MANAGING ADHD

There is no known cure for ADHD. The management or treatment focuses on controlling the symptoms but usually does not make them disappear. A multifaceted approach to management requires good communication among the teenager, family, physician, therapists, and teachers. This communication can become more difficult as the adolescent strives for independence.

Medication has assumed an increasingly important role in the treatment of ADHD. Most of the medications used in ADHD are stimulants, such as methylphenidate (Ritalin), dextroamphetamine (Dexedrine), and pemoline (Cylert). The use of stimulants seems paradoxical in a disorder in which hyperactivity often occurs. But these drugs work by stimulating attention so that the individual is better able to control his or her behavior and activity level. As the behavior improves, relationships with peers, siblings, teachers, and parents improve. The vicious cycle of misbehavior and negative feedback is broken, and the adolescent's self-image begins to improve.

As in John's experience, described at the beginning of this chapter, medication often does help control the ADHD, but it is not a panacea. Stimulants have definite limitations and side effects. Their use must be monitored closely by a physician who is familiar with ADHD. The medication improves attentiveness in up to 80 percent of children with ADHD, but it does not change learning or processing problems. Even when the behavior and attention improve, the learning problems will continue to require special educational techniques. For the teenager with ADHD since childhood, a medication begun in middle or high school cannot fill in the gaps in learning that occurred throughout the earlier years.

Ritalin is the most widely prescribed medication for ADHD. Its most common side effects are a decrease in appetite and stomachache. The peak effect of Ritalin usually occurs within one to three hours, but the total effect may last up to six hours. The doses can be adjusted so that they do not interfere with meals. Growth must be monitored very closely in children who take Ritalin, especially as they approach the growth spurt of puberty. If nutrition and weight gain are threatened, the dose should be decreased or a change in medication considered.

Some children and adolescents on Ritalin also have trouble falling asleep at night; this too responds to a change in the timing of the medication. Other side effects may include a jittery feeling or a faster heartbeat. Less commonly, Ritalin and other stimulants may precipitate motor tics like eye blinking. These medications usually are avoided in patients who have preexisting tic disorders like Tourette syndrome.

A side effect of Ritalin that is frequently bothersome to parents is a rebound phenomenon in which the symptoms of the ADHD become worse as the medication wears off. Doses are usually given to maximize the effectiveness of the medication during the school day. The wearing-off phase then occurs in the late afternoon or evening when the teenager is at home. Rebound symptoms may include hyperactivity, talkativeness, irritability, and moodiness. Although bothersome, rebound usually is short-lived, diminishing within an hour.

Dexedrine has side effects similar to Ritalin, but they tend to occur more often. Cylert differs from Ritalin and Dexedrine in the timing of its effect. While Ritalin usually wears off within three to six hours, Cylert does not begin to wear off until seven hours after ingestion. Advantages of Cylert, especially for the adolescent who does not want to take medication at school, are that one morning dose often is sufficient and rebound does not usually occur.

There are times when stimulants are ineffective, poorly tolerated, or not recommended (for children with seizures or tic disorders, for example). Tricyclic antidepressants such as imipramine (Tofranil) are the next line of treatment. They may be especially effective in the teenager with ADHD who is also depressed (Chapter 13).

Clonidine (Catapres) is another drug that has been used for ADHD. This medication also is used to treat high blood pressure or hypertension in adults. Although it causes a fall in blood pressure when used for ADHD, it is begun at a low dose and increased very gradually so that the effect usually is well tolerated. The most frequent side effects in adolescents are fatigue and dry mouth.

Regardless of which medication is used, its effectiveness and dose should be reevaluated several times a year. Many teenagers who have been on fairly stable doses will require lower doses or even no medication as they approach adulthood. Some will do well with "medication holidays" in which the drug is stopped for the summer or other school vacations. Whether or not the medication is discontinued, its effect *always* should be reviewed about a month after school begins each year. This review requires good communication between the adolescent, family, teachers, and physician.

Parents may worry that years of medication will result in addiction to the drug. No evidence proves that this occurs. The medication does not lose effect with prolonged use. As children grow, the dosage may need to be increased, but this is due to their greater body weight rather than a tolerance to the drug's effectiveness.

Medication, no matter how effective, will not be sufficient for the optimal management of ADHD. Even more important than the medication is a supportive educational and emotional network. "But how do we do this?" parents frequently ask. The old behavior modification techniques of childhood—stickers or other rewards for sitting still and reading four pages without interruption—are hardly appropriate for a teenager. During adolescence, encouragement and support should take different forms. Teenagers may still need help in specific study skills, but they also need more freedom to take responsibility for their schoolwork and social behavior.

It may help to remember that teenagers with ADHD are often uneven in their cognitive development. They may be quite advanced in one area, yet they may be failing in another. For example, an adolescent may have strong conceptual and language skills but may have great difficulty with memorization or following several instructions in a given sequence. This unevenness is frustrating for the creative, bright teenager whose ideas are soaring but who cannot write them down in an organized paragraph.

Many adolescents with ADHD tire quickly when they are in situations that require passive listening or prolonged sitting. They become restless and fidgety during lectures. They have trouble during study halls. This is not simply boredom. The foot bouncing, finger tapping, and wiggling in the chair are ways to arouse themselves in the face of inattentiveness and fatigue.

Studying for tests is trying for adolescents with ADHD because they have trouble determining what they do and do not know. Educators call this ineffective self-monitoring; in other words, they lack self-testing skills. They may do well in a class discussion but are unable to organize their thoughts for a written test. Their inattention to detail also hinders their performance. They tend to rush through tasks and resist checking or proofreading their work.

The school environment can become a critical factor for the teenager with ADHD, both in terms of learning and self-esteem. The pressures in the classroom and on the playing field are felt by all teenagers but may become overwhelming for the teenager who has trouble with focus and organization. If teachers, coaches, and guidance counselors are aware of the problem, they can help provide the structure and individual time that the adolescent needs. Most importantly, they can work with parents to emphasize strengths and boost confidence. Like all teenagers, those with ADHD need opportunities to develop autonomy, self-reliance, and a solid personal identity. So often these opportunities are restricted because of the inattentiveness or impulsiveness. With appropriate counseling and a focus on the positive, adolescents with ADHD can—and must—be allowed to experiment and function independently.

Children and adolescents with ADHD have wonderful qualities that *result* from their attention problems. For example, they may ignore details but, in the process, have a global view that is creative, free-thinking, and conceptually sound. They may not notice every tree, but they see the whole forest. They may have trouble with a paragraph, but their doodles evolve into an extraordinary architectural plan. Their innate restlessness can lead to initiative, ambition, and accomplishment. Adolescents with ADHD have difficulty with traditional learning modes, but they also have talents, individuality, humor, and skills that should be recognized and reinforced.

IV

SEXUALITY AND REPRODUCTION

15

Reproductive Development

Most adolescents study "sex education" in school. From the elementary grades through high school health classes, human reproduction is portrayed through drawings, diagrams, charts, models, and films. This approach conveys straightforward information that is basic and important, but it is not comprehensive. Human sexuality is far more than biological facts and functions. It involves emotions, communication, and concepts about ourselves and others.

Outside the classroom, teenagers have been learning about sexuality throughout their lives. As babies, they experienced touch and intimacy in the ways they were hugged, kissed, cuddled, and rocked. As children, they verbalized the universal question, "Where do babies come from?" They incorporated nonverbal cues by observing their parents' interactions, expressions of affection, and sexual attitudes. As teenagers, they begin to learn more from each other and from the popular culture. They pay careful attention to television, movies, music, and advertisements. In other words, sex education is lifelong and multidimensional. For some teenagers, though, the piecemeal nature of the information can be confusing.

Today's teenagers are bombarded with pressures to make early decisions about sexual behavior. They are living in a world where:

• Fifty percent of girls and 60 percent of boys aged fifteen to nineteen have had sexual intercourse.

• The proportion of adolescents who have first sexual intercourse at a young age is increasing. In 1982, 19 percent of girls had intercourse by age fifteen. By 1987, the percentage reached 27.

• Fifty percent of teenagers do not use birth control the first time they have intercourse. Only one third of all adolescents routinely use birth control.

• Sixty percent of sexually active girls aged fifteen to nineteen say that they have had two or more sexual partners.

• One million American teenagers become pregnant each year. Fifty percent of these pregnancies result in birth, 36 percent in abortion, and 14 percent in miscarriage. The United States has the highest teen pregnancy rate in the Western world, twice as high as England, France, and Canada.

Adolescence is a time of decision making. From choice of clothing to choice of contraception, teenagers make countless decisions that express their sexuality and define their identity. They need accurate information and the opportunity to ask questions, voice concerns, and practice decision-making skills. Teenagers' interest in sexuality should be encouraged as a part of normal development. Most teenagers welcome a straightforward discussion with their parents. Through open communication about the important topics in the following chapters, adolescents and parents can learn together and from each other. The best times for these discussions is now—before a problem arises.

Most human organs are alike in females and males. A male's liver resembles a female's liver. A female's heart may be slightly smaller, but its four chambers pump blood just as a male's does. The male and female reproductive organs are quite different, though, even before birth. With puberty, a girl begins to menstruate, her uterus grows larger, her vagina becomes longer and more elastic. A boy's penis grows, his testicles become larger, and he begins to produce spermatozoa (sperm).

Sexual development begins at different ages and proceeds at different rates depending on factors such as heredity and nutrition. The beginning and pace of puberty are controlled by two glands located in the brain. The hypothalamus gland triggers puberty by sending a hormonal message to the pea-size pituitary gland. The pituitary gland secretes hormones that control many glands and organs outside the brain, including the ovaries in females and the testes (testicles) in males. When the pituitary gland receives its message from the hypothalamus, it sends a hormonal signal through the bloodstream to the sex organs (the ovaries or testes). The ovaries respond by producing the female sex hormones (estrogen and progesterone). The testes respond by producing the male sex hormone (testosterone).

Some of the first signs that puberty is underway are the appearances of secondary sex characteristics: a boy's voice deepens and facial hair appears; a girl's hips widen and breast development begins. In boys and girls, hair grows under the arms and in the pubic area. Less visible, internal developments accompany these external manifestations of puberty.

Males

Testosterone is produced in the testes, a pair of oval glands located in a pouch of skin called the scrotum (Figure 15.1). One testicle is often slightly larger than the other or hangs somewhat lower. This asymmetry is normal and common.

Beginning at puberty, the testes produce millions of spermatozoa, the male sex cells. It takes about forty-six days for the testes to produce one sperm, but millions are produced simultaneously. A sperm is a microscopic cell shaped like a tadpole, which is carried in a clear or milky-colored fluid called semen. The sperm-containing semen is stored in two tubes (the vas deferens) and two small sacs (seminal vesicles).

Early in puberty, boys normally begin to experience wet dreams or nocturnal emissions. When the vas deferens and seminal vesicles become filled, the semen is released, or ejaculated, through the urethra, the tube that runs through the penis. Nocturnal emission usually begins a year or two after the first signs of puberty. The average age is thirteen, though it may occur normally as early as age ten or as late as age fifteen.

A male also ejaculates during sexual stimulation, intercourse, or masturbation. When a male becomes sexually excited, blood flows into the penis, making it larger and stiffer. During sexual intercourse, the erect penis ejaculates and releases semen into the vagina. The sperm travel through the female uterus into the fallopian tubes, which connect the ovaries to the uterus. If an egg is present in the fallopian tube, one sperm fertilizes the egg and pregnancy results.

Many boys wonder about the relationship between urinating and ejaculating. Urine and semen both travel through the urethra, but

MALE GENITALIA

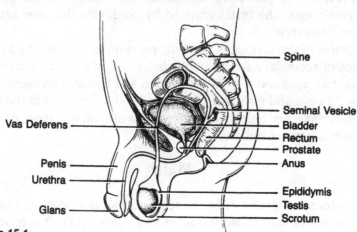

Figure 15.1

at different times. A male cannot urinate and ejaculate at the same time because a valve stops the flow of urine prior to ejaculation.

Boys sometimes worry about the size of the penis. Size has no effect on sexual drive, sexual pleasure, or the ability to reproduce. Some boys are self-conscious about whether they have been circumcised or not. Circumcision is the surgical removal of the foreskin, a layer of skin covering the tip of the penis. Many baby boys are circumcised by a physician a day or two after birth. Other boys, particularly in Jewish or Muslim families, are circumcised after leaving the hospital by a nonphysician who is especially trained in the surgical procedure and the religious ceremony accompanying it. Whether or not a male has been circumcised has no effect on his reproductive ability or sexual pleasure. Uncircumcised males should push back the foreskin while bathing to keep the area clean and to avoid infection.

As mentioned in Chapter 2, many boys in early adolescence notice enlargement of one or both breasts. This normal condition, called gynecomastia, is caused by an increase in the female hormone (estrogen) that occurs in all boys during puberty. Up to 20 percent of ten-and-a-half-year-old boys and over 60 percent of fourteen-year-old boys experience gynecomastia. It disappears within one year in 70 percent of boys and within two years in 95 percent. There is no evidence that gynecomastia is related to the development of breast cancer in males.

Females

A girl's first physical signs of puberty may appear as early as age eight or nine, when her breasts begin to develop, pubic hair begins to grow, body fat increases, or hips widen. During the year before her first menstrual period, she may notice a slight vaginal discharge of clear or whitish fluid. This is caused by the rising level of estrogen. It is entirely normal and usually is a sign that the first period will happen soon.

Before the first menstrual period occurs, a girl usually has progressed through three or four of the five stages of puberty (Chapter 2). She also has gone through the height spurt of puberty and may be near her final adult height. Though the age of menarche (the first menstrual period) varies considerably from one girl to another, the average age in the United States is 12.8 years, a full year earlier than two generations ago.

A human female has a pair of ovaries, one on each side of the uterus and connected to it by the fallopian tube (Figure 15.2). From the time she is born, her ovaries hold all the eggs she will ever have—as many as 300,000. Over the course of her life, only about

THE MENSTRUAL CYCLE

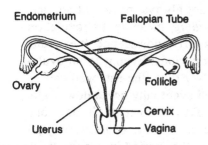

1. An egg matures in a follicle.

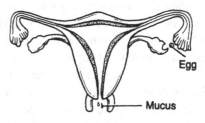

2. The egg leaves the ovary midmonth and enters the fallopian tube.

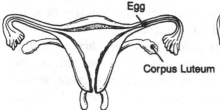

3. The egg travels through the tube to the uterus.

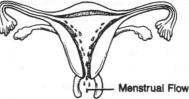

4. The unfertilized egg and uterine lining are shed as menstruation.

Figure 15.2

400 of these eggs will actually mature and leave the ovaries. During the typical menstrual cycle, the ovaries produce estrogen and progesterone, which thicken the lining of the uterus (endometrium). At the same time, an egg in the ovary develops within a small fluid-filled cyst called a follicle. About two weeks into the cycle, when the hormonal levels peak, the follicle ruptures and the egg is released from the ovary into the fallopian tube. This is called *ovulation*. There may be an increase in vaginal secretions around this time. The follicle remaining in the ovary is called the corpus luteum. As the mature egg travels along the fallopian tube toward the uterus, one of two things results: pregnancy or menstruation.

If there has been sexual intercourse, a sperm can fertilize the egg, which will then nestle into the endometrium. Early in the pregnancy, hormones produced by the corpus luteum help support the pregnancy. Over the next nine months, the fertilized egg will grow from one cell, to a tiny embryo, to a fully developed fetus.

If there has been no sexual intercourse, or if contraception (Chapter 19) has been used to prevent fertilization, the corpus luteum will shrink, and the egg will be discharged through the vagina along with blood and endometrial tissue. Unless the egg is fertilized by sperm and a pregnancy results, menstruation *always* follows ovulation two weeks later.

If a female menstruates, it does not always mean that she has ovulated. *Anovulatory menstrual bleeding,* meaning that ovulation did not occur, is very common during early adolescence. It explains why so many teenagers have irregular periods. Even without ovulation, the ovary produces estrogen. Over time, the estrogen causes the lining of the uterus to build up and eventually break down. The *breakthrough bleeding* that results looks like a period. It may vary from a day or two of light spotting to many days of heavy vaginal bleeding. The adolescent may have another period in two weeks or not for six weeks or two months. It takes one or two years for many adolescents to establish a regular menstrual pattern. Irregularity in early adolescence is common, but if periods are excessive or painful, a physician should be consulted (Chapter 17).

Many girls ovulate two weeks before their very first period. It is possible, therefore, to become pregnant before the first period has ever occurred. Because of this possibility, contraception should *always* be used, regardless of age or menstrual pattern. A missed period in a sexually active teenager should be considered a possible pregnancy until proven otherwise.

The menstrual cycle is counted from the first day of menstrual bleeding and lasts an average of twenty-eight days. Few females have menstrual cycles so regular that they can predict the period to the exact day. Most can predict their periods within a few days or a week. Many aspects of daily life affect the "menstrual clock" and alter the timing from month to month: tension, emotional upset, exercise, weight change, climate. Though twenty-eight days is the average span, it is common to have cycles as short at twenty days or as long as thirty-six days. During warm summer months, many females experience shorter menstrual cycles.

It is helpful to mark on a calendar when each menstrual period begins and ends. Without a written record, a girl may assume that her cycles are quite irregular. Calendar months vary from twenty-eight to thirty-one days. Even a perfectly regular twenty-eight-day cycle, therefore, will not always begin on the same day of the calendar month. The written record may help the adolescent see that her pattern is more predictable than she thinks. For example, one period may have begun at the end of March, the next early in May, and the third in the second week of June. She may have worried that she had no period in April and that these three periods began at different times during a calendar month. Yet, if she had noted the dates and counted the weeks, she would have seen that these periods were almost exactly five weeks apart (March 30, May 4, June 9). Keeping a written record not only helps a girl understand her own personal timetable, but it also can assist a doctor if any menstrual problems appear.

Over the centuries, diverse cultures have expressed various attitudes toward menstruation. In ancient times, when menstruation was not understood, negative connotations surrounded it. A menstruating woman was not supposed to touch plants because, it was believed, she would make them wither and die. Nor was she supposed to look into a mirror while she was menstruating—she would tarnish it and the next person to look into it would be bewitched. In the southern provinces of France, a menstruating woman was not to go near newly fermenting wine or flowers used for perfume for fear of tainting them. But not all cultures treated menstruation like "the curse," its old nickname. In some Native American tribes, for example, a girl was honored at menarche with songs and dances to celebrate her maturity.

Menstruation is a normal biological process that signals a young woman's good health and ability to reproduce. It is something to be discussed and understood by all older children and adolescents—female and male. No young girl today should be frightened or confused by her first period. It is the responsibility of her parents, school, and physician to prepare her for this very normal and important part of her development.

Some Questions That Teenagers Often Ask (or Are Afraid to Ask)

IS MASTURBATION HARMFUL?

Different cultures, societies, and families have different attitudes and beliefs about masturbation. There is *no* evidence, though, that masturbation is in any way harmful to the body. Sixty to 90 percent of adolescent boys and 40 percent of girls masturbate. It need not be a source of emotional conflict, guilt, or fear. Masturbation is a normal way to discover sexual feelings in private, often before the teenager decides whether or not to engage in sexual activity with another person.

WHAT HAPPENS DURING SEXUAL INTERCOURSE?

When a male puts his erect penis into a female's vagina, it is called intercourse. He often—but not always—ejaculates sperm during intercourse, which can make her pregnant (Chapter 19).

A male has to be sexually excited for his penis to become erect and hard enough to insert into the vagina. As the female becomes excited, her vagina becomes moist, which makes it easier for the penis to enter. A small organ near the front of the vaginal opening, called the clitoris, contains many nerves and is highly sensitive to touch (Figure 15.3). As a female's sexual excitement increases, the clitoris fills with blood and becomes more sensitive.

WHAT IS ORGASM?

Through sexual stimulation, males and females may reach a peak of excitement that ends with an orgasm, a feeling of great pleasure that releases sexual tension. A male's penis muscles contract and relax when he is sexually excited and his semen ejaculates in short spurts. When he ejaculates, he has an orgasm. Then his penis goes back to its normal size. A female has similar muscle contractions

FEMALE EXTERNAL GENITALIA

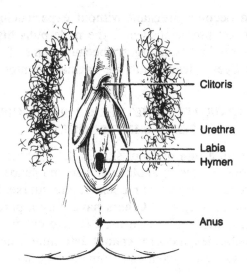

Clitoris

Urethra
Labia
Hymen

Anus

Figure 15.3

when she has an orgasm, though she does not ejaculate. She can become sexually stimulated when the clitoris is rubbed, or when the penis moves back and forth in the vagina. When either occur, the clitoris fills with blood and becomes firm as sexual tension builds to a climax; the release of this tension is an orgasm. Sexual partners often do not have orgasms at the same time. People respond differently to sexual stimulation, and intercourse does not always end in orgasm.

WHAT IS IMPOTENCE?

Impotence is a male's inability to have or keep an erection during intercourse. Tension or worry can prevent him from having an erection. Later, after he is relaxed, he will usually be able to have an erection. If he has repeated problems with impotence or is concerned about it, he should talk to a health professional.

A female also can have difficulties with intercourse or reaching orgasm. Nervousness can affect sexual arousal and vaginal secretions. If the vagina does not become moist, intercourse can be uncomfortable or even painful. Later, after she relaxes and becomes sexually excited, the problem usually will not recur. But if she is worried about it, she should talk to a health professional.

DOES A FEMALE HAVE TO HAVE AN ORGASM TO BECOME PREGNANT?

No. She can become pregnant without experiencing an orgasm. She also can get pregnant even if the male pulls his penis out of her vagina before he has an orgasm because some of his sperm may have already been released into her vagina (Chapter 19).

CAN A DOCTOR TELL WHETHER OR NOT A GIRL HAS HAD SEXUAL INTERCOURSE?

No. The hymen, a thin piece of skin in the opening of the vagina, varies from one female to another in size and shape (Figure 15.3). It is often broken or torn by first sexual intercourse. Some females are born without a hymen. Others have only a part of a hymen. Sometimes a hymen breaks during exercise or tampon use. With so many possibilities, a doctor cannot determine whether a girl has had intercourse simply from examining the hymen.

Adolescents have many other questions about sexual behavior and feelings, contraception, sexually transmitted diseases, etc. Some of these questions are answered in school, and many are answered by friends. A safe place to get honest, correct information can and should be at home. Parents can try, from childhood on, to create an environment that encourages open discussion. Adolescents can try to ask the questions, even if the first attempt seems awkward. The process of trying and talking brings teenagers and parents closer and helps to foster an understanding that persists through adulthood.

16

Sexual Identity

Yesterday, Barbara felt attracted to Scott, who sits next to her in biology class. Today, she feels attracted to Susan, who has been helping her with their history assignment. She begins to wonder about her sexual identity—"Am I heterosexual (attracted to the opposite sex)? Am I homosexual? Could I be both? Are these feelings wrong?"

During adolescence, the observations, feelings, and attitudes of childhood begin to translate into behaviors that help teenagers define themselves as sexual beings. The behaviors require daily choices, from minor ones about dress and hair style to more significant ones: Casual flirtation, or kissing, or intercourse? A same-sex best friend or a romantic, sexual relationship? These decisions can be very difficult.

The sexual experimentation of adolescence is a normal, but at times confusing, part of development. It is a process of flux in which personal identity may vary day to day but, over time, moves along a course of increasing clarity and definition.

One of the most sensitive areas of adolescent development is sexual identity. This actually begins long before puberty and involves two key issues: gender identity and sexual orientation. *Gender identity* is an individual's personal sense of being male or female. This usually is established in early childhood. *Sexual orientation* is an individual's attraction to others of the same or opposite gender. It too develops during childhood, but its expression is delayed until adolescence or adulthood. When this expression runs counter to the expectations of family, culture, or society, sexual orientation may be denied or suppressed. For many people, adolescence becomes the time to test and understand their sexual orientation.

Around age twelve to fourteen, many adolescents feel drawn to teenagers or adults of the same gender. This is normal in early adolescence. The attraction usually takes the form of a romantic crush or fantasy. Sometimes the feelings are played out in sexual behaviors. A young teenager can be very confused by same-sex attraction. It can be both frightening and appealing at the same time.

Most children and teenagers experience some sexual play with friends of the same gender. Usually, the play is secretive but not anxiety producing. For most, it is part of a developmental experiment resulting in a heterosexual orientation.

Some children and teenagers sense that the same-sex behavior represents more than fleeting play. This realization may contribute to a ready acceptance and a comfort with their homosexual orientation. For many, though, there may be a sense of difference and separateness. They may hide or deny their feelings because of shame, discomfort, fear, or early disapproval by others. For some young people, repression of homosexuality lasts a lifetime. For many others, it lasts into adulthood. An increasing number of homosexual teenagers recognize and accept their sexual orientation and establish a stable personal identity and a support peer network.

Sexual orientation is not as clear-cut as most people think. Nearly fifty years ago, *The Kinsey Report* on human sexual behavior showed that people fall along a continuum from exclusively heterosexual to exclusively homosexual thoughts and behaviors. At some time, most people have been attracted to others of the same sex. Some never act on these thoughts; others do. Some heterosexual teenagers experiment with homosexual behavior, especially when the setting provides the opportunity. Some homosexual adolescents experiment with heterosexual behavior, often in an attempt to follow the cultural norm. Whatever the sexual orientation during adolescence, it is part of the developmental process and may change or evolve with time.

Who and Why?

The prevalence of homosexuality depends on its definition. Five to 10 percent of adolescents identify themselves as homosexually oriented. By age nineteen, 17 percent of boys and 11 percent of girls report at least one homosexual experience. Half of these teenagers will become gay or lesbian adults. Gay refers to male homosexuals, lesbian to female homosexuals.

Most gay adolescents are aware of their attraction to other males by age fourteen. One study found that 77 percent of adult gay males had formed homosexual attachments by adolescence, and 86 percent had engaged in homosexual behavior by age fifteen. There is less information about lesbian adolescents, but homosexual prevalence in females probably is half that of males.

Why do some teenagers identify themselves as homosexual while others—such as siblings raised in the same environment, with the same parents, with similar friends and experiences—identify themselves as heterosexual? The answer remains unknown. Theories include genetic, hormonal, psychological, and environmental factors. Different studies support and refute nearly every theory that has been proposed. It is likely that many factors work together to define sexual orientation. The goal for families is to understand rather than explain, to support rather than blame. The first step is communication—parents and teenagers talking together about sexual orientation.

Family Reactions

As adolescents wrestle with sexual identity, both they and their parents may experience a whirlwind of conflicting emotions. For gay and lesbian teenagers, the effort to accept and express their sexual orientation coincides with fear of rejection or condemnation by parents, peers, and community. The family can do much to ease a difficult process for the adolescent. Parents and teenagers benefit from open discussion of their reactions and concerns. The discussion should include some basic concepts:

• It is important to accept the teenager's sense of being different. Attempting to talk the teenager out of this feeling, or calling it "a passing phase," will not help and may add to the turmoil.

• Talking about homosexuality will not cause homosexuality. Rather, the discussion may help alleviate anxiety.

• Homosexuality is *not* an illness or a disease. It is *not* a matter of making a "wrong" choice, because choice is rarely involved. As described earlier, sexual orientation usually is established long before puberty, so most teenagers do not make a conscious selection.

• Parents often feel guilty, angry, ashamed, or grief-stricken when teenagers identify themselves as homosexual. Parents do not "cause" sexual orientation. Their job remains what it has always been: to accept, love, and support their children as they are.

• Homosexual teenagers have many of the same problems and concerns as heterosexual teenagers. It is a mistake to link all problems encountered by gay and lesbian teenagers to their sexual orientation.

• Meeting with a counselor or therapist who is skilled in working with adolescents can help families cope with their reactions. While psychotherapy generally is unsuccessful if it attempts to change sexual orientation or gender identity, it can help teenagers understand and accept who they are.

• Males engaged in homosexual behaviors need clear and specific information about health risks and safer sex precautions. This is true for *all* adolescents, but especially for gay adolescents and heterosexual males who are experimenting with homosexual activities.

Special Medical Issues

Acknowledging a teenager's homosexuality has always been difficult in a homophobic society (one that rejects homosexuality as "bad" and accepts only heterosexuality as "good"). Since the early 1980s, families have faced an added challenge in accepting male homosexuality—the AIDS epidemic.

In addition to the risk of HIV infection, other medical problems are directly related to male homosexual behavior. The problems fall into two categories: rectal trauma and sexually transmitted diseases (STDs).

Anal intercourse causes stretching and frequently tearing of the rectal skin and lining. The resulting symptoms include rectal pain, especially on bowel movement, and rectal bleeding. Lubricants used during anal intercourse also may cause irritation or itching from allergic reactions.

The most dangerous problems associated with unprotected anal intercourse are STDs, including HIV infection (Chapters 21 and 22). Rectal itching, irritation, pain, discharge, or bleeding can be caused by infections such as gonorrhea and chlamydia. Perirectal (around the area of the rectum) ulcers or blisters may be caused by herpes simplex virus (HSV) infection, and perirectal warts by human papilloma virus (HPV). Diarrhea may be caused by sexually transmitted infection with any one of over ten different organisms, ranging from bacteria to viruses to parasites (Chapter 29).

Anyone who engages in anal intercourse or fellatio (oral sex)—whether as the inserter or insertee—is at risk for all sexually transmitted diseases. Two factors that are directly associated with this risk are failure to use condoms and the number of sexual partners. STDs spread quickly in the gay population because many infected males have no symptoms. The more sexual partners an adolescent has, the more times he is exposed to potential infection. The sexually active gay adolescent must remember three key points:

- *Always* use condoms.
- Limit the number of partners.
- See a doctor or nurse at least twice yearly for STD screening.

Finding a doctor or nurse with whom he is comfortable can be difficult for a gay adolescent. Do not let this be a barrier to much needed care or preventive screening. The names of health professionals who are skilled and comfortable providing care for gay youth often come from the gay community. Other places to call include local adolescent clinics or health departments. Additional resources that provide information nationwide are listed in *Resources* at the end of the book.

The medical evaluation of the gay adolescent begins with a thorough history (Chapter 3), including information about sexual intercourse with males and females, oral sex, number of sexual partners, condom use, previous STDs, and previous HIV testing. During the physical examination, the doctor will look closely for signs of STDs such as enlarged lymph nodes ("glands"), inflammation of the throat, rashes or skin lesions, rectal irritation or bleeding, discharge from the penis, and sores on the genitalia. The doctor will use a cotton-tipped applicator to swab the tip of the penis; the specimen

collected will be be sent to the laboratory to be checked for gonorrhea and chlamydia.

Blood tests may include screening for three STDs: syphilis,
hepatitis B, and HIV. Syphilis has increased among all sexually
active adolescents (Chapter 21), but is most common among homosexual males. Hepatitis B is a virus that infects the liver and can
progress to a chronic form of severe liver disease (Chapter 29). Up
to 50 percent of homosexual adult males have been infected with
the hepatitis B virus, and over 5 percent remain contagious throughout their lives. An effective vaccine against hepatitis B prevents
infection (Chapter 3). It is important that all gay adolescents either
receive the vaccine or have a blood test that proves that they are
already immune to the disease. This recommendation now holds
for *all* children and adolescents, but it is especially important for
gay adolescents, who are at very high risk of infection.

The decision to screen for HIV infection rests with the gay
adolescent, his physician and, whenever possible, with his parents.
Whether or not the test is ordered, and whether it is positive or
negative, sexually active teenagers *must* understand that they and
their partners are at risk and that safer sex precautions are more
than an option—they are essential (Chapter 22).

Transsexual and Transvestite Behaviors

Homosexuality is not the same as transsexuality or transvestism.
Homosexual adolescents are sexually attracted to people of the
same biological sex—males are attracted to males, females to females. Transsexual adolescents identify their own gender differently than their biological sex—biological males see themselves
as females and biological females see themselves as males. Most
transsexual individuals also are homosexual. However, most homosexual individuals are not transsexual.

Transsexuality is more common in males than females. Psychiatric treatment of transsexual adolescents has met with little success.
Gender identity, usually established during childhood, is resistant
to change by emotional or psychological means. Some transsexual
adults eventually have surgery to change their biological sex. This
type of surgery is not done during adolescence. Most teenagers are
trying to make major decisions about their lives and futures. They
are experimenting, considering, and changing. Some transsexual

adolescents will become adults who are comfortable with both their gender identity and their biological sex. Surgery should never be done until the individual is mature, stable with regard to gender identity, and quite certain of the decision.

Transvestite behavior is different from either transsexualism or homosexuality. Individuals who are transvestites dress as the opposite sex but have a gender identity that is consistent with their biological sex. For example, a transvestite man sees himself as a man but dresses as a woman. Many people who are transvestites—but not all—also are homosexual.

Homosexuality, transsexualism, and transvestism are more than words or semantics. They imply very important differences in the adolescent's sense of self and sexuality. The stereotypes that are commonly applied to gay or lesbian youth are incorrect and misleading. Most gay adolescents consider themselves and appear male. Most lesbian adolescents consider themselves and appear female. It is a mistake to assume that gender identity, appearance, biological sex, and sexual orientation are always the same. Each adolescent is unique, with his or her own blend and balance. Teenagers work hard to understand who they are. The parents' job is to accept that person, no matter what the blend or balance may be.

17

Menstrual Disorders

About half of all teenage girls experience menstrual problems, ranging from mild cramping, to irregular periods, to disabling pain, or heavy bleeding. Menstruation is a new and significant experience for adolescent girls. Many have not yet determined which symptoms are normal and which are not. Some girls are reluctant to voice concerns or ask questions about menstruation. The result may be an incorrect interpretation of their symptoms. Most concerns about the menstrual cycle cause needless worry, but some represent more serious problems that should be evaluated and treated.

This chapter addresses the most common menstrual disorders of adolescence. Before discussing the problems, the normal menstrual cycle is reviewed in order to help adolescents and parents differentiate the normal and the expected from problems that require medical intervention.

The Normal Menstrual Cycle

The *average* age of menarche (the first menstrual period) is 12.8 years for American girls. The age *range* when girls begin to menstruate is wide, from nine to sixteen years. Menarche usually occurs about two years after breast development begins and one year after the growth spurt. To illustrate how different—yet normal—two girls can be, consider Liz and Shana, both age fourteen. Liz's first period occurred two weeks before her twelfth birthday. When she was eleven, she grew four inches and gained twenty pounds. Shana has not yet begun to menstruate. Her height and weight have increased somewhat over the past year, but not dramatically. Liz worried that her period came too early and that she would keep growing too fast. Shana worries that she will never develop, that she will never begin to menstruate. Both girls are healthy and completely normal. Liz simply entered puberty earlier than Shana. Both will reach the same place—normal menstruation and normal adult height—by age fifteen or sixteen.

Most early menstrual cycles are "anovulatory," that is, they occur even though the ovary has not released an egg into the fallopian tube. The hormones estrogen and progesterone are produced by the ovary even when ovulation (release of the egg) does not occur. These hormones act on the endometrium (the inner lining of the uterus), causing it to thicken. Eventually, pieces of the endometrium slough off, and the uterus expels this tissue into the vagina. This "breakthrough bleeding" is very common during adolescence. It can appear as very light spotting or as heavy, prolonged bleeding. For most teenagers, ovulation begins within a year of menarche and the periods then follow a predictable cycle.

The menstrual cycle is measured from the first day of one period to the first day of the next. The length of a normal cycle varies between individuals from twenty-one to forty-five days. For any one individual, however, the cycle length is fairly constant. Once Shana began to menstruate, two months after her fifteenth birthday, her cycles averaged thirty days. Liz's averaged twenty-four days.

Normal menstrual flow lasts two to seven days and is usually heaviest on the first and second days. The average blood loss during a normal period is 30 to 40 milliliters, which is equal to a little over one fluid ounce or two to three tablespoons of blood. The quantity appears greater because the blood is mixed with endometrial tissue from the lining of the uterus and secretions from the vagina.

Tampon Use

When girls begin to menstruate, they often wonder whether to use sanitary pads or tampons. Sanitary pads or napkins are completely safe and protective yet may feel bulky or uncomfortable, especially during warm weather or exercise. Tampons also are safe and protective when used appropriately, but they do carry some risk of infection for some women. If tampons are used, the following recommendations may decrease the risk of infection: Always wash hands before insertion; change the tampon at least every four to six hours; use a sanitary napkin at night rather than leaving a tampon in place for a long time; remember to remove the last tampon at the end of the menstrual period.

Toxic shock syndrome (TSS) is a rare but potentially fatal disease that occurs predominantly in menstruating adolescents and young women under age thirty who use tampons. (It also can occur in non-menstruating women and in males; Chapter 34.) TSS is caused by a toxin-producing bacteria called *Staphylococcus aureus*. The bacteria can accumulate in the vagina during the menstrual period, particularly if tampons are not changed frequently. TSS has also been reported, though rarely, in women using the contraceptive sponge or diaphragm. The warning signs of TSS include the following:

- sudden high fever (over 101° F) during the menstrual period;
- rash that resembles sunburn;
- fall in blood pressure, usually accompanied by light-headedness or fainting;
- vomiting or diarrhea;
- severe muscle aching;
- redness of the eyes, mouth, throat, or vagina;
- disorientation, confusion, or lethargy.

Adolescents who develop any of these symptoms during menstruation should remove the tampon and see a doctor immediately. *If the doctor cannot be reached, the adolescent should go to an emergency room.* TSS is most effectively treated early in its course, so time is of the essence. The treatment usually involves hospitalization, the administration of fluids intravenously to support the blood pressure, antibiotics, and flushing of the vagina to decrease the toxin-producing bacteria.

Teenagers who have had TSS face about a 30 percent risk that it will occur again. They should use no tampons for at least six months and should try to limit use even beyond that time.

Amenorrhea

Amenorrhea is the absence of menstruation. There are two types: primary and secondary amenorrhea. *Primary amenorrhea* is delayed menarche (the first menstrual period). It is defined as any one of three conditions:

1. The absence of menarche by age sixteen with normal growth and pubertal development (breast development, pubic hair, etc.);
2. The absence of menarche by age fourteen with delayed puberty;
3. The absence of menarche two years after puberty is otherwise completed.

Secondary amenorrhea is the absence of menstruation after menarche has already taken place. Menstrual periods are often irregular during early adolescence, but they usually stabilize in length and regularity within a year or two after menarche. At about eighteen months after menarche, it is considered abnormal for the adolescent to miss three consecutive cycles or to have no period for at least six months.

All teenagers with primary or secondary amenorrhea should seek medical care. The first essential question is, "Am I pregnant?" If the adolescent has never had sexual intercourse, the answer is no. The adolescent who last had intercourse a few months ago and who had some bleeding a few weeks later may assume *incorrectly* that she cannot be pregnant. Spotting or even definite bleeding can occur early in a pregnancy. Any adolescent who has had sexual intercourse and has missed a period therefore must assume that she is pregnant until proven otherwise by a urine or blood pregnancy test.

Adolescents with primary amenorrhea who have had sexual intercourse also *cannot* assume that they are not pregnant. It is possible to conceive before the first menstrual period has ever occurred.

Consider Joan, a fifteen-year-old who began having intercourse one year ago. Joan has never had a menstrual period. Two weeks ago, she ovulated for the first time in her life. Her first menstrual period should have occurred today. But one day after she ovulated, Joan had intercourse. The egg, on its way from the ovary to the uterus, was fertilized in the fallopian tube by the sperm. Joan is pregnant. She has never had a period, so she does not know that she will "miss" her first period. Nevertheless, she is very definitely pregnant. Any sexually active woman who is not menstruating each month—even if she has never had a period—may be pregnant.

Once a pregnancy has been excluded, the physician will consider several other causes of amenorrhea. The possibilities differ, depending on whether the amenorrhea is primary or secondary. In the adolescent with primary amenorrhea, the family history and pubertal maturation are very important. There is an association between the ages at which mothers and daughters begin to menstruate. Mothers who menstruate late often have daughters who menstruate late, and vice versa. Menarche tends to occur at stage four of the five stages of sexual maturation (Chapter 2). A sixteen-year-old who is at stage two probably has amenorrhea because of a problem that has delayed puberty in general. Conversely, a sixteen-year-old who is at stage five has completed puberty on time and has delayed menarche for some other reason.

The most common reason for both primary and secondary amenorrhea is that the hypothalamus and pituitary gland in the brain are not sending appropriate hormonal messages to the ovaries. Consequently, the ovaries are not producing adequate amounts of hormones to result in menstruation. One way to measure how much has been produced is with a "progesterone challenge test." In this simple trial, the teenager is given oral progesterone tablets for several days or a single injection of progesterone. If her ovaries have been making estrogen and if her uterus has responded normally to it, she will have a menstrual period several days after she takes the medication. This "withdrawal bleed" lets the doctor know that the ovaries and uterus are normal and that the cause of the amenorrhea is in the brain.

The brain may not signal the ovaries appropriately when the teenager is experiencing emotional stress or when her body weight and body fat are too low. Periods commonly are delayed when she is feeling anxious about school, family, peers, or a changing environment (such as a new neighborhood, summer camp, or college). A girl who has not achieved a minimum amount of body fat will not begin to menstruate or, if she does not maintain an adequate level, menstruation will cease. This may be caused by intentional dieting, inadequate calorie intake during a time of rapid growth, weight loss due to illness, or exercise. Some athletes, for unclear reasons, do not menstruate even when they achieve a critical minimal weight and body fat.

The major risk of amenorrhea is osteoporosis, or thinning of the bone. Osteoporosis can begin as early as adolescence if the estrogen level is too low. Hormone replacement therapy, with either an oral contraceptive or a combination of estrogen and progesterone tablets, may be recommended for some teenagers with persistent amenorrhea.

Primary or secondary amenorrhea may be caused by chronic illnesses such as anorexia nervosa (Chapter 7), inflammatory bowel disease (Chapter 29), thyroid disease (Chapter 33), and diabetes mellitus (Chapter 33). Almost any disease can stress the body to the point that the hypothalamus does not stimulate the ovary to produce estrogen.

An uncommon cause of primary or secondary amenorrhea is a small tumor of the pituitary gland. The only symptom of this "pituitary adenoma" may be the amenorrhea. At other times, there may be a discharge from the breasts called galactorrhea. A good screen for pituitary adenoma is a blood test in which the level of a hormone called prolactin is measured. If the prolactin level is elevated, a brain X-ray or scan (CT or MRI) may be done. Pituitary adenomas usually grow very slowly or are stable in size. Because of this, they often can be managed with medication and need not require surgical removal.

The other causes of amenorrhea are quite rare. Some girls with primary amenorrhea may have congenital abnormalities or absence of the ovaries or uterus. Others may have been born with normal ovaries and uterus but experienced damage to them from injuries, infections, or medications during childhood. In some girls, the ovaries and uterus are normal, but the flow of menstrual blood is blocked by a membrane in the vagina called the hymen. As the blood collects, it can cause pain and swelling at the opening of the vagina. The problem is easily corrected by a minor surgical procedure in which the hymen is opened.

Whenever amenorrhea occurs—whether primary or secondary—it deserves medical attention and evaluation. The vast majority of adolescents with amenorrhea, though, do *not* have serious underlying problems. In most, periods will resume and become regular without treatment.

Dysmenorrhea

Painful menstruation—dysmenorrhea—is the most common gynecologic problem during adolescence. An estimated 75 percent of menstruating women have some degree of dysmenorrhea, which makes it the leading cause of school and work absence. Many medications can safely and effectively ease or prevent the very real discomfort experienced by millions of adolescents.

Dysmenorrhea is categorized as primary or secondary. The type is important because it determines treatment. The words primary and secondary are used differently when referring to dysmenorrhea than when referring to amenorrhea, as described earlier. *Primary dysmenorrhea* refers to painful periods without an identifiable abnormality in the uterus, ovaries, or fallopian tubes. Most dysmenorrhea during adolescence is primary. The major symptom is cramping type pain in the lower abdomen that begins just before or soon after the onset of menstrual bleeding. The pain may extend to the legs, lower back, buttocks, or rectum. Some young women also experience diarrhea, nausea, vomiting, fatigue, headache, or light-headedness. The discomfort is usually most severe on the first or second day of menstruation.

Many teenagers have no or infrequent dysmenorrhea during the early months or years following menarche. Dysmenorrhea tends to accompany ovulatory cycles and, as discussed earlier in this chapter, the early periods often do not follow ovulation. As ovulation becomes more regular, dysmenorrhea may increase and usually does not indicate an underlying problem. The pattern of discomfort typically stabilizes within two years of menarche, when ovulation and menstrual periods become more regular. If pain continues to become worse beyond this point, a doctor should be consulted.

Primary dysmenorrhea is caused by fatty acids that are produced in the uterus during menstruation. These "prostaglandins" stimulate the uterine muscles and blood vessels to contract. Prostaglandins probably also increase the sensitivity of the pain sensors in the uterus. The combination of these effects causes the cramping pain of dysmenorrhea.

For many young women, over-the-counter medications containing ibuprofen (such as Motrin, Advil, Nuprin) are effective in reducing dysmenorrhea. If these preparations are insufficient, a physician may prescribe ibuprofen in a higher dose or similar medications, such as mefenamic acid (Ponstel) or naproxen (Naprosyn).

All of these medications are "prostaglandin inhibitors" and work by blocking the uterine production of prostaglandins. The earlier the medication is taken during the menstrual period, the better it works. The first dose should be taken as soon as the bleeding begins. The medication usually can be stopped within two days, or whenever the cramping eases.

If the prostaglandin inhibitors do not control the dysmenorrhea, the physician may suggest an oral contraceptive ("the pill"). This controls the discomfort for 90 percent of women with dysmenorrhea. It works by preventing ovulation and reducing prostaglandin production over time, which means that the maximum effect of the pill may require several months. If the adolescent does not need the pill for contraception, it may be discontinued after four to six months and the symptoms of dysmenorrhea can be reassessed. If the adolescent is sexually active, the oral contraceptive can be continued indefinitely (Chapter 19).

When dysmenorrhea does not respond to prostaglandin inhibitors or oral contraceptives, or when dysmenorrhea begins with menarche and rapidly becomes worse over several cycles, there may be a structural abnormality of the ovaries, uterus, fallopian tubes, or vagina. This is called *secondary dysmenorrhea*. The doctor will begin the evaluation with a thorough menstrual history and a pelvic examination (Chapter 3). A pelvic ultrasound examination or diagnostic laparoscopy may be done to help identify the cause of the pain. Ultrasound is simple, painless, and can be done in the doctor's office. A microphone is placed on the abdomen or in the vagina and sound waves are transmitted through it. These sound waves bounce off the ovaries and uterus, creating a picture of these internal organs. Laparoscopy involves a minor surgical procedure and general anesthesia. A surgeon makes a tiny incision in the abdomen and inserts a lighted, hollow tube through which the internal organs can be visualized. Laparoscopy is done as a "short procedure," meaning that the teenager need not stay in the hospital overnight.

The most common cause of secondary dysmenorrhea during adolescence is endometriosis. This is a condition in which cells of the endometrium (the lining of the uterus) migrate to unusual places, such as the fallopian tubes, the ovaries, an intestinal wall, or the bladder. Endometriosis usually responds to treatment with oral contraceptives. It often improves as women get older, especially after childbearing.

Other causes of secondary dysmenorrhea during adolescence include benign uterine tumors (fibroids), uterine malformations, ovarian cysts (collections of blood or fluid), and pelvic inflammatory disease resulting from a sexually transmitted infection (Chapter 21).

Dysfunctional Uterine Bleeding

Heavy or prolonged bleeding that originates in the uterus and flows through the vagina is called dysfunctional uterine bleeding (DUB). It usually occurs with anovulation, when eggs are not released from the ovary and periods are irregular. DUB is very common in early adolescence, since over half the cycles that occur within two years of menarche are anovulatory. The unpredictable, often heavy nature of the bleeding can be frightening for an adolescent who is just trying to adjust to menstruation.

A common question of teenagers is how much bleeding is too much bleeding. Menstrual bleeding should not last more than eight to ten days. Over forty milliliters of blood loss per period, which translates into over fifteen soaked pads or tampons per period, is excessive. It is very difficult, though, for most women to assess how much blood they are actually losing. If there is any question, a doctor should be consulted.

DUB symptoms vary. One girl may have moderate bleeding every ten days. Another may have monthly periods that last two weeks. Another may spot all day, every day. Another may bleed so heavily for five or six days that she cannot leave the house, but then has no periods for three or four months. Whatever the pattern, all of these represent either heavy or prolonged bleeding.

DUB during adolescence usually indicates a slight imbalance in the levels of estrogen and progesterone. The imbalance either will correct itself or can be easily adjusted using hormonal medication. In the teenager, unlike the adult, surgery rarely is necessary for DUB.

Causes of DUB that may require surgery include ovarian cysts, uterine fibroids, and uterine polyps (benign growths of mucous membranes). Occasionally, the bleeding may be coming from a cut or scratch of the vagina rather than the uterus. A pelvic examination will help the physician determine where the bleeding is originating. The blood pressure, heart rate, and hematocrit (red blood cell count) will tell how much bleeding has occurred and how the body has adjusted to the loss. For example, Kim has lost a lot of blood over a long time. She has a low blood count (anemia) but normal blood pressure and heart rate. Her only symptom is fatigue. Joanna has lost the same amount of blood over the past two days. Her blood count is the same as Kim's, but she feels very dizzy and has a low blood pressure. Joanna's bleeding represents a medical emergency. Kim's bleeding needs evaluation and treatment but is not an emergency.

The first thing the doctor will do is decide how severe the bleeding has been. Questions will be asked about personal or family history of bleeding disorders and evidence of bleeding in other parts of the body (for example, easy bruising, gum bleeding, nosebleeds). Sexual history and contraceptive use also are important components of the medical history. Laboratory testing usually is done to determine the blood count and sometimes to check thyroid function since hypothyroidism (underactive thyroid) is associated with DUB. Adult women with DUB may require an endometrial biopsy (the removal of a small amount of uterine tissue) or a D & C (dilation of the cervix and curettage, or scraping, of the endometrium). These procedures rarely are necessary for adolescents.

A very important part of the history and examination for adolescents with DUB is evaluation for sexually transmitted disease or pregnancy. Teenagers with gonorrhea or chlamydia often have inflammation of the endometrium or cervix that causes bleeding. A miscarriage can cause heavy bleeding before the adolescent is even aware that she is pregnant. An ectopic pregnancy, in which the fertilized egg begins to grow inside the fallopian tube, can cause heavy bleeding and represents a surgical emergency.

DUB *always* deserves full medical evaluation because of its many possible causes—some of which the teenager may be reluctant to discuss with a parent.

DUB can be managed in several ways, depending on the severity of bleeding and the blood count. If the blood count is low and the teenager's blood pressure is unstable, emergency treatment is imperative. The adolescent will be treated with intravenous fluids and may require blood transfusions. Hormones will be used immediately to stop the bleeding and then will be continued for several months to regulate the periods.

In most situations, adolescents with DUB have no or mild anemia, the blood pressure is stable, and the cause is hormonal. DUB then is best managed with an oral contraceptive. It typically is prescribed in a high dose (several pills a day) for several days to stop the bleeding, followed by a single pill each day for several months to regulate the menstrual periods. If the teenager is anemic, iron tablets will be prescribed to help her replenish the red blood cells that she has lost. With the iron, her blood count will begin to increase within one to two weeks.

Adolescents with DUB should understand that the first menstrual period after they start taking hormones usually is heavy. The subsequent periods on the hormone therapy should become progressively lighter and more predictable. After about six months, the oral contraceptive can be stopped if the teenager does not need it for contraception.

When irregular bleeding persists for several years, the most likely cause is polycystic ovary syndrome (PCOS). In this disorder, many small cysts form in the ovaries and the hormonal levels remain out of balance. PCOS usually responds very well to ongoing treatment with an oral contraceptive. Many women with PCOS choose to remain on the oral contraceptive until they are ready to become pregnant.

DUB is a very common, yet complex, disorder of adolescence. Usually it is mild and ends on its own without treatment. DUB can be severe or peristent, though. Because of the many possible causes and outcomes of DUB, as well as the discomfort and anxiety that it can produce, it deserves early medical attention and treatment.

18

Disorders of the Male Genitalia

Routine health screening for the male includes examination of the reproductive organs, or *genitalia*. A teenager may be more at ease if he knows the terminology and what to expect (Chapter 15, Figure 15.1).

The *testes,* or testicles, are the two organs that produce sperm and the male sex hormone, testosterone. The physician will examine the testes to assess their size, shape, and position. Normally, the testicles are firm and move freely within the scrotum.

The *scrotum* is the pouch located below the penis that contains the testicles. The doctor will examine the skin of the scrotum and will insert a gloved finger into the scrotal skin to detect hernias (p. 42).

The *penis* is the male sex organ. The physician will examine its size and shape, the skin for any sores or lesions, and the foreskin in uncircumcised males.

The *urethra* is the tube running through the penis that carries sperm from the testes and urine from the bladder. The opening of the urethra at the tip of the penis will be examined.

The *prostate gland* secretes a milky fluid into the urethra, aiding the movement of sperm during ejaculation. The physician may examine the prostate by inserting a gloved finger into the rectum.

The *epididymis* is a convoluted tube attached to the testicle that collects the sperm. It leads to the *vas deferens,* or "seminal duct," where sperm are mixed with fluid (semen). The vas deferens leads,

213

in turn, to the urethra. The doctor uses the thumb and forefinger to feel the epididymis along the back of the testicle.

Testicular Cancer and the Self-Examination

During the physical examination, the doctor should show the teenager how to examine himself for testicular cancer. There is no blood test or X-ray that can be used to screen for testicular cancer. Early detection, which can mean complete cure, depends on regular self-examination. If the physician has not reviewed the examination, ask for a demonstration.

The self-exam should be done once a month. Each testicle is rolled between the thumb and three middle fingers until its entire surface is felt. The testicles should feel smooth and round with no lumps or painful areas. They should be roughly equal in size, though one may hang slightly lower than the other.

Testicular cancer typically appears as a hard lump in one testicle. Over half of adolescents have no symptoms at all; the remainder have an aching sensation in the groin or scrotum. Rarely, the tumor may become apparent after it has spread to the lymph nodes or bones, causing masses (lumps) or pain elsewhere in the body.

Some testicular tumors produce specific "markers" that can be measured in the blood. The most common markers are called alpha-fetoprotein and human chorionic gonadotropin, or HCG. If a marker is present on blood testing, its level will be followed to measure how well the tumor responds to treatment. As the tumor shrinks (or if it is removed surgically), the blood level of the marker falls.

Testicular cancer is very aggressive and spreads quickly if untreated. With treatment, the prognosis depends on the cells that make up the tumor and the spread, or stage, of the tumor. Seminoma, the most common cell type, has over a 95 percent cure rate if it is limited to the testicle. The treatment involves surgical removal of the testicle and radiation therapy. This high cure rate depends on early detection—through regular testicular self-examination. If a seminoma spreads beyond the testicle, the cure rate is below 85 percent. Tumors that are not seminomas are more aggressive, but cure rates up to 85 percent are reported with surgery and chemotherapy together.

Masses, Pain, and Swelling of the Scrotum

Any pain, lump, injury, discharge, or change in the size of the scrotum should be brought to a physician's attention. It should not be ignored, and care should not be delayed. Do not attempt self-diagnosis or self-treatment. Testicular and scrotal abnormalities can have serious consequences for future health and fertility. Most can be corrected if recognized early and treated appropriately.

The evaluation of a testicular or scrotal abnormality begins with a careful history of the symptoms and physical examination. Severe pain and swelling that start very suddenly represent a medical emergency because the blood supply to the testicle may be impaired. Pain that develops gradually and is associated with a discharge from the urethra suggests an infection, especially a sexually transmitted disease (STD). Laboratory tests that may help the physician make a diagnosis include cultures from the urethra, scans of the scrotum that indicate blood flow, and ultrasound techniques that provide information about both blood flow and size and shape of the scrotum.

Testicular torsion is the twisting of the cord that suspends the testicle inside the scrotum. The affected testicle is pulled into a higher and more horizontal position from its normal vertical, lower location. Torsion begins suddenly with severe pain on one side of the scrotum that may spread to the groin. Redness and swelling of the scrotum appear shortly after (or occasionally before) the pain.

Torsion is *an emergency* that requires immediate surgery to untwist the cord and save the testicle. If not corrected promptly, the blood flow is cut off, and the testicle will no longer be able to produce sperm. With surgery, the testicle is attached to the scrotum in its proper position with sutures (stitches) to prevent a recurrence of the torsion. The testicle is saved in the vast majority of cases treated surgically within six hours. The chance of saving the testicle is extremely poor if surgery is delayed beyond twenty-four hours. A testicle that has lost its blood flow eventually dies. It should be removed and, sometime later, can be replaced by a prosthesis (an artificial part) that will make the scrotum appear normal.

Testicular torsion occurs more frequently during adolescence than at any other time in life. This is probably because the testes are growing very rapidly during these years. Their heavier weight, along with the greater physical activity of adolescence, increases the chance that the testicle will twist on its cord. Most adolescents with testicular torsion also have an abnormality in the position of the testicle that has been present since birth.

Orchitis is an inflammation of the testicles caused by infection or injury. Mumps is a common cause of orchitis, which occurs in nearly a third of adolescent and adult males who contract the disease. For this reason, it is important that all children receive the mumps immunization early in life (Chapter 3). Mumps orchitis does not occur in people who have been immunized.

The symptoms of orchitis include fever and painful swelling of one or both testicles. A sign that mumps is the cause is painful swelling of the salivary glands at the jaw. Orchitis is treated by bed rest and elevating the scrotum. Antibiotics generally do not help. The pain and swelling improve within one to two weeks, but the testicle can be left permanently scarred and shrunken by the inflammation.

Epididymitis is an inflammation of the epididymis. It is usually caused by microorganisms associated with STDs such as chlamydia and gonorrhea (Chapter 21). The major symptoms of epididymitis include the gradual onset of pain and swelling of the scrotum. Other symptoms may include a discharge from the urethra, pus in the urine, difficulty or pain on urinating, and fever.

Epididymitis is treated with antibiotics and bed rest. Elevating the scrotum with a small pillow or towel helps relieve the pain and swelling. When epididymitis is caused by an STD, all sexual partners must be examined and treated.

Trauma to the testicles and scrotum is an infrequent consequence of athletic and motor vehicle injuries. The degree of injury ranges from minor bruising to rupture of the testicles. Ultrasound scans of the scrotum are used to help assess the cause of swelling and possible need for surgical repair. A ruptured testicle or large collection of blood in the scrotum typically requires emergency surgery. Do *not* apply ice after an injury to the scrotum. Ice can make matters worse by diminishing the blood supply and increasing the pain.

Varicoceles are enlarged (varicose) veins inside the scrotum. They appear after puberty, usually on the left side. Most varicoceles cause no discomfort and are detected on routine physical examinations. A large varicocele looks like a thickened blue vein under the skin of the scrotum. A smaller varicocele may not be visible but can be felt above the testicle.

Most varicoceles cause no long-term problems, but in some men fertility may be decreased later in adulthood. Surgery is recommended during adolescence if there is any discomfort, decrease in the size of the testicle, or change in the production of testosterone or sperm.

Hydroceles are accumulations of fluid in the membranes covering the testicles. They occur most often in infancy. If they appear during adolescence, they may accompany testicular torsion, epididymitis, orchitis, injury, or tumor. Most hydroceles cause no symptoms, but some teenagers experience heaviness or a lump in the scrotum. Surgical drainage of the hydrocele is done only if it is causing discomfort.

Spermatoceles are small cysts containing sperm, usually located above and at the back of the testicle where the epididymis is attached. They are harmless and usually do not require surgical removal.

Cryptorchidism, or undescended testicles, is found in 3 percent of newborn males but less than 1 percent of adolescent males. During fetal life, the testes normally develop in the abdomen and descend into the scrotum by birth. This descent may be delayed until the first few months after birth. Cryptorchidism that persists into childhood—and certainly adolescence—merits attention because of its strong association with testicular cancer. Surgery should be done as soon as possible (usually by a year of age) to move the testes into the scrotum. If the testes are absent or shrunken, a prosthesis can be placed in the scrotum for cosmetic reasons during adolescence.

An undescended testicle typically causes no symptoms and is discovered during a routine physical examination. If both testes have failed to descend, testosterone production usually is impaired and puberty is delayed.

Teenagers with a history of undescended testicles, whether corrected in infancy or later, should be aware of the increased risk of cancer and should perform testicular self-examination regularly.

Inguinal hernias cause swelling in the inguinal region, or groin, where the thigh and abdomen meet. A hernia is a rupture of a weak muscle that allows tissues usually contained within the abdominal cavity to protrude into the groin or scrotum. The swelling is most noticeable when a person coughs or strains to move the bowels. Most hernias do not cause pain. The danger is that the intestines will become trapped, or incarcerated, in the groin. This can cause severe pain, swelling, and eventual destruction of the trapped contents. An incarcerated hernia is an emergency that requires immediate surgery.

An inguinal hernia should be corrected surgically even if there are no symptoms. It will not heal on its own. It is always preferable to operate electively, before an emergency occurs.

Prostatitis

Inflammation of the prostate gland, or prostatitis, affects adults more than teenagers. The most common cause during adolescence is an STD such as gonorrhea or chlamydia. Less commonly, bacteria that cause urinary tract infections cause prostatitis in teenagers.

The symptoms of prostatitis include lower back or pelvic pain, a frequent urge to urinate, painful urination, difficulty emptying the bladder, and fever. The appearance of blood in ejaculated semen, or *hematospermia,* may be a sign of chronic prostatitis.

Prostatitis is treated with antibiotics taken orally for several weeks. If the teenager is acutely ill, he may be hospitalized for a few days to begin the antibiotics intravenously.

Conditions of the Penis

Circumcision, the removal of the foreskin, was performed on most newborn American males until the 1970s, when the American Academy of Pediatrics stated that there was no medical reason for its routine use. Doctors generally agree that the only proven benefit is that 10 percent of uncircumcised males may later require circumcision because of irritation or pain at the tip of the penis (see *balanitis,* p. 219). There is *no* proof that circumcision decreases the chance of STDs, urinary tract infections, cancer of the male genitalia, or cancer of the cervix in female sexual partners.

During the first few years of life, the foreskin normally cannot be pulled back, or retracted, to expose the glans (the tip of the penis). By school age, though, the foreskin is retractible in 90 percent of uncircumcised males. Retracting the foreskin while bathing helps to keep the glans free of bacteria.

If retraction is difficult, teenage boys should gently (never forcefully) slide the foreskin back to loosen the opening at the end. In some cases, the foreskin may be attached so tightly that it cannot move freely. This condition, called *phimosis,* can cause discomfort during urination or sexual activity. Phimosis is corrected by circumcision.

If the foreskin can be retracted but then cannot be moved forward over the glans, the condition is called *paraphimosis.* The pain and swelling from paraphimosis can be reduced by applying cold compresses, lubricating the area, and then applying gentle pressure to move the foreskin forward to its normal position. Circumcision is recommended to prevent its recurrence.

Balanitis, or inflammation of the glans of the penis, is more common among uncircumcised than circumcised males, particularly if they have phimosis. It can be caused by infections, irritation, and poor hygiene. The symptoms include redness, swelling, burning, and itching. A doctor should always be seen because treatment varies, depending on the cause. A yeast, or candida, balanitis will be treated with an antifungal cream, while a bacterial balanitis may require antibiotics. Circumcision may be recommended if the inflammation recurs frequently.

The skin of the penis and scrotum is thin and can be sensitive to the compounds in some spermicides or lubricants (Chapter 19). The symptoms can be relieved temporarily with topical creams, but the treatment requires identifying and avoiding the irritating substance.

Hypospadias is a birth defect in which the urethra ends before reaching the tip of the penis. The urethra may open on the shaft or at the base of the penis, and there may be a curve or bowing of the penis. Severe hypospadias is nearly always recognized and corrected surgically early in childhood. Mild hypospadias may not become apparent until puberty. The penis may appear straight when flaccid but curved during erection. Surgery can be performed to straighten the penis and, if necessary, to extend the urethra so that it opens at the tip of the penis.

Priapism is an involuntary, painful, continuing erection that happens without any sexual stimulation. It occurs when more blood flows into the penis than flows out. The most common cause of priapism in adolescents is sickle cell anemia (Chapter 35). A physician should always be seen immediately both to control the pain and to decrease the chance of permanent damage.

Impotence, the inability to have an erection, is uncommon during adolescence. When it does occur, teenagers are embarrassed and reluctant to discuss it. Impotence may have a psychological cause—anxiety about sexual function, fear of pregnancy or STDs, or other emotional conflicts. Or impotence may have a physical cause, such as the effect of a particular medication or underlying illness. Impotence in teenagers usually is a temporary problem. It helps to discuss it with a sensitive, knowledgeable physician.

Urethritis

The symptoms of *urethritis,* or inflammation of the urethra, include a discharge and redness at the tip of the penis and burning or pain on urination. The most common cause of urethritis is an STD such as gonorrhea or chlamydia (Chapter 21), in which the diagnosis is made by a culture taken from the tip of the urethra. "Nonspecific urethritis" is another STD, but the culture does not reveal any particular organism. It is treated with an oral antibiotic such as doxycycline.

When urethritis does not respond to antibiotic treatment or when other symptoms appear, the cause may not be an infection. *Reiter syndrome* is a disease of adolescents and young adults that involves urethritis, conjunctivitis (Chapter 25), and arthritis (Chapter 31). Frequently, there are small sores or ulcers in the mouth or genitalia and discolored spots on the palms or soles. The arthritis typically causes pain and stiffness of the knees, lower back, and feet. The cause of Reiter syndrome is unknown, but it often follows sexual contact or an episode of severe diarrhea (that may be sexually transmitted). About three quarters of people with Reiter syndrome have a protein in their blood called HLA-B27, suggesting that they may have an inherited predisposition to the disease.

Reiter syndrome has no known cure. The symptoms are controlled with anti-inflammatory medications such as aspirin, ibuprofen, or indomethacin. The symptoms frequently disappear on their own within weeks to months, but two thirds of people with Reiter syndrome experience recurrences.

19

Contraception

Birth control can be an awkward, controversial subject for parents and teenagers to discuss. Many parents wish teenagers simply would abstain from sexual activity or, at least, postpone it until their late teens or twenties. Their hopes are outweighed by widely publicized facts: 50 percent of girls and 60 percent of boys between ages fifteen and nineteen have sexual intercourse; 50 percent of teenagers do not use birth control the first time they have intercourse; only one third routinely use a method of contraception; a million American teenagers become pregnant each year; and sexually transmitted diseases (STDs) are widespread.

So, parents face a dilemma—do they acknowledge that their teenager has a fifty–fifty chance of being sexually active and discuss methods of contraception? Or do they look the other way, hoping their teenager abstains? The most prudent answer is, "Talk about it together." Adolescents who are knowledgeable about sexuality, contraceptive options, and STDs are more likely to protect themselves and their partners from unplanned pregnancy and infection.

Information about birth control does not promote or encourage sexual activity. It does not cause promiscuity. Parents and teenagers can and should talk together about contraceptive methods and how to use them. The discussion should consider sexual activity and birth control options within the framework of the family's own set of values. After the discussion, the teenager should be entrusted to make his or her own thoughtful, mature choices. Ideally, the decisions are made with support, but without pressure, from parents, partners, or friends. It is the adolescent, not the parent, who will or won't use a contraceptive method. The choice is only as effective as the teenager's willingness to use the method correctly and responsibly each and every time intercourse occurs.

For most teenagers, questions about sexual activity are daunting: Should I have intercourse? With whom? What types of sexual experiences do I want to have? Should I have one partner at a time? Is it okay to have sex with more than one person in the course of a few months? What if I get pregnant . . . or my girlfriend gets pregnant? Would I raise the child? Get married? Give the baby up for adoption? Have an abortion? Do I ever want to get married? Have children? How would this affect my future?

In a perfect world, teenagers would sit down, think through these questions, and incorporate their decisions into a long-range plan. But emotions and sexual situations often are unplanned. The questions may remain unasked and unanswered. Impulsive decisions, made in the passion or pressure of the moment, may feel uncomfortable the following day or week. Teenagers need education and counseling about contraception BEFORE they find themselves in situations that lead to spur-of-the-moment decisions. They deserve the opportunity and the time to consider their options and the consequences of their choices. Adolescents can behave responsibly and maturely when provided the information and resources to do so.

This chapter addresses several methods of contraception. Before detailing each method, one common denominator should be acknowledged: The most important word in the vocabulary of contraception is protection. Teenagers should think of birth control as a way to protect themselves and their sexual partners from unintended pregnancy and STDs. A woman should not assume that the man will provide for contraception by using a condom. The man should not assume "She'll protect herself." These assumptions are reckless. *Both partners are responsible for protection.* They must talk about it together, before having intercourse. And whatever method they choose, it works only if it is used consistently—every time they have intercourse.

Male Condoms

Condoms should always be used during sexual intercourse—each and every time, regardless of any other method of contraception that is used. The primary reason for this recommendation is the prevention of STDs. Other than abstinence, the condom is the only known way to decrease the risk of infection. It is not foolproof, but it *definitely* helps. The condom alone is not adequate protection against pregnancy, though. Teenage girls who rely only on the male condom face up to a 20 precent chance of pregnancy within one year. Using a vaginal spermicide (a cream or jelly that kills sperm on contact) along with the condom decreases the chance of pregnancy to less than ten percent.

Condoms are safe, inexpensive, easy to use, and readily available. They can be purchased through vending machines in both men's and women's public bathrooms, and in pharmacies and convenience stores. Family planning clinics often distribute condoms free, and some schools are beginning to distribute them.

A condom is a thin, elastic covering for the penis. A man wears it during sexual intercourse to catch his sperm and prevent them from entering the woman's vagina. Most condoms sold today are made of latex, although some are made of sheepskin. The latex types are recommended because they are more protective against STDs. If the packaging breaks or becomes dry and brittle, the condom should be replaced. Before use, a condom should always be checked for small holes or tears and replaced if there is any sign of damage. A condom should *never* be used more than once.

The condom should be put on the erect penis *prior* to any contact with a woman's genital area. It should be rolled all the way to the base of the penis, leaving a half inch of empty space at the tip of the penis to catch the semen. To create this empty space, the tip of the condom can be pinched closed as it is rolled on. This also prevents air from filling the empty space, which can create a balloon effect with tearing (Figure 19.1).

After intercourse, the man should withdraw his penis immediately from the vagina while holding on to the rim of the condom to prevent the semen from spilling. Before he throws away the condom, it is important to check it for breakage. If the condom appears to have leaked or torn, a spermicidal foam or gel (p. 225–27) should be inserted immediately into the vagina to reduce the risk of unin-

How to Use a Condom

Figure 19.1

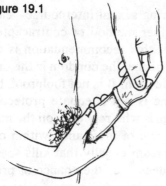

1. Pinch the tip of the condom. Put it on the erect penis.

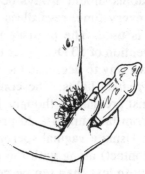

2. Unroll the condom to the pubic hair, leaving space at the tip.

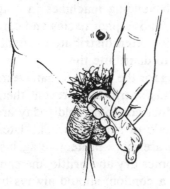

3. After sex, hold the condom on the penis as you move away from your partner.

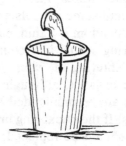

4. Throw the condom away: do <u>NOT</u> reuse it.

tended pregnancy. This should be done even if the condom contained a spermicide.

Given the risk of breakage, it is best to use backup protection with the condom, such as a contraceptive foam or gel, a contraceptive suppository, a contraceptive sponge, a diaphragm, or oral contraceptive pills. Extra protection against pregnancy is a wise choice, but these methods used alone do not prevent STDs. Use them—but use them with a condom.

Teenagers sometimes carry condoms around in a pocket or purse and wonder how long a condom is effective. Condoms can last as long as five years if they are stored in a cool, dry place. They may weaken, though, if exposed to heat or light. Some condom packages are dated, but that is the date of manufacture, not the expiration date. It is wiser to throw out old condoms and buy new ones than to risk using one that has been stashed in a bureau drawer for a year or two.

Some couples use lubrication (creams, gels) to ease the entrance of the penis into the vagina. Certain brands of condoms have their own lubrication. It is fine to use water-based lubricants such as K-Y jelly or contraceptive gels, foams, or creams, Do *not* use oil-based products like Vaseline, mineral oil, baby oil, or suntan oil. Such products can cause the condom to lose its protective properties against both pregnancy and infection.

Female Condoms

The female condom is a relatively new method of protection. It was developed to do the same things as the male condom: prevent pregnancy and protect against STDs, including HIV. A condom worn by a woman allows her control and protection even if her male partner does not wear a condom. Unfortunately, the female condom does not seem to provide as much protection against pregnancy and STDs as the male condom.

The female condom is a thin polyurethane vaginal pouch that has a closed ring at one end and an open ring at the other. The closed ring is pinched and inserted deep into the vagina. Once in place, the ring opens, stretching the closed end of the pouch over the cervix. The soft, thin sides of the pouch cover the vaginal walls and extend out of the vagina, covering the labia. The open-ring end of the sheath circles the woman's external genitalia, creating a barrier against the male's genitalia. The female condom comes in one size, does not require a prescription, and can be purchased in pharmacies.

Vaginal Spermicides

Spermicides are safe, easy-to-use methods of preventing pregnancy. They can be purchased in any pharmacy without a prescription. Condoms used with spermicides may reduce the risk of STDs more than condoms used without spermicides.

Spermicides consist of a sperm-killing chemical in a foam, jelly, cream, suppository or two-by-two-inch sheet (Figure 19.2). The suppository or sheet should be inserted into the vagina at least ten

Some Contraceptive Methods

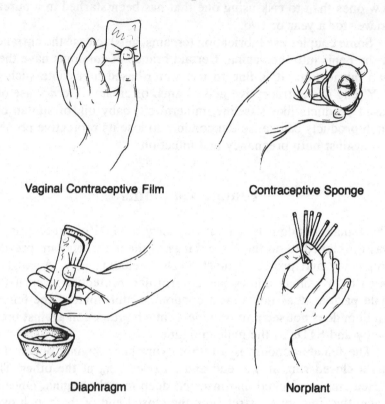

Vaginal Contraceptive Film

Contraceptive Sponge

Diaphragm

Norplant

Figure 19.2

or fifteen minutes before intercourse to allow time for it to dissolve and take effect. Foam, jelly, or cream are effective immediately after insertion.

Occasionally, spermicides may irritate the vagina or penis. Another form or brand of spermicide can be tried before discontinuing use altogether. Pain, itching, or discharge should not be attributed to the spermicide until an examination has excluded the possibility of an STD.

Using spermicides requires some planning. For example, it may be difficult to tell when the spermicide container is running out; keeping an extra on hand is smart. If using foam, it is important to shake the container vigorously—about twenty times—before use. Most spermicides are inserted with a plastic applicator that should be washed with plain soap and warm water after each use. Nothing else (like talcum powder) should be used on the applicator.

Three other points to remember about spermicides: (1) Hands should be washed carefully with soap and water before use; (2) a new application of spermicide is necessary each time intercourse takes place; (3) after intercourse, the spermicide should be left in place for at least six to eight hours.

Women often wonder if douching (cleansing or rinsing the vagina) after intercourse decreases the risk of pregnancy. Douching is *not* a reliable birth control method. Furthermore, if a spermicide has been used, washing it out of the vagina within six to eight hours of intercourse could actually increase the chance of pregnancy. Douching is not necessary for hygienic purposes, but if done, should be delayed at least eight hours to maximize the effectiveness of the spermicide. If a contraceptive sponge, diaphragm, or cervical cap is used, it should be removed prior to douching. If an oral contraceptive is used, it is safe—but not necessary—to douche any time without interfering with the contraceptive effect.

Oral Contraceptive Pills

Combination oral contraceptive pills are the most effective method of birth control. "Combination" means that the pill contains two types of hormones: estrogen and progestin. A progestin-only pill, called the minipill, is not recommended for routine use. The pregnancy rate for the minipill is much higher than for the combination pill, and irregular bleeding occurs frequently. All of the discussion that follows refers to the combination oral contraceptive, sometimes called "the pill."

The pill has been widely used by women since its approval in 1960 by the Food and Drug Administration. In the early years, pills contained higher doses of estrogen and progestin than they do today. These higher doses tended to raise concern about long-term health effects. The lower-dose pills that are now prescribed by physicians are as effective in preventing pregnancy, are safe, and are associated with far fewer side effects.

Oral contraceptive pills come in 28-day or 21-day packets. The 28-day packet contains twenty-eight pills, one for each day of the menstrual cycle. When one packet is finished, a new one is begun the very next day. The last seven pills of each packet contain no hormones and are included to help women remain on schedule. The 21-day packet contains twenty-one pills, one daily for the first three weeks of the menstrual cycle. The woman takes no pills for seven days and then begins a new packet. The menstrual period usually occurs during the fourth week, when the woman is taking either the last seven pills of the 28-day packet or no pills from the 21-day packet. Oral contraceptive pills should be taken at the same time each day to maximize effectiveness and minimize the chance of irregular bleeding. A good way to establish consistency is to link taking the pill to another daily routine, such as brushing teeth or going to bed.

Oral contraceptive pills work by preventing ovulation (release of an egg from the ovary). If there is no egg to meet a sperm, pregnancy cannot result. If a woman does not take a pill every day, it is possible that ovulation could occur. Even if this happens, though, the pill produces some other changes that may help protect against pregnancy. It alters the endometrium (lining of the uterus), making implantation unlikely, and thickens the cervical mucus, trapping the sperm. Even though ovulation is blocked, the estrogen and progestin in the pill have an effect on the uterus so that a monthly menstrual period takes place.

Different physicians recommend different starting days for the first packet of pills. Most suggest taking the first pill on the first Sunday after the beginning of the menstrual period. If the period begins on a Sunday, take the first pill that same Sunday. If the period begins on Monday through Saturday, take the first pill on the following Sunday. Some physicians prefer to use day five or day one of the period as the first day of the pill. All of this applies only to the very first packet of pills. After the first packet, each subsequent packet will automatically begin at the end of the twenty-eight-day cycle.

There is nothing magic about when to start the first packet of pills. No matter when it is begun, the pill is up to 5 percent less effective in preventing pregnancy during the first cycle than in later cycles. A back-up method of contraception therefore should be used during the first cycle.

ADVANTAGES OF THE ORAL CONTRACEPTIVE

About 50 million American women have used oral contraceptive pills. Thirteen million are using pills now. One reason for this widespread use is that the pill allows a woman to control her own fertility. Consistent use means no pregnancy. If the combination estrogen–progestin pill is reliably taken as prescribed, every day, the pregnancy rate is nearly zero (about 0.5 percent). Among teenagers, pregnancy rates up to 18 percent have been reported because of missed pills or discontinuation. The oral contraceptive works, but *only* if it is taken correctly.

Unlike other methods of birth control, the pill's use and effectiveness are not linked to the timing of intercourse. If it is taken correctly, it provides full pregnancy protection all the time, every time. But the pill does *not* protect against STDs, so condoms should always be used, even if the woman is taking the pill.

Many young women find that oral contraceptives have benefits in addition to contraception. For example, they regulate the menstrual period, decrease the amount of blood loss, shorten the duration of flow, and diminish menstrual cramping. Oral contraceptives have long-range medical adavantages, as well. They decrease the chance that gonorrhea or chlamydia, if contracted, will progress to cause pelvic inflammatory disease (Chapter 21). They also decrease the likelihood of benign (noncancerous) breast lumps or cysts and may protect against cancer of the ovary and uterus. Some adolescents with acne find that their skin improves when they are on the pill.

MINOR SIDE EFFECTS

The pill has side effects for some women. There may be breakthrough bleeding, or vaginal bleeding that occurs between periods. If this happens, it is usually in the first few cycles after beginning the pill, often in the second week of the packet. The woman should continue to take the pill every day. The bleeding is not dangerous, is common, and usually stops by the third cycle. If irregular bleeding is heavy or persists beyond three cycles, a physician should be consulted. It is always possible that the bleeding is caused by something other than the pill. If no other cause is found, a different type of combination estrogen–progestin pill might be prescribed that would diminish the bleeding. For example, pills that vary the amount of estrogen and progestin over the month may be indicated.

Some women experience nausea during the first pill cycle or during the first day or two of subsequent cycles. It may help to take the pills after dinner or with a bedtime snack rather than on an empty stomach in the morning. The nausea usually disappears within two or three cycles. If it does not, the doctor may suggest trying a pill that has a lower dose of estrogen.

Many teenagers worry about weight gain on the pill. This is uncommon with the low-dose pills that are prescribed today. Breast enlargement and breast tenderness also have become less common with the lower-dose pills.

After an adolescent has been on the pill for months or even years, she may notice progressive lightening or even complete absence of her periods. If a period is missed, pregnancy must be considered and a pregnancy test should be done. If the test is negative, the amenorrhea (absence of menstruation) is probably caused by the low dose of estrogen in the pill. The teenager should continue the pill because periods often will begin again after one or two cycles. If the amenorrhea persists, the physician may suggest a pill with either more estrogen or less progestin.

Some women notice that their skin and hair may change when they use oral contraceptives. Skin color may darken, usually above the lip, on the forehead, or under the eyes. There may be some hair loss from the scalp, or body and facial hair may increase and darken. These changes are uncommon and are not harmful, but may cause concern about appearance.

Many women experience less premenstrual irritability while on the pill. Others notice vague changes in their mood throughout the month. If the feelings persist, a different type of pill might be tried. Usually the feelings diminish on their own, without a change in the pill.

MAJOR SIDE EFFECTS

Some side effects are merely inconvenient or annoying, while others can signal medical risk. If any of the following symptoms occur, a physician should be contacted immediately:

- severe abdominal pain;
- severe chest pain, cough, shortness of breath;
- leg pain or swelling;
- severe headaches;
- vision loss or blurring;
- speech problems;
- numbness or weakness in an arm or leg.

Teenagers should know the major risks associated with oral contraceptive use, but they should also understand that these risks are very rare in adolescents—especially adolescents who do not smoke cigarettes. In fact, the risk of death is far greater among sexually active fifteen-to-nineteen-year-old girls who use no contraception (35 deaths per 100,000 girls) than among girls who use the pill and do not smoke (3 per 100,000). Among girls who use the pill and do smoke, the risk of death is intermediate (12 per 100,000). The reason for these differences is that using no contraception can lead to pregnancy, and pregnancy carries medical risks, including death. Cigarette smoking increases the risk of blood clots, which are associated with pill use. For that reason, pills generally are not recommended for women who smoke heavily (over fourteen cigarettes a day).

On the rare occasions when blood clots do form, they are most common in the legs. This is called deep vein thrombosis. The danger is that a piece of the clot will break off and travel through the bloodstream to the lungs ("pulmonary embolus"). Any calf or thigh pain or trouble breathing therefore must be reported immediately to a physician.

Another rare type of blood clot that may be linked to pill use occurs in the brain ("stroke"). The symptoms or warning signs of a stroke include headache, numbness or weakness of an arm or leg, trouble speaking, and confusion. The risk of stroke in healthy adolescents who are on the pill is practically zero. The greatest risk is in women over age thirty-five who smoke and have high blood pressure. Because both high blood pressure and migraine headaches are associated with stroke, women with these problems should consider a contraceptive method other than the pill.

An important concern of women who use the pill is their future risk of cancer. The final word is not in. Most studies have found no increase in breast cancer among women who have used the pill. Some studies have found higher rates of cervical cancer among pill users, but it is not clear that the pill causes the cancer. It is possible that women who use the pill are less likely than nonusers to insist that their partners use condoms. Nonuse of condoms may result in higher STD rates, which are associated with higher cervical cancer rates (Chapter 21). Condoms should *always* be used, regardless of pill use.

Another concern of women who use the pill is their future risk of heart attack ("myocardial infarction"). Pill use during the teens and twenties appears to carry no risk. Among women over age thirty, smoking and pill use seem to compound the risk of a future heart attack. For this reason, the pill is not recommended for older women, especially if they smoke.

MISSED PILLS

Oral contraceptive pills are only effective if they are taken regularly. Young women often worry, "What if I forgot to take my pill yesterday . . . or for three days? Could I get pregnant?" If one pill was missed, it should be taken as soon as remembered and the next pill should be taken at its regular time. For example, Jill forgot to take her pill last night at her usual time of 10:00. She remembered when she woke up today at 7:00. Jill took last night's pill this morning, and will take today's pill at 10:00 p.m. as usual. Missing one pill probably does not interfere with protectiveness, but it is best to use a backup method of contraception for the rest of the cycle.

Missing two or more pills does affect the protectiveness, and a backup method must be used. Very often, the teenager will remember that she has missed the pills when unexpected bleeding begins. If a young woman misses two pills in a row, two pills should be taken together today, two pills tomorrow, and one pill as usual to complete the cycle. If three or more pills in a row have been missed, she should take one pill daily until Sunday (the day when most pill cycles begin), throw away the rest of the packet, and start a new packet that Sunday.

The more often pills are missed, the higher the risk of pregnancy. Any time a period is missed, pregnancy must be considered, and a pregnancy test should be done.

Norplant

The newest forms of contraceptive devices involve hormone-containing implants that can prevent pregnancy for years at a time. Norplant, the best known of these, is a set of six progestin capsules, each about the size of a matchstick (Figure 19.2). After injecting a local anesthetic (numbing medication), a physician inserts the capsules under the skin on the inside of the woman's upper arm. The procedure is done in the clinic or office and takes ten or fifteen minutes. Nothing else needs to be done to prevent pregnancy, but condoms always should be used to prevent STDs.

Norplant protects a woman against pregnancy for five years before it needs to be replaced. It is a very effective form of contraception with less than a 0.7 percent pregnancy rate. If the woman changes her mind and wants to become pregnant, the capsules can be removed at any time.

Norplant offers continuous, long-term, effective birth control without pills, creams, or devices. It has some disadvantages, though. It does nothing to protect against STDs. Some women dislike the fact that the capsules are slightly visible. Norplant costs more than other methods of contraception initially. A common, bothersome side effect during the first six to twelve months is irregular bleeding. This includes frequent periods, prolonged or heavy periods, very light periods, or no periods at all. If there is unexplained vaginal bleeding beyond six months, a health care professional should always be consulted.

Depo-Provera

Depo-Provera is an injectable method of contraception that was approved by the U.S. Food and Drug Administration in 1992. It has been used in other countries for many years. A medication called medroxyprogesterone is injected into the muscle of the upper arm and provides over 99 percent protection against pregnancy for three months. The injection *must* be repeated every three months to provide ongoing protection. The most common side effect is irregular bleeding, though most women become completely amenorrheic (no periods) after a year of continuous use. Other less common side effects include weight gain and headache.

Vaginal Barrier Methods

For centuries, women have protected themselves against pregnancy by inserting devices into their vaginas to prevent sperm from reaching an egg. These forms of birth control are called barrier methods because they put a barrier between the sperm and the egg. The barrier may be a vaginal sponge, diaphragm, or cervical cap. When used correctly, these barriers provide a reliable way to prevent pregnancy and they offer an extra measure of protection against STDs when used in conjunction with spermicides and condoms. Regardless of which barrier method is chosen, oil-based lubricants should not be used.

VAGINAL SPONGES

These small polyurethane pillows contain a spermicide called nonoxynol-9. Sponges come in one size and can be purchased over-the-counter. The sponge (Figure 19.2) has a concave, dimpled side to fit over the cervix and keep the sponge in place. It also has a loop for easier removal.

Before intercourse, the sponge should be moistened with about two tablespoons of clean water and squeezed once before insertion. It is inserted into the vagina by sliding it along the back wall until it reaches the cervix. The dimple side of the sponge should face the cervix and the loop should be away from the cervix for removal later. For the next twenty-four hours, the sponge protects against pregnancy by releasing spermicide and trapping the sperm within it. It remains effective for up to twenty-four hours even if intercourse occurs more than once during that time. The sponge should be left in the vagina for at least six hours after last intercourse. It is then pulled out of the vagina by its string and thrown away.

The sponge is 78 to 87 percent effective in preventing pregnancy. In other words, of every 100 women who use the sponge alone for one year, 13 to 22 will become pregnant. It is highly recommended that the man use a condom, even if the woman uses the sponge, to prevent both pregnancy and STDs.

The risks of the sponge are allergic reactions (usually causing vaginal itching), fragmentation of the sponge on removal, and—rarely—toxic shock syndrome (Chapter 17). Teenagers who use the sponge should know the warning signs of toxic shock syndrome and should use another method during the menstrual period.

DIAPHRAGMS

Diaphragms are soft, dome-shaped latex cups that cover the cervix. They are used with spermicides and they come in several sizes and shapes (Figure 19.2). The diaphragm is washed after each use and can be used repeatedly for up to two years. A woman must be fitted for a diaphragm by a health care professional to assure the proper size and effectiveness. She also must be taught how to insert it, check its position in the vagina, remove it, and wash it.

Before the diaphragm is inserted, one to two teaspoonsful of spermicidal cream or jelly are applied to its rim and to the concave side that will face the cervix. Some women use a plastic "introducer" with some styles of diaphragm; most women find it easier to insert it with their hands. After inserting the diaphragm, the woman must place her finger deep in the vagina to check that the soft cup is covering the cervix.

The diaphragm must be left in the vagina for at least six hours after the last intercourse. While it is in place, an additional applicator-full of spermicide must be inserted before having intercourse again. After removal, the diaphragm should be washed with soap and water. It should be checked frequently for holes.

The major problem with the diaphragm is nonuse. Many women either stop using it altogether or do not use it every time they have intercourse, so its effectiveness in preventing pregnancy varies widely, from 77 to 97 percent.

The risks of the diaphragm include allergies to the latex or spermicide, vaginal discharge if worn longer than the recommended twelve hours, urinary tract infection, and, very rarely, toxic shock syndrome (Chapter 17). As with the sponge, the teenager should use another method during the menstrual period.

CERVICAL CAPS

This contraceptive resembles a small diaphragm with a tall dome. The cup-shaped cap fits over the cervix. A seal between its rim and the surface of the cervix holds it in place.

Before insertion, the cap should be filled one third full with spermicidal jelly or cream. To develop proper suction, the cap is best inserted a half hour before intercourse. It can remain in place and provide effective contraception for forty-eight hours, regardless of how often intercourse takes place within that time. Extra spermicide need not be applied with repeated intercourse, but the position of the cap should be checked each time.

After intercourse, the cap should not be removed for six to eight hours. To remove it, find the cap rim on the cervix, press the rim until the seal against the cervix is broken, hook the finger around the rim, and pull it out sideways. The cap should be checked for holes or cracks, washed with soap and water, and dried.

The pregnancy rates with the cervical cap are similar to those with the diaphragm. Both require a prescription for the correct size and education about how to use them. The risks of the cap include irritation of the cervix with vaginal discharge and odor. There have been rare cases of toxic shock syndrome (Chapter 17) reported with use of the cervical cap.

Intrauterine Device

A generation ago, the intrauterine device (IUD) was a popular method of long-term birth control. After insertion of the IUD into the uterus by a physician, a woman was 98 percent protected against pregnancy for several years, until the IUD was removed. In the 1970s, IUD-related problems led to lawsuits and the removal of several types from the market. A few types of IUDs are available today, but they are recommended only for women who have previously given birth. Most physicians do not consider IUDs appropriate for teenagers, even if they have given birth, because of the risk of pelvic inflammatory disease (Chapter 21) and subsequent infertility.

Morning-after Pills

Things do go wrong. Pills can be forgotten. Condoms can break. Cervical caps and diaphragms can shift out of place. One act of unplanned, unprotected sexual intercourse can lead to pregnancy. Then a woman may wish she could turn back the clock.

High-dose estrogen, taken within seventy-two hours of unprotected intercourse, does lower the likelihood of pregnancy. This treatment is called postcoital contraception, or the morning-after pill. The treatment does cause side effects. Nausea is common, and vomiting can be severe. Other symptoms of the medication include fluid retention, weight gain, breast tenderness, headache, and irregular vaginal bleeding. The morning-after pill is an option if an accident occurs, but it *never* should be relied upon as the only method of contraception.

The decision to have sexual intercourse is a major step for an adolescent. With this decision comes the dual responsibilities to prevent unwanted pregnancy and STDs. Teenagers who are knowledgeable about their options *can* make choices that will protect themselves and their partners. Parents and health professionals can counsel and guide, but the decisions ultimately rest with the adolescents themselves.

20

Pregnancy

Ann is fifteen, nauseated, and irritable. Her breasts are tender. Her period is late. She waits one week. Then two weeks. Afraid that she is pregnant, Ann makes an appointment at a clinic. The test is positive. She has just told Jim. They are frightened and confused. How can they tell their parents? Should she have the baby? What about school? Who can they talk to?

Pregnancy is a major life event at any age. For teenagers, pregnancy involves decisions, changes, and responsibilities that traditionally are reserved for adulthood. It touches every aspect of their lives. It affects the girl's physical and emotional health, her sexual partner, their families, and their future.

Beyond each individual situation, teenage pregnancy presents critical issues for society as a whole:

• The United States has the highest adolescent pregnancy rate of all developed nations—twice as high as England, France, and Canada, three times as high as Sweden, and seven times as high as the Netherlands.

• Four of every ten girls become pregnant by age nineteen.

• One million fifteen-to-nineteen-year-olds become pregnant every year.

• Another 30,000 girls *younger than fifteen* become pregnant each year.

• Twenty-two percent of births to adolescent mothers are repeat births.

• Two thirds of teenage mothers are single parents. Out-of-wedlock births to teenagers have increased fourfold since 1960.

• Less than 25 percent of teenage pregnancies are planned, yet only 32 percent of teenagers with unplanned pregnancies used contraception.

What happens to the one million teenagers who become pregnant each year? Forty-seven percent deliver babies, 40 percent have abortions, and 13 percent miscarry. The result is 1.3 million children living with 1.1 million teenage mothers. Half of all adolescent mothers and over 80 percent of those who are unmarried live below the poverty level. These teenagers and their children face a future of struggle and limitations.

What factors contribute to teenage pregnancy? The answer differs for each adolescent, but some general conclusions can be reached from studies of large numbers of adolescents. The two most important predictors of teenage pregnancy are beginning sexual activity at an early age and inconsistent use of contraception.

Adolescents today enter puberty and become fertile at younger ages than in the past. A century ago, the average age of menarche (first menstrual period) was nearly seventeen; today it is 12.8 years. This means that teenagers begin to ovulate at a younger age than ever before. Young adolescents typically have not yet thought much about their futures and often do not fully link today's behaviors with tomorrow's consequences. This developmental immaturity contributes to their haphazard use—or nonuse—of contraception. Girls who begin having intercourse at age fifteen or younger are twice as likely to become pregnant within the first six months as are girls who wait until age eighteen or nineteen. The older a teenage girl is, the more likely she is to use contraception at first intercourse and consistently thereafter.

Most sexually active teenagers—66 percent—never, or only occasionally, use any form of birth control. Many teenagers deny their vulnerability and fertility. They hold onto the myths: "It can't happen to me" or "I've had sex before and didn't get pregnant" or "It can't happen the first time." *Pregnancy can happen the first time and anytime thereafter.* Twenty percent of teenage pregnancies occur within one month of first sexual intercourse, and 50 percent within six months. Despite this, only one in seven adolescent girls has received contraceptive care from a family planning clinic or doctor's office before initial sexual intercourse. Most adolescents wait at least nine months before obtaining contraceptives.

The major reasons for inconsistent contraception are probably immaturity and denial, but society's portrayal of sexuality may contribute. Films and television depict sex as glamorous and spontaneous without mentioning the planning, protection, or potential consequences: pregnancy and sexually transmitted diseases (STDs). Teenagers also cite the difficulty of obtaining contraceptives. They do not know where to get them and are too embarrassed to ask; they worry about cost; they fear parental discovery. Some teenagers say that they know the *names* of the contraceptive methods but do not know how to use them. Many fear side effects. Some say that their sexual partners refuse to use contraceptives or believe that most methods inhibit sexual pleasure.

Many male adolescents say that contraception is the female's responsibility, and indicate little concern if pregnancy results. Only 15 percent of male teenagers in one survey said that they always used contraceptives, and only 35 percent said they sometimes used them.

Many teenagers are well-informed about birth control but say that they want to become pregnant. Their reasons include wanting to demonstrate their love of each other, to secure their relationship, to have a child to love and to be loved by in return, to prove their fertility, to establish their independence, and to rebel against their families.

While researchers have not identified a psychological characteristic that unifies all pregnant teenagers, they have found some common characteristics. Compared to sexually active teenagers who use contraception effectively, pregnant teenagers are more likely to experience low self-esteem, poor school achievement, poverty, poor family relationships, violence, abuse, neglect, and substance abuse. Stereotypes can be misleading and simplistic, though; many teenagers with none of these features become pregnant.

Recognizing Pregnancy

The most common early sign of pregnancy is a missed period. *Any adolescent who misses a period and has had sexual intercourse within the past month must have a pregnancy test, regardless of the contraception that she or her partner has used.* Other symptoms of pregnancy may include breast tenderness, nausea (especially in the morning), fatigue, and weight gain. If pregnancy is suspected, do not wait. It will not go away. Have a pregnancy test done as soon as possible at a clinic or doctor's office. The test and the result can remain confidential. It is up to the adolescent to decide who she tells and when.

Urine pregnancy test kits can be purchased in pharmacies without a prescription. These tests usually can detect pregnancy by the time the first period is missed. The false-positive rate (a positive pregnancy result when the woman is not really pregnant) is very low. *Every woman with a positive result should assume she is pregnant and should schedule an appointment at a clinic or doctor's office.* The false-negative rate (a negative result when the woman really is pregnant) is about 5 percent. A false-negative test usually occurs early in a pregnancy. If the test is negative at the time of the missed period, it should be repeated in two weeks. If it is still negative, the adolescent should see a doctor.

Occasionally some spotting (light vaginal bleeding) may occur around the time of the expected period, even when the woman is pregnant. This bleeding usually happens when the fertilized egg implants in the lining of the uterus. Very light bleeding, lasting only a day or two, should not be considered a period. If the woman had intercourse within the preceding month, it may reflect an early pregnancy.

Consequences of Pregnancy

A positive pregnancy test brings about immediate, profound challenges for a teenager. Her educational, vocational, and social future may be compromised. She must decide whether to continue the pregnancy, raise the child herself, or place the baby for adoption. She must decide how and when to tell the baby's father, her family, friends, and school. She must arrange prenatal (pregnancy) care and then follow a routine of clinic visits, prenatal vitamins, good nutrition. Her current-day activities and her future prospects may undergo dramatic shifts.

Maternal morbidity (illness) and mortality (death) are higher for adolescent mothers than for mothers over age twenty. Pregnant teenagers are at high risk for anemia (low blood count), nutritional deficiencies, inappropriate weight gain, and high blood pressure. The risks are highest among the youngest teenagers who do not receive adequate prenatal care. Many problems during pregnancy and at delivery can be prevented or minimized by early detection and treatment.

Infant mortality is also higher for adolescent mothers than older mothers. Nearly 6 percent of babies born to mothers younger than fifteen die in their first year of life, a rate more than twice that of infants born to women over twenty. The babies of teenage mothers are more likely to be premature, to have low weights at birth, and to have ongoing problems that require hospitalization during the first five years of life. Some studies suggest that babies born to teenagers have lower intelligence, slower social and emotional development, and more behavioral problems than do babies born to adult mothers. Like the maternal risks, the infant risks are reduced markedly if the mother receives good medical care during pregnancy.

The social consequences of pregnancy for many teenagers are serious. Adolescent mothers complete fewer years of school, hold lower-status jobs, and are more likely to be impoverished as adults than are older mothers. The most important predictors of social difficulties are young age at first pregnancy, school dropout, and repeated pregnancies during adolescence. In recent years, many schools have developed programs to help teenagers stay in school during and after pregnancy. These schools have established on-site child care programs and classes for young mothers in parenting skills and vocational training.

The school dropout rates for fathers under age seventeen are also high: 40 percent for unmarried fathers and 60 percent for married fathers. Teenagers who marry because of pregnancy also are three times more likely to divorce than couples who marry in their twenties. Whether or not the couple marries, fathers should be encouraged to participate in the care of their children. Several studies have demonstrated that children do better when their fathers are involved in their upbringing. There are far fewer programs available for teen fathers than teen mothers. Consequently, young fathers need the support of their family, friends, and community.

Choices

"Should I have the baby? Should I give it up for adoption? Should I have an abortion?" Faced with the crisis of an unplanned pregnancy, a young woman needs emotional support and information before making this important decision. She will be influenced by family attitudes, age, education, socioeconomic status, and culture, but the decision ultimately is hers.

Everyone involved with the adolescent during this process should recognize and accept the ambivalence and the confusion that she may be experiencing. A decision that seems clear-cut to a parent or partner often is far more difficult for the young woman whose body, emotions, and future are on the line. The decision-making process for the teenager can be smoother if several things occur:

• She should see a doctor or family planning counselor immediately to discuss openly and confidentially her feelings about the pregnancy. Later, if she desires, her family and partner can be included in a discussion.
• She should be informed about all aspects of teenage pregnancy, and she should explore all options. She needs facts about prenatal care, labor and delivery, infant care, abortion, adoption, foster care, and school programs for pregnant adolescents and young mothers.
• She should realize that the decision and the resulting responsibilities are hers. They can—and should—be shared with her partner and family, but she should take the leadership role in reaching a decision.

Once she makes a choice, she needs help in identifying and obtaining the necessary health care. Most of this care will be available within her community; some (such as abortion services) may require travel outside the community.

She may benefit from psychological counseling during and after the decision-making process. Over the coming months, her relationships with her parents, the child's father, and her friends may change. She may consider dropping out of school. She may wish she had made a different decision. She may cope better with these challenges if she has psychological and emotional support.

Continuing the Pregnancy

Of the half million teenagers who give birth each year, 96 percent keep the babies and 4 percent place them for adoption. Every newborn infant, no matter where the future home will be, deserves the benefit of good health care. This care begins long before the baby enters the world, in the first trimester (the first three months) of pregnancy.

Prenatal care for adolescents should be age-appropriate and multidisciplinary; that is, it should address her educational, economic, and psychological needs as well as her medical care. Prenatal clinics designed especially for teenagers exist throughout the country. These programs follow the adolescent closely, contact her if she fails to keep an appointment, pay attention to the unique nutritional needs of teenage mothers, prepare her for labor and delivery, teach her basic parenting skills, and help her with contraceptive decisions after delivery. All of these many components of prenatal care are managed by a team of health professionals: a doctor, nurse, nutritionist, and social worker. Frequently, groups of pregnant teenagers meet with a health professional to discuss issues such as anesthesia during labor and delivery, fetal monitoring during labor, breast feeding, and newborn care.

Some adolescents prefer to go to a private practice obstetrician, a nurse midwife, or a prenatal care clinic that sees women of all ages. *The single most important thing is that all pregnant women get prenatal care.* Where they get the care is less important than getting it. Not all communities have adolescent prenatal programs, but *all* communities have access to some prenatal care. The best chance for a comfortable pregnancy, a smooth delivery, and a healthy baby is medical supervision by a health professional early in, and throughout, the pregnancy.

Unfortunately, far too many pregnant adolescents postpone or never receive prenatal care. Two thirds of mothers under age fifteen, half of those fifteen to seventeen, and 40 percent of those eighteen to twenty do not seek medical care in the first trimester of pregnancy. These mothers are at high risk for undetected problems that may result in early labor, premature delivery, and babies who have not grown or developed as they should. Many of these problems can be prevented and, if they do occur, can be treated early with excellent outcomes for mother and baby.

The first prenatal visit will include a thorough history of the teenage mother's health, her family's medical history, and the health history of the father and his family. It is very important that the adolescent mother talk about—and stop—her use of cigarettes, alcohol, and illegal drugs. All of these substances can affect the growth and development of the fetus. The first visit also will include a thorough physical examination and a pelvic examination (Chapter 3). Using the date of the last menstrual period and the size of the uterus on pelvic examination, the doctor or nurse will tell the adolescent approximately when she can expect to deliver the baby.

Laboratory tests will include blood and urine tests, cultures for STDs, and a Pap smear (a test for cervical cancer; Chapter 3).

In follow-up medical visits, the adolescent should discuss with a health professional all the various aspects of pregnancy: nutrition, the changes that are taking place within her body, sexual activity, protection against STDs, and avoidance of tobacco, drugs, and alcohol. Pregnant teenagers should visit the doctor or clinic every two to four weeks until the eighth month. The visits should be every two weeks in the eighth month and then weekly until birth.

Most adolescents are advised not to diet while pregnant. The ideal weight gain for a teenager over the course of her pregnancy is about twenty-eight pounds. She should plan to increase her daily food intake by about 200 to 300 calories. It is best to increase these calories by eating more protein rather than more fat or carbohydrate. If the adolescent eats a balanced diet, the only vitamin supplements usually recommended are iron, folic acid, and sometimes calcium. Moderate exercise is good for the mother and baby, but prolonged aerobic exercise should be avoided.

Drugs of many kinds—over-the-counter, prescription, illegal— can endanger the baby's health. Before taking *any* medication during pregnancy, check with a doctor. Even medications that have been used safely throughout adolescence may be dangerous to the developing fetus. For example, tetracycline is commonly prescribed for adolescent acne. During pregnancy, tetracycline can affect the baby's bone growth and discolor the baby's teeth as they form before birth.

Cigarettes, alcohol, and illegal drugs are especially dangerous during pregnancy. Nicotine in tobacco increases the risk of miscarriage or premature delivery and can impair the baby's growth. Alcohol can cause mental retardation, learning difficulties, and physical abnormalities. Marijuana and LSD increase the risk of birth defects. Crack and cocaine can cause miscarriage, prematurity, birth defects, and developmental problems in the baby.

The pregnant adolescent should take special precautions to protect herself and her baby from STDs. She should insist that her sexual partner use a condom each and every time they have intercourse. She should consult her doctor about any sign of infection: vaginal discharge or itching, sores in the vaginal area, abdominal pain, discomfort with urination. She also should be aware of danger signs that require immediate medical attention: vaginal bleeding, severe abdominal pain, fever. Do not wait if any of these symptoms occur; the pregnancy may be endangered and prompt medical care is imperative.

During the pregnancy, the adolescent must learn about childbirth and infant care. She must make plans for at least two lives after the birth, her own and the baby's. Whenever possible, the baby's father should be involved in these plans. Teenage parents need all the help they can get from their families. They need encouragement to finish school, help with child care, financial support, and guidance. When their own parents provide love and support, a new young family stands a far better chance for a healthy beginning.

Adoption

Deciding to have a child results in a new life, full of potential. Deciding to raise a child affects both the life of the infant and the rest of life for the adolescent. Some teenagers feel that the best decision for their babies and themselves is adoption. The decision should belong to the adolescent—not to her parents or physician.

Once an adolescent has decided to place the baby for adoption, she may feel confused about whom to contact or where to go. A good place to begin is with the doctor or nurse who is providing prenatal care. Prenatal clinics usually have names and addresses of agencies that handle adoptions. Another good source for information is the adolescent's church or synagogue because many religious groups have special services to help pregnant women find homes for their babies. The community's department of human services or child welfare may also provide names of both local agencies and nationwide agencies with local offices.

Making the telephone call does not commit the adolescent to proceeding with adoption. The first contact or call should be viewed instead as a chance to gather information and make an informed decision. The control and the outcome remain with the pregnant adolescent.

Abortion

One quarter of the abortions in the United States are obtained by teenagers. Of the one million teenagers who become pregnant every year, more than 400,000 have abortions. Teenagers are less likely than women in their twenties to have first-trimester abortions and more likely to delay the procedure into the second trimester, when it becomes more dangerous and traumatic. An adolescent should never be rushed into making a quick decision about pregnancy options, but she should know that if she chooses abortion, it is far safer when performed during the first trimester.

Some teenagers, fearing parental reaction, may delay obtaining an abortion because they assume that their parents will be informed or that they will need parental consent (Chapter 10). Other adolescents may think, incorrectly, that abortions are easy to arrange—they will schedule the procedure whenever they can fit it into their busy lives. Abortions can be difficult to obtain, especially in small towns and rural areas. One fourth of all abortions in the United States are performed in just five cities (New York, Los Angeles, Chicago, Washington, D.C., and San Francisco). Many hospitals around the country have discontinued abortion services because of high costs and a declining number of physicians trained to perform the procedure. Only 13 percent of the obstetrics/gynecology training programs in the United States require new doctors to learn abortion techniques.

If an adolescent is having trouble finding an abortion service, she should *never* allow herself to be pushed in the direction of an illegal, unsafe abortion. The risks of death, bleeding, infection, and infertility are very high for women who have illegal abortions. Abortions should be performed *only* by licensed physicians who are trained in the procedure and equipped to handle complications.

The type of procedure depends on the stage of the pregnancy. During the first trimester, the preferred method is called vacuum or suction curettage, a procedure that involves local or general anesthesia followed by removal of the fetal tissues from the uterus. The adolescent usually will have the procedure done in the morning, will remain in a recovery room for a few hours, and will go home in the afternoon. After the abortion, she will have vaginal bleeding for several days, which is like having a heavy period. If she plans to use birth control pills, she usually will be told to start them on the first Sunday following the procedure.

In the second trimester of pregnancy, other procedures are performed. Up to sixteen weeks of pregnancy, the cervix may be dilated and the contents of the uterus removed. Between sixteen and twenty weeks, the risk of serious injury to the cervix or uterus increases. Procedures that induce uterine contractions therefore may be considered.

As long as abortion has been legal in this country, it has been considered a relatively safe procedure. Even under the safest conditions, though, abortion carries risks and complications. The overall death rate for women from abortion is low, but the rate increases with the length of time from conception. Compared to older women, teenagers have a lower death rate, but a higher complication rate because they are more likely to postpone the abortion into the second trimester. The complications include infection, bleeding, retention of blood clots or fetal tissue in the uterus, tears of the cervix, and injury to the uterus.

When first-pregnancy, first-trimester abortions are performed by skilled physicians, there is no evidence of a long-term increase in subsequent miscarriages, infertility, or poor pregnancy outcomes. The evidence is less clear for women who have had two or more abortions, especially when performed in the second trimester.

Studies on the psychological consequences of abortion during adolescence vary in their results. Most indicate that abortion is a stressful experience for teenagers, but that the reaction diminishes with good support throughout and after the procedure. One follow-up study found that teenagers who had abortions were no more prone to psychological problems two years later than teenagers who never had abortions. A caring family and partner, along with good medical follow-up, can do much to ease the strain for the adolescent.

Pregnancy, parenting, adoption, and abortion are realities for many adolescents. Whatever the decision and the outcome, the teenager's life has been changed by the experience. She needs all the love, support, encouragement, and guidance that her family and friends can provide. Surrounded by this network, she can make a decision that is right for her and that allows her to move ahead with hope and purpose.

21

Sexually Transmitted Diseases

The current epidemic of sexually transmitted diseases (STDs) is a major health threat to adolescents—a threat that includes the risk of infertility, cancer, and death. STDs represent the most widespread, devastating, and expensive set of communicable diseases facing American youth.

AIDS, the acquired immunodeficiency syndrome, is the most frightening and well-known STD. Vast public attention has focused on AIDS and the virus that causes it, HIV, the *human immunodeficiency virus.* HIV can be transmitted through both heterosexual and homosexual contact, from a pregnant mother to her fetus, through intravenous drug use, and through blood transfusion prior to 1985. HIV and AIDS are discussed in great detail in Chapter 22. This chapter is about the other STDs. It discusses how to prevent, recognize, and treat the most common STDs among American adolescents: chlamydia, gonorrhea, genital herpes, human papilloma virus (HPV), trichomonas, and syphilis. It also describes the "sequelae," or complications, that result from these very serious infections.

Adolescents and young adults (under age twenty-five) make up more than half of the twenty million STD cases reported annually in the United States. A quarter of these infections occur in teenagers who have not yet finished high school. One third of all reported cases of gonorrhea occur in only four years of the whole life span—ages fifteen to nineteen. STDs are a grim and very real part of adolescence today.

248

STDs can be prevented. Most are curable. If infected, teenagers *must* go to a clinic or doctor's office. Self-treatment will not work. Delay will make it worse. STDs can be a matter of life and death.

Risk Factors

Adolescents are at greater risk for STDs than are people of other ages. Most of this risk comes from the sexual behavior of teenagers. Some of the increased risk is attributable to biology. The cells of the vagina and cervix change during adolescence and, in the process, become slightly more resistant to infection. A younger girl who has intercourse with an infected male is more likely than an older girl to become infected. Subsequently, she may pass the infection on to another male or to her baby if she becomes pregnant.

Most of the risk of STDs, though, is related to sexual behavior rather than to physiology. Adolescence is a time of sexual initiation and experimentation. Teenagers are more likely than adults to take sexual risks without considering the long-term consequences. Many have a strong sense of denial and invulnerability—"It can't happen to me." Many believe that they will never have sex with an infected partner. Even after the symptoms of an STD appear, adolescents tend to deny and delay treatment: "It's just a yeast infection." "It's just a scratch." "I don't know where to go for help."

Teenagers are more likely than adults to have spontaneous rather than planned sexual intercourse. In spontaneous situations, precautions may not be taken to prevent infection. Many adolescents avoid talking to their partners about sexual issues such as abstinence, condom use, contraception, and sexual history. An illusion of safety arises from not asking and not knowing.

The epidemic proportions of STDs, combined with adolescent behaviors and attitudes, can be a volatile mix. But teenagers *can* protect themselves. STDs are very prevalent, but they are also *preventable*. The more information teenagers have about STDs, the better prepared they are to avoid them. Once they accept that sexual activity carries risks with debilitating, even fatal outcomes, they may be more willing to abstain or to practice safer sex.

Prevention

A major factor in prevention is knowledge about how STDs are spread. STDs are infections caused by the transfer of body fluids from one person to another during sexual contact. STDs do not spread in the same way as the common cold or the flu. The viruses that cause colds and influenza can survive outside the body—in water, air, and food; on telephones, doorknobs, and eating utensils. In other words, they are all around us and are easily spread. STDs are *not* all around us and are *not* spread through casual contact like opening doors, shaking hands, hugging, or sitting on a toilet seat. STDs are spread by sexual contact with an infected person. This "contact" means that secretions from the penis, vagina, or mouth of the infected person touch a mucus surface or broken skin of the partner. The more contact, the higher the risk of spread. This is why it is much more risky to have sexual intercourse than to kiss or touch a partner's genitals.

Safe sex has become a well-known term in the nationwide effort to educate the public about preventing STDs. Yet, many health professionals argue that the term is misleading. The only truly safe sex practice is abstinence from sexual intercourse.

For many teenagers, abstinence is perfectly acceptable. They feel secure about postponing sexual activity until they are older or until they have a long-term relationship with a partner who is STD-free. Until then, they can say to a boyfriend or girlfriend, "I'm not ready," or "If you care about me, respect my wishes," or "We can show that we love each other in ways other than intercourse."

Fifty percent of adolescents do abstain from intercourse. For the teenager who does *not* abstain—whether once or frequently—prevention each and every time is vital. Safe sex is not an absolute guarantee against STDs. There are *safer* sex methods, though, that reduce the likelihood of getting or spreading an STD. The first line of defense is a condom.

CONDOMS

Condoms can help prevent STDs. A condom is most protective if it is used *before* the man's penis comes into any physical contact with his partner's vagina, anus, or mouth. The correct way to use a condom is described in detail in Chapter 19.

Condoms do provide some protection against STDs, but they must be used each and every time. Adolescents should *never* have intercourse without a condom, no matter what other method of contraception is used.

CHOOSING A SEXUAL PARTNER

Another safer sex precaution is the selection of a sexual partner. Teenagers may be shy or hesitant to ask a new partner about condom use, infections, or number of previous sexual partners. Such reluctance is normal and natural. A teenager enjoys the attention of a new boyfriend or girlfriend and fears losing it by asking intimate questions. But questioning does not have to sound like an inquisition. If phrased honestly and in a tone that promotes mutual benefit ("We need to know something about each other before we start this . . ."), the discussion can promote understanding and trust. A teenager who senses that a partner is being dishonest or secretive still has time to avoid exposure and decrease the risk of infection.

Low-risk sexual activities are preferable with new or unknown partners. Low-risk refers to avoiding exposure to bodily fluids (semen, blood, mucus). High-risk sexual activities include any unprotected vaginal intercourse, anal intercourse, and oral-genital contact.

NUMBER OF PARTNERS

Limiting the number of sexual partners reduces the risk of getting an STD. The ideal is no sexual intercourse or sex with one partner who is completely faithful and has had no sexual activity with anyone else. Such an exclusive (or monogamous) relationship may last three months, six months, or a year, but it is safer than having sexual contact with several people over the same period.

The term "serial monogamy" refers to a series of one-partner relationships. After one relationship ends, a new one may begin with someone else, but it also is a monogamous relationship. Sexually active teenagers commonly are monogamous at any given time. But, because they begin their relationships at a young age, they often have had more than one partner by the time they reach adulthood. The more partners over a lifetime, the higher the risk of STDs.

LOOKING FOR SIGNS OF INFECTION

Sexually active teenagers should check their bodies often for signs of infection. Sexually active females should have routine gynecologic examinations, with cultures from the cervix every six months and a test for cervical cancer (Pap smear) every year. Sexually active males should have regular examinations, with cultures from the tip of the penis every six to twelve months. If symptoms of an STD develop, sexual activity should stop completely until the cause has been diagnosed and treated. The disappearance of symptoms without treatment does *not* mean that the infection is gone. A doctor *always* should be consulted, even if the symptoms go away. Remember that STDs travel together; where there is one STD, there is risk of another.

Signs and Symptoms

STDs can have many different signs and symptoms. In males and females, there may be sores, bumps, blisters, or growths on the genitals, lips, mouth, throat, or rectum. Rashes may appear anywhere on the body. Lymph nodes ("glands") in the groin, neck, or under the arms may enlarge and become tender. Fever, itching in the genital area, or burning on urination are other signs. Joints can become achy or swollen. In males, there may be a discharge from the penis. In females, there may be a vaginal discharge, irregular bleeding from the vagina, or pain during intercourse.

PELVIC INFLAMMATORY DISEASE

One of the most common and serious symptoms associated with STDs in females is abdominal pain. This may indicate that the infection, usually from gonorrhea or chlamydia (see below), has spread through the uterus and into the fallopian tubes, causing "pelvic inflammatory disease" (PID). Women with PID face severe illness in the short term and the risk of infertility and chronic pain in the long term.

The infection that causes PID can be treated with antibiotics, but the inflammation can lead to permanent scarring of the fallopian tubes. This may prevent fertilization of the egg or may block passage of the fertilized egg to the uterus. If the fertilized egg begins to develop outside the uterus, an "ectopic pregnancy" results. The developing fetus cannot survive, and the resulting miscarriage can be life-threatening for the mother.

The symptoms of acute PID include lower abdominal pain, vaginal discharge, fever, irregular vaginal bleeding, nausea, vomiting, and diarrhea. Up to one fifth of women with PID have inflammation around the liver that causes pain in the upper abdomen, right shoulder, or right back. Another 15 to 20 percent may develop a *tubo-*

ovarian abscess (TOA), a collection of pus around the fallopian tube or ovary.

Most teenagers with PID—and all teenagers with TOA—need to be hospitalized for intravenous antibiotic therapy. Even after treatment, over 20 percent of women with PID will experience some ongoing pain; 20 percent will be infertile; 5 percent will have an ectopic pregnancy. With each episode of PID, the risk of a long-term problem increases.

It is essential that all women with PID receive early treatment and complete the prescribed course of antibiotics. A repeat pelvic examination and cultures are done after treatment to be certain that the infection is cured. All sexual partners must be examined and treated, even if they have no symptoms.

VAGINITIS

Inflammation of the vagina with discharge, itching, or pain is called vaginitis. After puberty, vaginitis is usually caused by an infection with yeast (candida), bacteria, or an organism called trichomonas.

Yeast infections of the vagina are *not* related to sexual activity. Some women are more prone to yeast infections than others. The characteristic symptoms of itching, redness, and a thick, white, odorless discharge tend to flare before the menstrual period. Candida vaginitis may be brought on by taking antibiotics or an oral contraceptive. It usually responds quickly to over-the-counter creams or suppositories containing miconazole (Monistat) or clotrimazole (Lotrimin, Mycelex). It is not necessary to take medication by mouth to cure candida vaginitis. If the infection recurs or does not clear up, a doctor should be seen.

Vaginitis caused by bacteria (bacterial vaginosis, or BV) is associated with sexual activity. BV causes a thin, white vaginal discharge that has a foul odor. It is generally treated with an antibiotic called metronidazole (Flagyl) that is taken by mouth. Vaginal creams and suppositories usually are ineffective.

Vaginitis caused by *Trichomonas vaginalis* is associated with sexual activity. In most men and half of women, the infection causes no symptoms, goes untreated, and consequently spreads quickly. Many women with trichomonas vaginitis eventually develop a malodorous, yellow vaginal discharge with redness and itching of the vagina. Trichomonas, like BV, is treated with metronidazole (Flagyl) taken by mouth. All sexual partners must be treated, even if they have no symptoms.

CYSTITIS

Sexual activity increases the risk of infections of the urinary bladder (cystitis) in females (Chapter 30). The symptoms usually appear within twenty-four hours of sexual intercourse and include burning or pain on urination, urinary frequency or urgency, and urine that is bloody, cloudy, or foul smelling. The infection is caused by bacteria and is treated with antibiotics. Cystitis should be treated immediately because the pain can become severe and the infection can spread to the kidneys. Sexual partners do not require treatment.

An adolescent with recurrent cystitis after intercourse should remember to urinate before and after intercourse. She should avoid using a diaphragm, which may be associated with cystitis. If the episodes persist, some physicians suggest a single tablet of a low-dose antibiotic immediately following intercourse or a three- to six-month trial of a daily antibiotic.

URETHRITIS

Infections of the male urethra, the tube leading through the penis (Chapter 15, Figure 15.1), usually are caused by STDs. The most common infections are gonnorrhea and chlamydia, but urethritis can also be caused by trichomonas, herpes, and yeast. The symptoms of urethritis include pain on urination, discharge from the penis, redness at the tip of the penis, and sometimes swelling of the lymph nodes in the groin. Early diagnosis and treatment are imperative because the infection spreads rapidly to sexual partners, male or female. The acute symptoms may disappear without treatment, but the infection remains, will spread, and can cause long-term complications in the male, such as scar tissue in the urethra, infections in the epididymis (epididymitis, Chapter 18), and spread of gonorrhea through the bloodstream. The specific treatment depends on the cause of the infection. Usually antibiotics by mouth or injection are necessary.

Some Common STDs

The most prominent STDs have changed over the course of the twentieth century. In the early and mid-1900s, textbooks referred mostly to gonorrhea and syphilis. By the 1980s, attention focused on three STDs caused by viruses: HIV (Chapter 22), genital herpes simplex virus (HSV), and human papilloma virus (HPV). Gonorrhea remains very common, but *Chlamydia trachomatis* infection has become an even more prevalent bacterial STD. Syphilis declined during the early 1980s, but in 1985 began a rapid climb that doubled its prevalence in some groups of adolescents. The result for American teenagers is an epidemic of STDs—some new, some old, but all dangerous and frightening.

CHLAMYDIA

Chlamydia trachomatis infection is the most common STD caused by bacteria. It is two to three times as prevalent as gonorrhea and affects 8 to 35 percent of sexually active teenagers. Adolescent females are at particularly high risk of infection with chlamydia because of the immaturity of the cells lining the vagina and cervix. About half of all infected teenagers have no symptoms and remain untreated unless routine screening tests are done. These test include swabs from the female cervix or male urethra that are then sent to the laboratory for culture or special stains.

When chlamydia does cause symptoms, different parts of the body may be involved. In males, it can cause urethritis (see above), epididymitis, and prostatitis (Chapter 18). In females, chlamydia can cause cervicitis (inflammation of the cervix), PID, and TOA (see above). After anal intercourse, chlamydia can cause rectal pain and discharge. After oral–genital intercourse, it can cause pain and inflammation of the throat. Chlamydia also is associated with inflammation of the area around the liver and can result in pain of the right upper abdomen, back, or shoulder. Joint pain and swelling (arthritis, Chapter 31) and redness and discharge from the eyes (conjunctivitis, Chapter 25) also are associated with chlamydia.

The long-term complications of chlamydia in females include chronic pelvic pain, infertility, and ectopic pregnancy. Chlamydia is associated with chronic arthritis in 2 percent of males. Babies born to infected mothers can have severe conjunctivitis and pneumonia.

Chlamydia infections are treated with an oral antibiotic such as doxycycline, tetracycline, or erythromycin for seven to fourteen days. All sexual partners should be treated.

GONORRHEA

Gonorrhea is caused by a bacteria called *Neisseria gonorrhoeae*. The highest rates of gonorrhea occur in females aged fifteen to nineteen and males aged twenty to twenty-four. Simultaneous infection with chlamydia is common in both females and males. Like chlamydia, gonorrhea is spread through sexual contact. In females, it can involve the cervix, uterus, fallopian tubes, and liver. In males, it can infect the urethra, epididymis and prostate. In both males and females, gonorrhea can infect the rectum, throat, skin, joints, blood, and brain. Infants born to infected mothers may have severe conjunctivitis (Chapter 25).

Gonorrhea is more likely than chlamydia to produce symptoms in males. Ninety-five percent of infected males develop a yellow discharge from the urethra, often with pain on urination. If untreated, the symptoms eventually disappear, but the infection persists. Fifty percent of females with gonorrhea, like chlamydia, have no symptoms. It is very important that all sexually active adolescents, whether or not they have symptoms, have regular screening examinations for gonorrhea. The diagnosis usually is made by culture of the bacteria from a swab taken from the cervix or the male urethra.

The most common complication of gonorrhea is PID (see above), with subsequent risks of liver inflammation, tubo-ovarian abscess, chronic pain, infertility, and ectopic pregnancy. Another complication that develops in one percent of infected males and females is *disseminated gonococcal infection (DGI)*. The bacteria spread through the bloodstream to infect distant sites, such as the skin or joints. The symptoms of DGI include fever, chills, joint aching or swelling, and painful skin lesions or sores. Rarely, DGI may involve the spinal cord, brain, or heart.

Gonococcal infections are treated with antibiotics. Some infections, such as urethritis or cervicitis, are treated with a single injection of an antibiotic or with an antibiotic taken by mouth. Others, such as PID or DGI, may require hospitalization and intravenous antibiotics. In *all* types of gonococcal infections, cultures should be repeated after treatment to be certain of a cure. All sexual partners must be evaluated and treated.

HERPES

Up to twenty million Americans are infected with genital herpes, and an additional half million new cases are reported each year. In some people, infection produces no symptoms—they harbor the virus in an inactive state for years or even a lifetime. Only the active state produces symptoms and spread of the virus.

Herpes is actually a family of viruses that cause different types of infections. Genital herpes always is transmitted sexually and usually is caused by herpes simplex virus (HSV) type 2. Oral herpes usually is *not* transmitted sexually and is caused by HSV type 1. The characteristic signs of oral herpes are cold sores of the mouth or lips.

The signs of genital herpes include sores or blisters of the cervix, vagina, or penis; vaginal or penile discharge; painful urination; fever and fatigue; and swollen glands in the groin area. Some people describe unusual shooting pains in the pelvic area beginning two or three days before the other symptoms.

Genital herpes is transmitted mainly through sexual contact, but the virus has been found to live for some time on inanimate objects, such as towels, toilet seats, or bed linens. Herpes is spread through direct contact. It can be passed from mouth to genitals by way of the hands or oral sex, but the virus cannot spread through the bloodstream from a cold sore in the mouth to the genitals.

If there are signs of active genital herpes, it is important to abstain from sexual activity until the sores are totally healed (usually three to four weeks for a first attack and one to two weeks for a recurrent attack). Strict hygienic measures can prevent the spread of the virus. Do not use the same towel, wash hands after touching the genital area, and maintain personal cleanliness. When sexual activity does resume, always use condoms with spermicides. If transmission from one person to another does occur, the first signs appear within two to twenty days. As mentioned above, though, many people have no symptoms and do not know that they are infected.

Herpes is particularly dangerous to newborn babies. It can damage the nervous system, internal organs, skin, and eyes. If a pregnant woman has herpes sores at the time of delivery, the baby can become infected as it passes through the vagina. To prevent this possibility, the baby is usually delivered through a surgical incision in the abdomen (cesarean section). After the birth, the new mother must wash her hands frequently and take extra precautions to minimize the chance of infecting the baby.

At the present time, there is no cure or vaccine for genital or oral herpes. Pain and itching can be relieved by ointments, pain relievers, or warm baths. A doctor may prescribe an oral or topical (applied to the skin) medication called acyclovir (Zovirax) to accelerate healing during a first attack. The medication helps less during recurrent episodes and must be started early to have any effect. When an episode ends and the sores heal, the herpes virus does not disappear. The virus retreats to nerve tissue where it remains dormant until some stress—physical or emotional—reactivates it.

GENITAL HUMAN PAPILLOMA VIRUS (HPV)

The most commonly recognized sign of infection with HPV is genital warts, or painless growths in the genital area. HPV also causes lesions that can only be seen with special techniques. These invisible lesions can develop on the vagina or cervix, penis, or rectum. HPV infection in females often is detected on the Pap test (Chapter 3). All patients with persistently abnormal Pap tests should have culposcopy, an office procedure that includes a magnified examination of the cervix and a biopsy of any abnormal-appearing area.

Over sixty different types of HPV exist. About twenty types have been associated with genital infections and five types with cancer of the cervix. Given the high rates of HPV infection among teenagers, it is essential that all sexually active girls have Pap smears performed yearly—and more frequently if an abnormality is found.

The treatment of HPV infection depends on the location and extent of disease. None of the treatments are self-administered. All require visits to a clinic or doctor's office. Genital warts can be treated with medications that are applied to the skin with a swab. When this does not work, other types of therapy, such as freezing the wart (cryotherapy) or laser removal can be tried. The goal of all forms of treatment is cure, or complete eradication of the virus.

SYPHILIS

During the 1980s the incidence of syphilis increased dramatically among many groups of sexually active teenagers. The organism that causes syphilis, *Treponema pallidum,* is spread during intercourse, kissing, and touching open, infected sores. The earliest sign of syphilis is a painless ulcer, usually in the genital area, called a chancre. If the infection is untreated, the chancre will disappear within a month. During the next, or secondary, stage of syphilis, other symptoms may appear: a rash anywhere on the body, fever, fatigue, sore throat, swollen glands (especially in the groin), headache, achiness. Without treatment, the secondary stage of syphilis disappears within weeks or months. Many years later, the tertiary (third) stage may develop, with progressive damage to the heart and central nervous system.

Most adolescents with syphilis have no symptoms. When eventually diagnosed, the discovery usually is made by a routine screening blood test (called VDRL or RPR). If one of these tests is positive, a second blood test (FTA-ABS or MHA-TP) is done to confirm it. Syphilis in teenagers is treated with either penicillin by injection or with doxycycline or tetracycline by mouth. After treatment, blood tests must be repeated every three months to prove cure. All sexual contacts must be evaluated and treated.

Treating STDs

Whenever symptoms of STDs appear, medical attention should be sought immediately. Depending on the type of STD, a physician may prescribe a particular course of antibiotics. But treatment of STDs is more complicated than simply taking medication. Compliance with the prescription and follow-up is essential to cure the infection. Some teenagers who have side effects, such as stomach upset or nausea, may stop taking their medication. This will not cure the STD. Complete compliance—taking the entire course of medication as prescribed—is crucial. If side effects are bothersome, the medication can be taken with food rather than on an empty stomach. If symptoms persist, or if teenagers have questions about the medication, they should contact their doctor or nurse. If instructions are not clear, they should be reviewed and explained.

Treatment of an STD involves more than one individual. When one person has an STD, all sexual partners are at risk. Even if they have no symptoms, all partners must be evaluated and usually treated. STDs are very serious. Teenagers cannot allow embarrassment to get in the way of treatment.

While on medication for an STD, adolescents must abstain from all sexual activity. The doctor or nurse will explain how long the treatment will last and when a follow-up examination will take place. Once the STD is cured, the teenager needs to be even more cautious, protective, and aware of safer sex behaviors.

22

HIV and AIDS

Enormous public attention and medical research have focused on the AIDS epidemic. Within a decade, AIDS became the leading cause of death among people between the ages of seventeen and fifty-five. By the early 1990s, AIDS cases among adolescents were increasing at a rate of over 75 percent every two years.

Even more alarming than the number of teenagers with AIDS is the number of teenagers infected with the AIDS-causing virus. That virus—HIV—can take years to ravage the body's cells. During the time between infection and illness, young people may not know that they carry HIV. Many adults who die today from AIDS were infected with HIV in their teens. Many teenagers who are infected today with HIV may die of AIDS as young adults.

The major causes of HIV infection in the 1990s are two specific risk behaviors: unprotected sexual intercourse and intravenous drug use. Teenagers *must* understand the facts in order to prevent HIV/AIDS and save lives. To begin, some basic information:

AIDS starts with a specific virus: *HIV, the human immunodeficiency virus.* A *virus* is an infectious organism that lives and reproduces in host cells. Many viruses are easily defeated by the *immune system,* the body's defense mechanism against harmful microorganisms. The cells of the immune system produce *antibodies,* or protein molecules that recognize and counteract foreign molecules.

The body reacts to HIV differently than it does to other viruses. Infections such as the common cold, flu, or chicken pox are suc-

260

cessfully conquered by a healthy immune system. HIV, over time, destroys the immune system, leaving the body unable to fight other infections and cancers. Once HIV invades the body's cells, it remains there for life.

HIV is the organism that causes *AIDS*, the *acquired immunodeficiency syndrome*. AIDS is "acquired" from someone else and it renders the "immune" system "deficient," or unable to fight disease. As a "syndrome," it is a cluster of different conditions and diseases that eventually are fatal. The average time between HIV infection and the development of AIDS is over ten years. Three of ten people with HIV, though, develop AIDS within five years.

People infected with HIV who have no symptoms are said to be asymptomatic. They look and feel healthy. There are many more people with asymptomatic HIV infection than with AIDS. Asymptomatic individuals with HIV may not know they carry the virus and, therefore, do not recognize that they can give it to someone else.

AIDS was first described in 1981, and HIV was isolated in 1983. Since then, the number of cases has skyrocketed among homosexual men, intravenous drug users, heterosexual men and women, and newborn babies. Estimates about the number of HIV-infected people change constantly, but one fact remains constant: HIV/ AIDS is an equal opportunity disease. It shows no gender, age, ethnic, or geographic discrimination. Anyone can get it.

Young people between the ages of sixteen and twenty-eight are at the highest risk for HIV infection. One fifth of people with AIDS are in their twenties. Teenagers infected with HIV tend to be asymtomatic longer than older people, meaning that they have more time to transmit the infection before symptoms lead them to diagnosis and recognition.

How HIV Is Spread

Specific *behaviors* put people at risk for HIV and AIDS, not the "groups" to which they belong. Being a homosexual male, for example, does not mean one has or will acquire HIV. The virus survives in and is transmitted by blood, semen, or vaginal fluids. Behaviors involving the exchange of infected blood or semen can transmit HIV. There is no evidence that HIV is spread through other body fluids such as tears, saliva, or urine. HIV is transmitted in the following ways:

• Vaginal, anal, or oral intercourse, both heterosexual and homosexual, without the protection of condoms, and sometimes even when condoms are used.

• Sharing needles or syringes during drug use, including body-building steroids. It is not possible to get HIV if a brand-new, sterilized needle and syringe is used every time drugs are injected. The risk comes from using the same needle or syringe that has been used previously by someone with HIV.

• Tattooing or body-piercing (ears, nose, and elsewhere). HIV can be transmitted through these routes, but only if the needle or syringe was used previously on an HIV-infected individual. Tattooing presents an especially high risk because tattoo dye needles are injected into the skin many times, increasing the chance that the virus will enter the body if the needle is contaminated.

• Transmission from mother to child before or during birth.

• Transfusion of blood or blood products prior to 1985, when routine HIV testing of transfusion products began in the United States.

• Transmission to health care workers who have accidentally stuck themselves with needles previously used on patients infected with HIV.

Sexual intercourse is the primary method of HIV spread from one person to another. If HIV is in a male's semen or in a female's vaginal fluids, the infection can be passed to a partner during intercourse. Oral sex is less likely to spread HIV, but it is possible.

How HIV Is *Not* Spread

It is equally important to understand how the virus is *not* transmitted. During the 1980s, the fear of AIDS led to much misinformation about HIV transmission. The virus is not transmitted by casual, everyday contact. HIV cannot survive in air, water, or on objects that have been touched by someone with HIV. It cannot survive outside the body, and it cannot be spread through unbroken skin.

Specifically, HIV is not spread by:

• shaking hands;
• hugging or dancing;
• sharing food utensils, dishes, or cups;
• using common gym equipment, showers, toilets, water foun-

tains, or swimming pools;
- sharing a room, workspace, or telephone with a person who has HIV;
- coughing and sneezing;
- insects or animals.

The question of kissing is often raised by adolescents. Kissing the face and lips is safe, and even deep tongue, or "French," kissing is a highly *unlikely* route of transmission. Another common question concerns masturbation. HIV is *not* transmitted by self-masturbation. Touching the genitals of a sexual partner is safe if there are no open sores or cuts on the hands.

There is also confusion about blood transfusion. You cannot get HIV by donating (giving) blood. Before 1985, it was possible to get HIV by receiving a blood transfusion. Since 1985, the United States has tested all blood products for HIV. This means that it is nearly impossible today to get HIV from a blood transfusion received in the United States.

Many people who are not HIV-infected worry because they have engaged in risk behaviors. If they are tested and the result is negative, some people wrongly presume that they are immune to the virus and can continue the same high-risk behaviors. Others with negative test results still worry excessively that they might become infected in the future. People who do not know the facts may become so fearful about contracting HIV that they will not use public toilets, water fountains, or restaurants. These fears are both debilitating and unnecessary. Concerns about HIV should be discussed with a doctor, nurse, or experienced counselor. Local health departments and AIDS hotlines also are available to help. (See the end of this chapter and the Resources section at the end of the book.)

Prevention

The only fail-safe way to prevent HIV infection and AIDS is abstinence from sexual intercourse, intravenous drug use, and all needle-sharing. Many young people are abstaining from, or postponing, sexual intercourse. Still others are engaging in "safer sex," or lower-risk sexual activities that do not involve exchange of body fluids.

Adolescents who are having sexual intercourse or oral sex must protect themselves and their partners each and every time they have sex. This means that they must use condoms every time they have vaginal, anal, and oral intercourse. Condoms that are most protective against HIV are made of latex. (Chapter 19 explains the proper use of condoms.)

Every adolescent who is sexually active is responsible for his or her own protection. Four key factors determine an individual's risk of getting HIV:

• Whether a condom is used each time intercourse occurs. If a teenager has vaginal intercourse just once with an infected partner, the chance of becoming infected is at least ten times greater when a condom is not used than when one is used correctly.

• The total number of sexual contacts the individual and the current partner have had. The more partners, the greater the danger of contracting HIV. A 1990 national survey by the Centers for Disease Control found that 19 percent of all high school students reported four or more sex partners. Among seniors, the number increased to 29 percent.

• The likelihood of HIV infection in the sexual contact. It is far more dangerous to have unprotected sexual intercourse with someone who has engaged in high-risk behaviors than with a partner who has not. For example, it is very risky to have sex with someone who uses—or has ever used—intravenous drugs.

• The type of sexual activity. Anal intercourse is the most risky. Oral intercourse is less risky than vaginal intercourse. Kissing is nearly zero risk. Hugging and touching are zero risk.

Adolescents who are involved in monogamous sexual relationships often wonder if they need to use condoms. The answer is yes. Monogamous means a long-term relationship with only one sexual partner. If neither partner has ever injected drugs or engaged in high-risk sexual behaviors, the monogamous couple has a low risk of HIV. Condoms should still be used, though, because one breach of monogamy places both teenagers at risk.

The only form of contraception that usually protects against HIV and other STDs is the condom. *All* other forms *must* be used with the condom. Sexual intercourse without a condom is high-risk behavior, no matter what else is done. Withdrawal before ejaculation does not protect against HIV. Douching after intercourse does not protect against HIV. Asking your partner about testing does not protect against HIV. Some partners with HIV do not answer truthfully. Others who have no symptoms may not know they are infected.

HIV is spread very easily through intravenous drug use. Adolescents who are unable to stop shooting drugs must use brand-new needles and syringes (still in the original wrappers). If drug use continues with used needles and syringes, they should be cleaned twice with bleach and then flushed twice with clean, boiled water. Holding a needle over a lighted match or boiling the equipment in water are ineffective methods.

HIV Testing

There is no single, universal test that is used to detect and confirm HIV infection. Most of the available tests are blood tests. Some can give false results. Some are done to confirm other tests. The currently used tests include:

The EIA (enzyme immunoassay) test identifies HIV by detecting antibodies to the virus. This test is highly sensitive, meaning that it picks up all people with HIV if it is done long enough after the infection is contracted. It can take up to three months for the body to make enough antibodies against HIV to be detected by the test. A positive test should always be repeated to confirm that it is correct. If the duplicate EIA test is positive, a confirming test should still be done.

The Western blot test is more specific than the EIA and is used to confirm the presence of HIV antibodies. An inconclusive Western blot test is repeated every few weeks for several months because the concentration of antibodies tends to increase over time.

PCR (polymerase chain reaction) detects very tiny amounts of the HIV genetic material that are present soon after infection. It becomes positive before the EIA or Western blot tests.

Antigen tests screen for HIV antigen and may be positive weeks before antibody tests. Different types of antigen tests represent different parts of the virus. The most common antigen test is called the p24. A positive p24 result can be a poor prognostic sign, indicating more rapid progression to AIDS.

HIV culture is a sensitive, specific method of confirming HIV infection. The virus is grown in the laboratory from samples of infected cells or body fluids. The test is time-consuming, expensive, and not widely available.

Deciding to Test

When teenagers suspect HIV, they face difficult decisions about whether and where to go for testing. The test itself is a simple procedure. The decision to have the test done can be very complex. Before being tested, teenagers should seek counseling and ask questions. The issues to consider include consent, confidentiality, the pros and cons of knowing the test result, and where to turn if the result is positive.

The legal rights of minors regarding HIV testing vary from state to state. All states have provisions that allow minors to consent to diagnosis and treatment of sexually transmitted diseases. Some states have specific laws about consent for HIV testing; most do not. Laws governing the confidentiality of an HIV test result also vary from state to state. Chapter 10 discusses these issues in more detail, but the bottom line is that teenagers should talk with knowledgeable HIV/AIDS counselors before screening tests are done.

Some teenagers who have engaged in high-risk behaviors do not want to be tested for HIV infection. They may fear a positive result and the prospect of a fatal illness. They may minimize the possibility of a positive result because they have no symptoms. They may think that they cannot or will not change their behavior regardless of the test result. They may think that a positive result will bring rejection by family and friends. They may be reluctant to go to their family doctor and may not know of a free, convenient, confidential testing center. Once they find a testing center that they trust, many high-risk adolescents do proceed with testing. Many clinics will protect the teenager's right to privacy. It is far better, though, to involve a supportive parent or other adult both before and after the test is done.

The reasons to test—or not to test—should be considered carefully. Knowing the result may be better than the anxiety and fear of not knowing. If the result is negative, teenagers not only will be relieved, but hopefully will avoid future risk behaviors. If the result is positive, they can make informed decisions about their future sexual relationships and can tell past sex partners of their risk of infection. A positive result also can mean early medical care that may prolong the time before the development of AIDS. Physicians and testing centers should always provide extensive counseling when the test result is positive. This helps the teenager understand the options for treatment and provides an important source of emotional support during a difficult time.

Where to Go for Testing

AIDS hotline numbers and agencies are listed in the Resources section at the end of the book. A local telephone directory or information operator usually can provide the phone numbers of local and state health departments that are knowledgeable about HIV testing. Public health departments can recommend reliable testing facilities. Hospitals and public testing sites generally should be used because some private agencies do not meet federally approved standards for HIV test procedures. Kits for home tests are unreliable and should not be used.

When making the first phone call, teenagers should give their age and ask several questions, such as: Will a parent have to accompany me? give permission for the test? be told of the result? Is the testing free? If not, how much will it cost? Will a bill be sent in the mail? Will the test result go in my medical record? Is it sent to my parents? their insurance company? my school? my sexual partner? my family doctor? Do you have counselors to help me talk to my sexual partner and my parents? How and when will I be told of the test result? Is the testing anonymous (meaning that a person's name is not used to label the test)?

Counseling

Both before and after testing, a counselor should explain the procedures and potential results, including the possibility of false or inconclusive results. If the teenager is unsure about having a test, the counselor can review the pros and cons. The counselor also can help the teenager make plans about what to do after the result is in, whether it is positive or negative.

After testing, a counselor should provide the test result in person, even if it is negative. Counseling sessions should allow teenagers ample opportunity to express their feelings, ask questions, review their understanding of risk behaviors and HIV transmission, and learn about the next steps in seeking preventive care, medical treatment, and emotional support.

The Test Result

A positive result means HIV infection is present in nearly 100 percent of cases. It does *not* mean AIDS. In fact, most people do not have AIDS at the time of testing. There is no way to predict exactly when AIDS will develop in someone who is HIV positive. For some, it may take six months; for others, three to five years; for still others, over ten years. The longer one has HIV, however, the sooner AIDS is likely to appear.

A false-positive test result, meaning that the test is positive in someone without HIV, occurs in less than 1 percent of cases. The improved methods of testing have made false-positive results exceedingly rare. A positive test result should be questioned if the teenager has absolutely no risk factors for HIV. Remember that even one episode of unprotected sexual intercourse constitutes a risk factor.

A false-negative result, meaning that the test is negative in someone with HIV, can occur soon after infection, before there are measurable levels of antibodies or antigens. The time between infection and a positive test result may be as short as two weeks or as long as six months. If a teenager has engaged in *no* high-risk behaviors in the six months before testing, a negative result is correct. Occasionally a test result is called inconclusive. Another blood sample should be collected and the test should be repeated.

A true-negative result, meaning that the adolescent does not have HIV, provides an opportunity to reconsider the behaviors that may have led to the testing. A teenager who had unprotected sex or injected drugs cannot afford to let a negative test become an excuse to continue the behavior. A negative result should be a new beginning. If risky behaviors continue, testing should be repeated at three- to six-month intervals.

A true-positive result means that HIV infection is present. The only exception is an infant who can have HIV antibodies from an infected mother but is not actually infected with the virus itself. Over time, the antibodies will clear and the baby will have a negative test. As difficult as it is to accept a positive test result, the teenager must seek early medical care and emotional support.

Where to Turn and What to Do If the Test Is Positive

Many people—teenagers and adults—initially deny that they are infected when an HIV test is positive. Temporary denial is a normal way to deal with the feelings of powerlessness, fear, and anger.

Prolonged denial can have serious consequences, such as delayed treatment and continued behaviors that place others at risk.

A counselor can help the teenager and family cope with the infection and its ramifications. By providing information, a counselor helps the teenager with HIV take some control of events. It is crucial to locate a counselor soon after receiving the test result. Test sites have, or can identify, counselors trained in helping HIV-infected adolescents. A good counselor can put the teenager and family in touch with other services and support groups.

The question "Who do I tell?" is one of the first thoughts to arise after a positive test result. For most teenagers, the answer is parents. Some adolescents find it easier to have the counselor present when the parents are told; others may prefer that the counselor tell the parents alone, with the teenager out of the room. Adolescents who are unable to tell a parent must confide in an understanding adult who can help them address difficult questions and decisions. Parents or other adults who are told should be given the name and phone number of the doctor or counselor who has been involved in the testing. This gives them an opportunity to ask questions and seek emotional support.

A teenager with HIV also faces the challenge of telling sexual partners or those with whom needles were shared. If the teenager is unwilling to tell these people directly, a health professional can be asked to do so without revealing the teenager's identity.

Once family and past sexual or drug contacts are informed, the adolescent has to decide whom else to tell at school, work, or within the community. One consideration in this decision is the fact that many people still do not understand the facts about HIV and may be fearful or distant toward someone with the infection. It is useful to discuss legal rights with someone familiar with state laws about HIV and AIDS. Local Civil Liberties Union branches, Legal Aid Societies, and AIDS hotlines can provide assistance about legal rights. It is illegal to discriminate against people with HIV or AIDS. They cannot be fired as long as they can perform their jobs. They cannot be denied housing or medical services.

The issue of school attendance can be complex. No law guarantees HIV-infected students a place in school. The Centers for Disease Control suggests that they be allowed to stay in school as long as they pose no risk to other students. Most states and localities agree with this policy, but many communities have committees to consider individual circumstances.

Although much fear, bias, and misinformation about HIV still exists, public understanding is increasing. It can be helpful and reassuring to confide in someone at school (a nurse, counselor, or teacher) because there will be times when classes must be missed for doctors' appointments or illness.

Protecting others is very important. A teenager with HIV should:

- inform sexual partners;
- abstain from sexual intercourse or always use condoms;
- use backup contraceptive methods to prevent an unplanned pregnancy that could put an infant at risk of HIV and AIDS;
- never donate blood, sperm, or any body organ;
- never share drug needles and syringes.

Teenagers with HIV, their families, and friends often worry about accidental bleeding from even the smallest cut. The risk to others is exceedingly small. Clean the soiled clothing or objects by dry cleaning or with soap and water followed by a solution of one-half cup household bleach and four and a half cups of water. Then wash the hands thoroughly with soap and running water.

After a positive test, a teenager who feels perfectly strong and healthy may see no need to seek medical care. Even when there are no symptoms, a doctor should be seen as soon as possible because early care can prolong health. If a teenager does not want to see the family doctor, the testing center can provide names of local physicians, clinics, or hospitals with experience in caring for young people with HIV.

The importance of establishing continous health care cannot be overemphasized. Some of the reasons include:

- HIV makes the body more vulnerable to both common and uncommon infections and illnesses. Some can be prevented. Others require early diagnosis and special or more prolonged treatment.

- As new medical treatments become available, a doctor may prescribe them in an attempt to postpone AIDS and prolong life.

Medical Treatment of HIV Infection

When a teenager with a new diagnosis of HIV is first examined, a physician will do a full health screening with particular attention to the medical history. The doctor will ask about past sexual contacts, drug and alcohol use, and blood transfusions prior to 1985. A history of sexually transmitted diseases, viral and bacterial infections, pneumonia, or persistent diarrhea is important because these illnesses may indicate problems with the immune system. The doctor also will ask about more generalized symptoms such as fever, weight loss, fatigue, rashes, headaches, vision changes, abdominal pain, and vaginal discharge or abnormal bleeding.

The physical examination will provide information about lung and heart function, body weight, and the size of the lymph nodes, liver, and spleen. The genital area and rectum will be examined for signs of STDs. In females, a pelvic examination and Pap smear (Chapter 3) will be done. A stool sample will be examined for blood. The physician will also look for specific signs that may indicate a decline in immune function, such as skin or mouth sores, plaques on the sides of the tongue, and fungus infections of the mouth and throat.

During the course of HIV infection, up to 80 percent of people develop some neurologic or psychiatric problems. A baseline examination of the brain and nervous system (Chapter 32) therefore is important. The doctor will check sensation, muscle strength, reflexes, and coordination. Questions will be asked to test memory, orientation, judgment, and concentration skills.

Diagnostic tests are done to measure the status or progression of HIV, to determine when to begin treatment, and to monitor the response to treatment. Blood tests are done to measure cell counts, assess liver function, and detect hepatitis and syphilis. A skin test will be done for past tuberculosis exposure and, if it is positive, a chest X-ray will be done (Chapter 27). Many doctors also will order a blood test for past exposure to toxoplasma, a parasitic infection carried by cats or in undercooked meat. Up to 40 percent of healthy, HIV-negative adolescents have positive tests for toxoplasma, but the infection poses no risk to them. Past infection does pose a risk to the HIV-positive person, though. A positive test in an adolescent with HIV may lead to the prescription of medication that will protect against reactivation of the toxoplasma.

Another blood test, called the CD4+ lymphocyte count, is used to predict the risk of "opportunistic" infections, which take advantage of a weakened immune system. The CD4+ count measures the number of helper T cells, which are white blood cells that help fight infections and tumors. As the CD4+ count drops, the chance of opportunistic infections increases. Teenagers should understand, though, that there is variability between measurements of the

CD4+ count. It changes over the course of the day, and it can decrease transiently after minor illnesses such as the common cold. The count, therefore, should be used as a guide, not as the only determining factor of prognosis or treatment.

ANTIVIRAL MEDICATIONS

Throughout the 1980s, adolescents were not included in clinical trials that led to treatment of HIV with antiviral medications. The treatment recommendations for adolescents with HIV infection and AIDS therefore generally follow the standards of care for adults. In 1992, several clinical trial sites were funded to enroll teenagers over age thirteen. Information specific to teens will become available as these trials are completed.

Antiviral medications block the replication of HIV in human cells and slow the progression of infection. HIV progresses by replicating itself in host cells of the human body. The virus inserts copies of its own genetic material into the cells of the immune system, weakening their ability to fight infection. During its long latency period, HIV can change its own structure to protect itself against antiviral medications. Presently, there is no vaccine to prevent HIV infection, and there is no cure that eradicates the virus after infection. Current treatment therefore attempts to slow the progression of HIV by decreasing its ability to replicate within the cells.

The most widely used drug for HIV infection is referred to by many names: zidovudine, ZDV, azidothymidine, AZT, and Retrovir. The most accurate name is zidovudine. Even before symptoms appear, it is given to people with HIV infection whose CD4+ counts fall to 500 or less. It may also be given to people with higher counts who develop symptoms associated with the infection. In many cases, zidovudine will result in an increase in the CD4+ count.

Zidovudine controls the virus but does not cure it. There are problems associated with its use, including side effects, cost, and resistance to its effect. The standard dose of zidovudine is 500 mg daily, or 100 mg five times daily. When teenagers begin zidovudine, they are checked by a doctor every two weeks for three months and then every one to three months. During the first few weeks of treatment, many people experience nausea, difficulty sleeping, or headaches; usually these symptoms diminish with time. A serious side effect that may require decreased dosage, or even discontinuation of the medication, is suppression of the bone marrow. This suppression causes low blood cell counts. People on zidovudine should have complete blood counts checked within one month of starting the medication and then every three months.

Another medication, dideoxyinosine (ddI) is related to zidovudine. It is used when HIV is progressing despite zidovudine treatment or when the side effects of zidovudine are intolerable. The side effects of ddI include headache, diarrhea, trouble sleeping, abdominal pain due to pancreatitis (inflammation of the pancreas), and numbness and tingling of the arms or legs.

Dideoxycytidine (ddC) is another drug that inhibits HIV replication and is an alternative to zidovudine or ddI. It also has side effects, including rash, fever, and numbness of the arms or legs.

PREVENTING OPPORTUNISTIC INFECTIONS

Opportunistic infections that are rare among healthy people take hold aggressively when someone is infected with HIV. Several medications are used to prevent these infections from the beginning.

The most common opportunistic infection of people with HIV is *Pneumocystis carinii pneumonia (PCP)*, a severe parasitic infection of the lungs. PCP can be prevented by consistent use of oral co-trimoxazole, trimethoprim-sulfamethoxazole (Bactrim, Septra), aerosolized pentamidine, and oral dapsone. PCP was the major cause of death in people with HIV until preventive treatment became a routine part of management.

Immunizations are important for people with HIV to prevent bacterial and other viral infections. There is no evidence that vaccination causes any further weakening of the immune system. Teenagers with HIV should ask their family doctor if their childhood immunizations are up to date. They should be fully immunized against pneumococcus, influenza, hepatitis B, polio, diphtheria/tetanus, measles, and *Haemophilus influenzae*.

Females with HIV face special problems and require regular examinations to prevent infection. They tend to be diagnosed later than men or children and, therefore, may have more advanced disease. Gynecological infections, such as vaginal candidiasis and pelvic inflammatory disease (PID, Chapter 21), can be severe and difficult to treat in women with HIV. The prevalence of human papilloma virus (HPV) and abnormal Pap tests (Chapter 21) are significantly increased in females with HIV. Pelvic examinations and Pap tests therefore should be done twice yearly in teenagers with HIV.

If a female with HIV is pregnant, she may transmit the infection to her infant. There is a 20 to 40 percent chance that the baby will become infected during pregnancy or delivery or through breast milk. Pregnancy does not affect the progression of the mother's HIV infection, nor will the pregnancy be at risk of complications because of HIV. A baby infected with HIV, though, probably will die of AIDS at a young age. The young mother, also infected with HIV, may not live to care for her ailing child.

Acquired Immunodeficiency Syndrome (AIDS)

Most people with HIV infection do not have AIDS. Even symptoms such as fatigue, skin rashes, and weight loss do not necessarily mean AIDS. Specific criteria, defined by the federal Centers for Disease Control, must be met for a diagnosis of AIDS. These "AIDS-defining conditions" are not caused by HIV per se, but by opportunistic infections and diseases that take advantage of the body's immune deficiency. The conditions primarily affect the lungs, digestive tract, brain and nervous system, skin, and eyes.

LUNG CONDITIONS

Fever, cough, and shortness of breath are worrisome symptoms in someone with HIV. Immediate evaluation by a physician is *essential.* The evaluation may include a thorough history, physical examination, chest X-ray, measurement of oxygen in the blood, and cultures of the sputum (or phlegm). In some cases, bronchoscopy (Chapter 27) will be done to diagnose the exact cause of the lung problem. A correct diagnosis is very important for both treatment and prognosis. If PCP is discovered, the adolescent meets criteria for AIDS. Bacterial or viral pneumonia on the other hand, does not necessarily mean AIDS.

PCP usually requires hospitalization and treatment with intravenous trimethoprim/sulfamethoxazole or pentamidine. If the pneumonia is very severe, corticosteroids also are given to decrease lung inflammation. If the pneumonia is very mild, the adolescent may be treated at home with high-dose oral trimethoprim/sulfamethoxazole, oral dapsone, or aerosolized pentamidine. After the

PCP is cured, the adolescent must remain on lifelong medication to prevent recurrent infection.

Tuberculosis is another common and very serious lung infection in people with HIV. Unlike PCP, tuberculosis is not an "AIDS-defining condition." However, HIV-infected individuals, with or without AIDS, are at high risk for a form of tuberculosis that is resistant to many antituberculosis medications. This makes treatment of the tuberculosis difficult and, at times, impossible.

Mycobacterium avium-intracellulare (MAI) is an infection that resembles tuberculosis. When it spreads throughout the body in someone with HIV, it is considered an AIDS-defining condition. MAI is extremely difficult to treat.

Recurrent, severe bacterial pneumonias in people with HIV, especially children and young adolescents, are AIDS-defining illnesses. They are treated with antibiotics, usually in the hospital. Fungal and viral pneumonias also are common in people with HIV, but are not AIDS-defining illnesses unless they spread throughout the body.

DIGESTIVE CONDITIONS

Any part of the gastrointestinal tract, including the liver, may be involved in AIDS. The most common problems are esophagitis, abdominal pain, diarrhea, and poor appetite.

Esophagitis is an inflammation of the esophagus (the food pipe from the throat to the stomach). The symptoms include a burning sensation in the middle of the chest, difficulty or pain on swallowing, and hiccough. The most common cause of esophagitis in someone with HIV is a yeast infection (candida esophagitis). This is an AIDS-defining condition and requires treatment with an antifungal medication such as ketoconazole, fluconazole, or amphotericin B. Other AIDS-defining causes of esophagitis include cytomegalovirus (CMV), which is treated with ganciclovir, and herpes simplex virus (HSV), which is treated with acyclovir.

Diarrhea is a frequent problem for adolescents with AIDS. Common causes of the diarrhea include bacteria such as *Salmonella* or *Shigella,* parasites such as *Giardia* or *Entamoeba*, fungi such as Cryptosporidium, and viruses such as CMV or HSV. The diarrhea is often accompanied by other symptoms, such as cramping, bloody stool, fever, and weight loss. Diarrhea in an adolescent with HIV or AIDS can cause rapid dehydration and malnutrition. A doctor should be contacted immediately.

BRAIN AND NERVOUS SYSTEM CONDITIONS

HIV can cause disease in the brain and nervous system either directly, through its own effects, or indirectly, through opportunistic infections. The symptoms of neurologic disease include persistent headache, lethargy, confusion, change in behavior or personality, unexplained fever, weakness or paralysis of a part of the body, numbness or tingling, burning pain in the legs and feet, and seizures. A teenager with HIV who has any of these symptoms should have a very thorough evaluation by a physician. This may include a lumbar puncture (a needle inserted into the spinal column to withdraw a sample of spinal fluid) and an X-ray or scan of the brain (CT or MRI).

AIDS-related neurologic problems include the following:

• HIV encephalopathy, also called AIDS-related dementia, is a progressive disorder of the brain that causes personality changes, progressive loss of short-term memory, social withdrawal, difficulty speaking, impaired muscle coordination, and seizures. It is important to rule out other treatable causes for these symptoms because HIV encephalopathy has no specific treatment.

• Toxoplasmosis is a parasitic infection that causes a ring-shaped lesion in the brain that can be seen on a CT or MRI scan. It is treated with pyrimethamine for a few weeks and sulfadiazine for life; relapses are common.

• Cryptococcal meningitis is a fungal infection of the lining of the brain that is diagnosed by lumbar puncture. It is treated with antifungal medications given intravenously, such as amphotericin B or fluconazole. After intensive initial therapy, it is necessary to continue lifelong maintenance medication because relapses are common.

• CMV and HSV both can cause infections of the brain. CMV is treated with ganciclovir, and HSV is treated with acyclovir.

• Syphilis should be treated very aggressively in adolescents with HIV or AIDS. Early syphilis in someone with HIV can cause an acute infection of the brain, a problem that is not seen in HIV-negative adolescents. It requires high doses of antibiotics for several weeks.

SKIN CONDITIONS

Rashes, skin lesions, and skin infections often are early indications of HIV infection. Herpes zoster, tinea infections, seborrheic dermatitis, and psoriasis (Chapter 24) all may appear when the CD4+ counts are still normal. As the counts fall and immune function deteriorates, other skin problems begin to appear.

Kaposi sarcoma is a type of skin cancer that produces purplish-brown lumps or blotches of the skin or mouth. When the lesions are few in number, they usually are not treated. If they increase in number or if they appear in the intestinal tract, lungs, or other organs, Kaposi sarcoma is treated with chemotherapy or radiation therapy. In some cases, antiviral medications such as zidovudine may help shrink the lesions.

Thrush, or oral candidiasis, appears as painless white patches on the tongue or inside of the cheek. It is caused by a yeast infection and usually responds to antifungal medications that are swished in the mouth (liquid nystatin) or allowed to dissolve in the mouth (clotrimazole lozenges). Vaginal candidiasis can be severe and persistent in women with HIV. It often does not respond to the vaginal antifungal creams that are used effectively by women without HIV and may require oral fluconazole or ketoconazole.

Ulcers or sores of the genitalia, mouth, or rectal area are common in people with HIV and may be caused by another virus such as herpes or by a fungus. Culture of the lesion should be done to determine the cause and appropriate medication.

Shingles, or varicella zoster, can be a recurrent, painful skin problem for people with HIV. It is a viral infection of the nerve endings in the skin that causes painful blistering of the skin. Shingles is treated with high-dose acyclovir.

EYE CONDITIONS

The frequency of eye problems increases as the immune system fails in people with HIV. All adolescents with HIV—even if there are no eye symptoms—should have regular eye examinations by an ophthalmologist who understands the course and complications of HIV and AIDS.

Retinitis, an inflammation of the retina (Chapter 25), is often seen with HIV and AIDS. It is usually caused by another virus, CMV. Retinitis may begin gradually in one or both eyes with floating spots in the field of vision or painless loss of vision. If untreated, blindness can develop quickly. The treatment for CMV retinitis is intravenous ganciclovir or foscarnet.

Caring for the Adolescent with AIDS

The most important aspects of caring for a teenager with HIV or AIDS are love and concern. Family and friends can best help the teenager if they are supported by a strong network that includes doctors, nurses, social workers, and counselors.

Most teenagers with HIV continue to live at home and attend school. They may do fine throughout adolescence or may experience increasing bouts of illness. Caring for anyone—but especially a teenager or child—with HIV or AIDS is very difficult. Loved ones, while coping with their own sadness and emotional stress, must monitor medications, watch for signs of illness, provide good nutrition, take time off from work for medical appointments, and worry about the future. Many families are heroic in their efforts to provide loving care. Many persevere in the face of rejection by friends, relatives, and neighbors who fear and do not understand HIV and AIDS. Teenagers and their families need the support and physical presence of others. Phone calls help but are not enough. Social support—in the form of visits or shared meals—helps the family remain connected to the community. If this support is not forthcoming, families can ask for help through their churches, synagogues, local Red Cross, social service agencies, or AIDS counseling groups.

A key to forming a strong support network is identifying a doctor or medical center that is experienced and comfortable in the treatment of teenagers who have HIV and AIDS. Medical care should be a team effort by health professionals who can help with other, related issues such as school, jobs, emotional counseling, nutrition, and preventive care.

As AIDS progresses, many adolescents can no longer get adequate medical care while living at home. They may enter a hospital for short stays and then transfer to a hospice or nursing care facility. Hospices provide care for people during the last stages of illness. Some hospice programs offer at-home care; many are located in community facilities. Hospice programs provide the comprehensive involvement of a team of physicians, nurses, nutritionists, social workers, and other health professionals. They help the adolescent and family deal with both the medical and emotional aspects of progressive illness.

Many different health professionals provide counseling for the emotional pain of AIDS. Counselors may combine one-to-one meetings, family sessions, and group discussions. Some meetings are designed to support individuals with HIV and AIDS, while others help parents, siblings, or friends.

Towns, cities, and states have medical and counseling services for those affected by HIV and AIDS. There are several places to begin: the family doctor, hospital social service department, clergy, local or state health department, or local medical society. An individual's identity need not be given when calling hotlines or public agencies for information. Libraries usually have brochures and lists of local HIV and AIDS services. If local resources are difficult to identify, the National AIDS Hotline provides information, education, free brochures, and referrals to local service organizations. The toll-free number, open twenty-four hours a day, seven days a week, is 1-800-342-AIDS. Similar hotlines are available in Spanish (1-800-344-SIDA) and for the hearing-impaired (1-800-AIDS-TTY). Other resources are listed at the end of the book.

23

Sexual Abuse

A thirteen-year-old boy is forced to undress by a neighbor . . . A fourteen-year-old girl is horrified when an uncle touches her breasts . . . A seventeen-year-old girl is raped by her date . . .

Teenagers are victims of abuse—sexual, physical, and emotional—more than individuals of any other age. The facts are:

- One in four girls and one in eleven boys are sexually abused before age eighteen;
- Half of all reported rape victims are adolescents;
- Nearly 70 percent of runaway adolescents have a history of sexual abuse;
- The rates of adolescent sexual abuse have risen nearly four-fold over the past twenty years in some U.S. cities.

Sexual abuse of children and adolescents has received increasing public attention, and the topic is discussed more openly than ever before. Victims are more likely to report abuse, yet health officials believe that most episodes still go unreported. This is especially true for a child or adolescent who knows the perpetrator and fears the consequences of disclosure.

The prevention of sexual abuse is discussed in schools, homes, and the media. Sometimes sexual abuse can be avoided or prevented; often it cannot. Teenagers are at high risk of abuse, and they must learn how to deal with dangerous or threatening situations. All adolescents should discuss the subject with parents or other trusted adults before episodes occur. They should know what to do, who to call, and where to go if they fear—or experience—abuse.

Just what is "sexual abuse?" For teenagers and adults, the many terms and degrees of involvement are confusing. First, some definitions:

• *Sexual contact* can be one or more events with or without the use of physical force. It often begins with touching but can progress to intercourse. Sexual contact may happen once with a stranger, or it may be a long-term pattern over months or years with a relative, family friend, or other known adult. Three out of four abused children and teenagers know the abuser. In half the cases, the abuser is a relative.

• *Sexual activity* is any form of sexual stimulation, including looking at the genitals, exhibitionism (undressing in public, for example), touching, oral–genital contact, insertion of objects into the vagina or rectum, or sexual intercourse.

• *Consent* means giving permission. Someone who is intoxicated, unconscious, or mentally disabled cannot give consent. Legally, minors cannot give consent for sexual activity.

• *Force* refers to physical violence or verbal threats (such as, "I'll kill you if you tell anyone," "I'll say you're making it up," "It will really hurt your mother if she finds out . . .").

• *Sexual abuse* refers to sexual contact or sexual activity that is accompanied by physical or psychological force. Sexual abuse is a power issue: one person dominating another. In cases involving children and teenagers, the adult abuser takes advantage of the victim's immaturity. The abuser may intimidate, deceive, coerce, or exploit a minor by wielding a position of authority or by misusing a trusted relationship. Sexual abuse can also occur between same-age peers, if, for example, a teenage boy forces a teenage girl to have sexual activity against her will.

• *Sexual molestation* refers to sexual contact other than intercourse that occurs without consent. Sexual molestation usually falls under the same criminal laws as rape.

• *Rape* is sexual intercourse without a person's consent, occurring with force or the threat of force. Rape is more narrowly defined as penetration of the penis into any oral, genital, or anal opening. Partial penetration of the genitalia or ejaculation of semen is sufficient evidence of rape.

• *Statutory rape* is sexual intercourse with a female below the age of consent—sixteen in most states.

• *Date rape* refers to sexual intercourse between two people in a dating situation but against one's will. Date rape has become a major concern of many teenagers. They fear it and are confused about its precise meaning.

• *Incest* is sexual intercourse between close relatives (for example, parent-child, brother-sister, uncle-niece, grandfather-granddaughter).

Protection Against Sexual Abuse

Most parents tell their children to be cautious about whom they date and where they go: "Be careful," "Don't hitchhike," "Never get into a car with a stranger." Simply saying "Be careful" is not enough to prevent sexual abuse. Teenagers do not have the experience of adults. They may underestimate the potential danger of a situation. Many deny that they could be victimized. Teenage girls *and* boys need to understand that sexual abuse *can* happen to them.

Adolescents may not realize that some sexual behaviors may provoke others. For example, kissing and touching may incorrectly signal a willingness to have sexual intercourse. Teenagers must explain clearly—before the passion heats up—just what they are and are not willing to do. When a verbal "no" is ignored, adolescents should try to protect themselves by screaming, running, or fighting. All teenagers need to understand that no means no. Stop means stop. Going beyond that expressed boundary constitutes assault, whether it happens on a first date or in a long-standing relationship.

Risky situations warrant special precautions. When teenagers— boys or girls—are with people or in places where victimization is possible, they should walk purposefully, stay in pairs or groups, avoid dimly lit areas, lock car doors when driving, stay inside the car if bumped by another car, and try to get to a safe setting immediately. Learning self-defense techniques before these situations occur can be reassuring even if nothing happens and life-saving if something does.

Most sexual abuse happens to females, but males are far from exempt. As previously mentioned, one in eleven boys becomes a victim of some form of sexual abuse before his eighteenth birthday. Among reported cases of rape, 96 percent are females and 4 percent are males. Teenage boys are less likely than girls to report sexual abuse. They may be embarrassed by the typically homosexual nature of the assault. They usually know the abuser. They often have been coerced or threatened rather than physically forced. Whatever the reason, sexually abused boys frequently live in silence, suffering the fear and humiliation alone.

In the majority of cases involving male victims, the abuse began in childhood. By the time the boy reaches adolescence, the abusive activities may stop, but his earlier trauma may be expressed through social withdrawal or problem behaviors such as aggression or drug use. First-time episodes of abuse during adolescence happen less often to boys living with their families. When the abuse does begin in adolescence, the victims frequently are boys who have run away from home, who have voluntarily begun homosexual activities, or who have become entangled in the criminal justice system.

Recognizing Sexual Abuse

Some children and adolescents will report sexual abuse immediately to a parent or another trusted adult. Many will not. Sexual abuse is such a devastating experience that many young victims keep it a secret because they feel ashamed, "dirty," embarrassed, frightened, or guilty. These feelings often are fostered by an abuser who threatens further harm if the secret is told or who makes the victim feel responsible for the abuse. Many young people hide, deny, or repress sexual abuse, although it is *never* their fault.

Adolescents who are hiding their trauma may show other, related signs of distress: nightmares, running away, disruptive or "acting out" behaviors, eating and sleeping disturbances, stomach pain, headaches, fatigue, sudden changes in friendships, unusual fears (of crowds, of being alone, for example), unexplained crying, anxiety, or nervousness. Other victims mask their pain with hidden symptoms, particularly if the abuser is a relative or family friend with whom the victim believes she must maintain a "normal" relationship.

When young victims do disclose a past experience of sexual abuse, they may reveal it unintentionally in a moment of fear or anger. They may confide in friends, who tell their own parents, who then report it to the authorities or to the victim's family. Some common misconceptions can confuse parents or friends who suspect or know of sexual abuse. The facts are:

• The victim did *not* provoke or cause the incident. Victims do not ask for abuse by wearing short skirts, low necklines, or heavy makeup. No one invites harm. Abusers seek vulnerable targets regardless of their appearance.

• Abuse is more than a sexual act; it is a *violent assault.* Even if physical force or a weapon was not involved, the abuse violates the victim's dignity, integrity, and sense of control.

• Children and teenagers rarely lie about sexual abuse. An accusation should be taken seriously when an adolescent describes abuse.

What to Do If Sexual Abuse Occurs

The following suggestions fall into several categories, depending on the nature of the abuse and when it happend.

Sexual abuse should *never* be minimized, whether or not it involved intercourse, whether it occurred yesterday or years ago. If it took place within the past seventy-two hours, the adolescent should see a physician immediately. If the abuse happened before this, a physician should still be seen, but emergency care is not as necessary. A physician or a therapist can help a young victim cope with the past trauma and lingering concern. Adolescent victims sometimes hold on to unnecessary worries or mistaken information about the effects of abuse on their future sexuality or reproductive ability.

Rape

Rape is a medical emergency and a psychological crisis. It is one of the most dehumanizing traumas anyone can experience. For an adolescent whose sexuality is evolving, rape can profoundly affect self-esteem and identity. Extreme care and sensitivity must be expressed by all adults involved with the young person.

Even if months have passed, an adolescent rape victim should see a physician immediately. He or she should be told clearly what will happen during a physical examination. A parent, trusted relative, or friend should stay with the victim throughout the examination. Police should not be present in the examining room. The victim, or her companion, should insist that the examination is conducted in a private area by a doctor who is experienced in treating rape victims.

The doctor will ask several questions, such as when, where, and how the assault happened, the date of the victim's menstrual period, whether she has showered or douched since the attack, and whether she has been using birth control. The doctor will observe her emotional state, behavior, and appearance (torn clothing, for example).

Before beginning a physical examination, the physician will explain that rape is a crime which must be reported by law in most areas. The victim usually has the right to consent to an examination and treatment without release of evidence to the police. Victims are generally encouraged, however, to allow collection of legal evidence in case they later decide to press charges. At the time of the examination, the victim should not be pressured into making quick decisions. She should be allowed to ask questions or stop the examination at any time. It is critical that she begin to regain some sense of control over what is done to her body. If the examining physician wants to have photographs taken of injuries, the victim may give or refuse permission. A female victim has the right to a female photographer and a male victim, a male photographer.

The doctor will look for external signs: scratches, bruises, bleeding, and foreign matter (such as grass, dirt, fibers, hair, dried blood or semen). Swabs from inside the mouth may be taken. The external genitalia will be examined for blood, secretions, cuts, scars, and bruises. If there is bleeding, pain, or signs of penetration or injury, a pelvic (internal) examination will follow. In the case of a male victim, a rectal examination will take place.

Cultures (small samples of tissue or discharge) and blood samples will be taken to the laboratory to test for sexually transmitted diseases (STDs). A urine or blood sample will be tested for pregnancy. The doctor may recommend "morning-after pills" to prevent the possibility of pregnancy. Antibiotics will be given to protect against STDs, even before the laboratory results are back.

A thorough postrape examination also should include counseling and emotional support. The doctor can offer the phone numbers of rape crisis centers or a referral to a psychotherapist. In some instances, medication may be prescribed to alleviate anxiety or difficulty sleeping. Many doctors and hospitals distribute written material for victims to take home and read as the immediate crisis begins to subside.

Follow-up medical examinations should be scheduled for two to three weeks to review the initial laboratory results and two to three months to collect additional blood tests. Some STDs, such as syphilis, do not become apparent for several weeks. A young victim may be reluctant to return for care that is linked to the traumatic event. The follow-up visits are very important to assure that all STDs have been fully treated. The visits also give the physician a chance to evaluate how the adolescent is doing emotionally.

Incest

Incest involves complicated psychological and family factors. Sexual abuse by a relative seems to have more serious, long-term emotional effects than sexual abuse by a stranger. Incest has many combinations. The most frequent, and probably least harmful, is the sex play of young siblings. The combination with the most serious consequences is father (or stepfather) and daughter. Step-relatives are more frequently involved in incest than blood relatives.

A common pattern of incest begins when the girl is ten to twelve years old. It starts with exhibitionism or voyeurism (looking at the child undressed), moves on to touching the genitals, and then to vaginal or anal intercourse. Children and teenagers usually conceal incest because they fear parental rejection or disbelief, or destruction of the family unit.

The signs of incest include those previously mentioned for sexual abuse in general. The adolescent victim also may take on new roles within the family. For example, a girl who is abused by her father may become highly protective of her younger sisters. She may take over household duties or assume the role of mother if she senses discord between her parents. She may feel that the future of her family depends on her silence. An unspoken conspiracy may envelop the family. Sometimes the other parent (usually the mother) knows of the incest but is unable to confront it. Sometimes she denies or represses the knowledge. In other situations, she has no knowledge or suspicion of the incest.

As the secrecy unravels, the whole family needs help. The immediate crisis requires separation of the adolescent victim and the adult perpetrator. First and foremost is the adolescent's safety, and this usually means family disruption. Blame and accusation will polarize the family, so care must be taken to evaluate the situation as calmly as possible and to seek medical and psychological treatment immediately.

Incest is a criminal offense and must be reported according to local legal requirements. It is extremely difficult for one family member to accuse another of an assault, but the abuse *must stop.* The victim and the abuser require counseling, and other family members can benefit from individual or family therapy.

It may take a long time for a young victim of sexual abuse to readjust. Individual reactions differ from victim to victim and between victim and parent. Parents typically react initially with anger and retaliation. They focus on identifying the offender. Young victims may react initially by withdrawing. They may refuse to press charges. They just wish the nightmare would go away.

The emotional response to sexual abuse, particularly rape, seems to change over time. Immediately after the incident, a victim typically responds with shock, disorientation, crying, hysteria, stoicism (toughing it out), insomnia, vomiting, or refusing to eat. Over the next few days or weeks, she appears to be coping, "getting back to normal," denying or minimizing her emotions. She also may withdraw from social interaction and show signs of mistrust. Eventually, she may experience mild to severe depression or gradual acknowledgment of the abuse event.

As the victim of sexual abuse gradually works through the aftershocks of the event, she needs consistent reassurance that she was not at fault. She may feel vulnerable, guilty, ashamed, and helpless for some time. She may need to talk about the incident over and over again. She can best cope with the crisis if family, friends, and therapist patiently listen to her. Their empathy can help her regain her sense of control and self-esteem.

MEDICAL
CONDITIONS
DURING
ADOLESCENCE

24

The Skin, Hair, and Nails

The body's largest organ—the skin—is critical for survival. It protects underlying tissues from infection, irritants, and harmful ultraviolet light. Its many nerve endings warn the brain of heat and cold, pain and pressure. It limits fluid loss and helps regulate body temperature.

The skin also contributes heavily to self-image and social interaction. Some part of the skin—on the face, arms, hands, legs—is always visible. It affects how teenagers feel about themselves and react to each other. A blemish or a rash that seems trivial to a parent can precipitate a bout of insecurity and even social withdrawal for a teenager.

This chapter discusses common adolescent conditions of the skin, hair, and nails. Some warrant attention primarily for their effect on appearance. Others may endanger health or signal disease elsewhere in the body. Pay attention to visible changes. Early recognition of skin problems can mean early diagnosis, treatment, and cure.

Acne

Acne occurs in 80 percent of adolescent girls and 90 percent of boys. It tends to begin earlier and last longer in girls but may follow a more severe course in boys. For most teenagers, acne is intermittent, mild, and easily managed. For others, it can be severe and persistent. Five percent of teenagers with acne have inflammation severe enough to cause permanent scarring.

There are many myths about acne. It is *not* caused by dirt, diet, masturbation, or sexual activity. Excessive, vigorous scrubbing will *not* cure it and can make it worse. Chocolate, nuts, pizza, french fries, and other greasy foods do *not* cause acne, though they should be limited for other health reasons (Chapter 5).

Acne is related to the hormones of puberty. These hormones stimulate the sebaceous glands of the skin to produce a fatty substance called sebum, which interacts with bacteria to cause pimples. Acne appears in areas that have many sebaceous glands, such as the face, back, and chest.

Acne can take different forms. "Comedones" are blackheads and whiteheads without much redness or inflammation. Inflammatory acne consists of red, often tender pimples. More severe inflammatory acne occurs when large pus-filled cysts develop under the surface of the skin. Rarely, the inflammation can be so severe that high fever and generalized illness develop.

Most teenagers are unable to identify a specific cause of their acne. The following factors can cause acne or make it worse and should be avoided: oil-based cosmetics and creams, certain medications or chemicals, and illegal steroids used for muscle-building. Some teenagers notice flares of acne with emotional stress or with menstruation. These flares are all the more frustrating because of their frequency.

Mild acne or an occasional outbreak can be managed by gentle, twice-daily cleansing with a mild soap (such as Dove, Camay, Neutrogena), followed by over-the-counter medications applied to pimples once or twice daily. More severe acne should be evaluated and treated by a doctor. Remember that no medication works instantly. Talk with your doctor about when to expect a response, then hang in there and continue the treatment.

The methods used to treat acne include the following:

• *Cleansing agents* (such as Stridex pads, Noxzema, Clearasil face wash or antibacterial soap bar). The skin should be cleaned *gently*. Overuse or rubbing, especially if the cleanser contains alcohol, will irritate the skin and make the acne worse.

• *Over-the-counter topical agents* (meaning they are applied to the skin). Gels, creams, and lotions containing benzoyl peroxide or salicylic acid reduce oil buildup and fight surface bacteria. A small patch of skin should be tested before the treatment is applied to larger areas. Some dryness of the skin is expected; excessive redness or peeling should be avoided.

Benzoyl peroxide is typically the first topical medication tried for acne. Most over-the-counter preparations vary from 5 percent concentrations (Oxy 5, Vanoxide) to 10 percent (Oxy 10, Clearasil). It is best to begin with lower concentrations applied once daily for a week or two. If the medication is tolerated, then it can be applied twice daily or a higher concentration can be tried.

• *Topical retinoic acid (Retin-A)*. This prescription medication is applied to the skin as a gel, liquid, or cream. It works by increasing skin turnover so that comedones move to the surface and open. After the first week or two, some redness or dryness usually occurs. After three or four weeks, the acne can appear worse as the comedones break up. Teenagers may become discouraged or tempted to discontinue use at this point. Improvement usually is seen within one to two months of beginning treatment.

A few important guidelines should be followed when using Retin-A. First, wear hats and sun block when outside because Retin-A increases the likelihood of sunburn. Second, treat the skin gently because the treatment can be irritating. Try to allow half an hour between cleansing and applying the medication. Third, this is a prescription medication; it must be used with a doctor's knowledge and supervision.

• *Antibiotics* can be applied either topically or taken orally. Antibiotics are only used for inflammatory acne, not for whiteheads or blackheads. Topical preparations containing antibiotics such as erythromycin or clindamycin have few side effects but also tend to have limited effectiveness in the treatment of adolescent acne. Oral antibiotics, such as tetracycline or minocycline, can be very effective but should not be used for prolonged periods. All antibiotics, whether topical or oral, require a doctor's prescription.

• *Oral Retinoic Acid (Accutane)* is very effective in the treatment of severe acne but can cause many side effects. When prescribed appropriately, Accutane results in significant, prolonged improvement for up to 60 percent of adolescents. *However,* it is important to understand its risks and to work with a physician familiar with its use. The most serious side effect of Accutane is harm to a developing fetus. For that reason, *all females using Accutane must use contraception consistently and effectively* while taking it and for at least one month after stopping it. Other possible serious side effects of Accutane include abnormalities in liver tests or blood counts, elevation of cholesterol or triglycerides, and headaches. Less serious but bothersome side effects include dry mouth, dry skin and lips, skin redness, conjunctivitis (Chapter 25), nosebleeds, hair thinning, joint and muscle pain, and sensitivity of the skin and eyes to light. Teenagers using Accutane should avoid exposure to the sun and should always use a sunscreen when outside.

Accutane typically is prescribed for four to five months. Shorter courses may improve the acne for a while, but it tends to flare much more quickly than when the medication is prescribed for the full recommended period.

• *Hormonal therapy.* In a small proportion of adolescents with acne, the cause may be related to disorders of the endocrine (hormone-producing) system. Treating acne with hormonal intervention must be done cautiously. For some teenage girls, estrogen can suppress the activity of the sebaceous glands, but it rarely is sufficient treatment alone. Estrogen is never prescribed for boys because it causes female characteristics such as breast development. Other hormones, such as corticosteroids, are rarely indicated in the treatment of acne.

• *Acne surgery.* A physician sometimes will remove comedones using a small needle or extractor. Teenagers are often tempted to squeeze or puncture whiteheads and blackheads on their own. If done too often or too vigorously, scarring can result. If large cysts form, a doctor can inject them with a steroid-type medication that decreases the redness and swelling within one to two days.

Young adults with acne scars may want to discuss surgical rehabilitation with a doctor. The possibilities include dermabrasion (scraping the skin's surface layers to remove scars) or collagen implants for depressions in the skin tissue.

Disorders of the Sweat Glands

There are two types of sweat glands. Eccrine sweat glands function throughout life, are located throughout the skin, and help the body regulate its temperature. Apocrine sweat glands begin to function at puberty, are located under the arms and in the genital area, and are stimulated by activity or stress. Body odor occurs when the secretions from both types of glands—but especially the apocrine—interact with bacteria on the surface of the skin.

The major site of body odor is under the arms. Prevention is aimed at decreasing both the secretions from the apocrine glands and the bacteria on the skin's surface. Daily bathing or showering with antibacterial soaps, use of antiperspirants, and clean clothes generally solve the problem.

Foot odor is another common problem for teenagers. It usually responds to daily use of antibacterial soaps, absorbent socks that are changed daily, and rotation of pairs of shoes. Shoes that "breathe"—because they are ventilated or are made of canvas or leather—are less likely to promote foot odor than those made of man-made products like vinyl. An antiperspirant foot spray (Dr. Scholl's, Drysol) also is helpful.

A disorder of the apocrine glands that begins during adolescence is called *hidradenitis suppurativa*. The glands under the arms or in the groin become so blocked by secretions and bacteria that eventually they rupture and form cysts or pus-filled abscesses. Hidradenitis suppurativa tends to run in families and is exacerbated by obesity, hot weather, tight clothing, and shaving. The condition can be very painful and, if untreated, can spread to involve nearby glands. A doctor should always be consulted if hidradenitis suppurativa is suspected. Treatment includes antibacterial soaps, topical or oral antibiotics, and injection of cysts with medication to decrease inflammation and scarring.

Dermatitis

The general term for skin inflammation is dermatitis. The types of dermatitis that commonly affect teenagers are atopic dermatitis, contact dermatitis, and seborrheic dermatitis.

Atopic dermatitis, or eczema, is a chronic, allergic reaction to one or more substances in the environment. Sometimes these substances are readily identified, such as animal hair or pollen. Often the cause is unknown. Signs of atopic dermatitis include itching; dry, cracked skin; redness; and scaling or crusted plaques. The affected skin may also weep, or ooze. Atopic dermatitis frequently begins in childhood and may be associated with asthma or hayfever. Most adolescents with atopic dermatitis have a family history of atopic dermatitis, allergies, or asthma.

Atopic dermatitis frequently improves during adolescence but usually does not clear completely. Typical skin areas of atopic dermatitis are the inner surface of the elbow, the inner wrist, the hands, behind the knees, the feet, and the neck.

A cornerstone in the treatment of atopic dermatitis is use of mild soaps (Neutrogena, Dove, Camay) and moisturizers (Keri Lotion, Moisturel, Lubriderm). Irritants, such as harsh soaps, detergents, dry air, very hot water, and alcohol should be avoided. Corticosteroid creams applied to the skin help control the redness, scaling, and itching. Low-dose corticosteroid creams (like 1 percent hydrocortisone) are available without a prescription. If this is insufficient, a doctor can prescribe a more potent cream or ointment.

Contact dermatitis appears on areas of the skin that have directly touched an irritating substance, such as poison ivy, or a substance to which the adolescent is allergic. Substances that often cause contact dermatitis because of allergies are nickel in coins or jewelry, rubber (as in the soles of shoes), wool, perfume, detergent, insect repellent, soaps and shampoos, body lotion, nail polish, and cosmetics.

The signs of contact dermatitis include itching, redness, blistering, scaling, cracking, or oozing. When the offending substance is identified and eliminated, the signs disappear quickly in most cases. Over-the-counter preparations that help relieve symptoms include low-potency corticosteroid creams, calamine lotion, and Burow's solution (or Domeboro packets). Antihistamines, such as Benadryl, are available without prescription and help diminish itching but may cause fatigue.

If the itching and irritation continue, a doctor may prescribe a more potent corticosteroid cream or ointment to apply to the skin. In severe cases, a five- to ten-day course of oral corticosteroids (prednisone) prescribed by a doctor can bring quick relief. Whatever the treatment, the dermatitis will not go away or stay away until the substance causing it is identified and removed.

Seborrheic dermatitis is a chronic inflammation of the skin in areas where the oil-producing sebaceous glands have become overly active—the scalp, forehead, eyebrows, nose folds, outer ears, armpits, navel, and groin. The symptoms include dandruff, scaling of the skin, dryness or oiliness, redness, and itching.

Medicated shampoos available without prescription (for example, Ionil, Pentrax, Selsun Blue, Sebulex, Zincon) usually help the dandruff of seborrheic dermatitis. Topical corticosteroid creams are appropriate for other parts of the body. High potency corticosteroid preparations prescribed by a doctor should not be used on the face, under the arms, or on the genitalia. No steroid preparation should be used for more than one to two weeks without a doctor's knowledge.

Fungal Infections of the Skin

Fungal, or tinea, infections of the skin typically involve the head, torso, genital area, hands, and feet. A doctor may make the diagnosis by physical examination, by shining a special light on the rash, or by examining some scales from the rash under a microscope. The most common types of tinea infections include the following:

• *Tinea capitis* is a fungal infection of the scalp. It causes inflammation, crusting, scaling, and hair thinning and brittleness. It may appear as localized patches or may involve the entire scalp. Tinea capitis spreads from person to person through shared hats, hairbrushes, and combs. Some forms can spread from animals to people. Treatment involves application of an antifungal cream (like Lotrimin, Monistat, or Micatin) and use of a medicated shampoo (like Selsun Blue). In some cases, an oral antifungal medication, called griseofulvin, is prescribed for several weeks.

• *Tinea corporis (ringworm)* is a fungal infection of the arms, hands, face, neck, or trunk. It starts as a small, red, scaly spot that slowly expands to resemble a ring with a dark, raised outer edge. Ringworm responds well to antifungal creams applied twice daily for several weeks until the rash has completely disappeared.

• *Tinea cruris (jock itch)* is a fungal infection of the groin, inner thighs, lower abdomen, or buttocks. It is more common in males and in warm weather. The symptoms include itching, burning, and a red, slightly raised rash. Antifungal creams applied once or twice daily usually are effective within several days. Tinea cruris can be prevented by good personal hygiene, loose-fitting pants, and antifungal powders (like Cruex).

• *Tinea pedis (athlete's foot)* is a fungal infection of the feet. It spreads easily in locker rooms and shared showers. Drying the feet well after showering and wearing shoes that "breathe" help to prevent it. The symptoms include itching, scaling, cracking, and redness between the toes or on the soles of the feet. The infection is treated with an antifungal cream continued for several weeks. Once cured, a medicated powder like Tinactin helps to prevent reinfection.

• *Tinea versicolor* is a fungal infection that causes patchy color changes of the upper back and shoulders, upper arms, neck, and chest. On pale skin, the patches appear tan; on suntanned skin, they look pale or white. The darker patches vary widely in size and shape but typically are flat with a very fine scale that may be invisible until the area is scratched. Treatment involves antifungal creams or Selsun Blue shampoo applied to the skin. The skin color may not return to normal for several months, even after the infection has cleared. This is because light patches need sun exposure to tan and tanned patches need time to fade.

Lice and Scabies

Lice are small insects that infest the scalp, eyebrows, eyelashes, trunk, or pubic hair. They produce severe itching, inflammation, and small reddish bumps. Scratching can lead to open sores, bleeding, and crusting. Treatment involves medicated creams or shampoos, anti-itch lotions, and hot-water washing of all clothing and bedding. Household members and sexual contacts should be treated even if they do not have signs of infection. Classmates and close friends should be examined and treated if there is evidence of infection.

Head lice are more common among younger schoolchildren than adolescents. The lice lay tiny white eggs called nits on the scalp. The nits stick to the hair and do not flake off easily like dandruff. The adult lice and nits are killed by using a medicated shampoo or lotion (such as Kwell, R&C, or RID) according to the directions on the package. After treatment, combing the wet hair with a fine-tooth comb will remove the dead nits.

Unlike head lice, body lice do not live or lay eggs on the body. They live on bed linens, mattresses, pillows, towels, and clothing but rely on the human body for food. The only evidence of their visit is a rash on a hairless part of the body, such as the back. The rash itself does not need to be treated. It will go away on its own once all bedding, towels, and clothing are thoroughly cleaned.

Lice in the pubic area cause small bites and bumps, intense itching, and nits clinging to the pubic hairs. They are usually sexually transmitted, and all sexual partners *must* be treated, even if they have no symptoms. The treatment involves two applications of a shampoo, lotion, or cream (such as Kwell) one week apart.

Scabies is a rash caused by microscopic insects that burrow under the skin's surface. The condition is very contagious and causes intense itching that is often worse at night. Scabies generally appears on the wrists, between the fingers, in the genital area, under the arms or buttocks, and around the navel or nipples. It may look like red, raised, threadlike lines under the skin; round, raised, red bumps; or blisters on a reddened base.

Scabies is transmitted through close physical or sexual contact with someone who is infected and through contact with infected clothing. Because it is highly contagious, treatment should include family, close friends, and sexual partners. Several types of creams and lotions (Kwell, Scabene) are available without prescription. The infected person should be treated twice, one week apart. Other people without signs of infection, but who have had contact with the infected person, should be treated twice. Clothing and bedding must be dry-cleaned or washed in hot water. Even after effective treatment, the itching may persist for a while. Sexual and close physical contact should be avoided until treatment is completed and there is no sign of infection.

Impetigo

Although more common among younger children, impetigo does affect adolescents and is highly contagious. It is a bacterial infection of the skin, appearing first as a small pimple that becomes pus-filled, ruptures, and leaves a thick yellow scab or crust that does not heal. The first pimple usually appears on the face; as its scab is scratched or rubbed off, impetigo spreads by the hands to other areas.

Impetigo requires treatment with an antibiotic. Until it is under control, children and teenagers should avoid skin contact with others and should not share towels or clothing. If impetigo is suspected, a doctor should always be contacted.

Pityriasis Rosea

Pityriasis rosea is a common skin rash of adolescence. It begins as a single, one- or two-inch pink or red patch, usually on the chest, abdomen, or back. This is called a herald patch because it warns of the rash that will follow within the next few days or weeks. The rash of pityriasis rosea consists of small pink lesions that are either flat or slightly raised and have a very fine scale. It typically affects the trunk, upper arms, and lower neck more than the face, scalp, feet, and hands. The rash is symmetrical, meaning it affects both sides of the body. Treatment involves antihistamines (such as Bena-dryl or Atarax) if itching is bothersome, but there is no other spe-cific treatment. The rash disappears on its own within six to eight weeks. Pityriasis rosea probably is caused by a viral infection. It is neither serious nor contagious, but the adolescent should see a doctor to be sure that the rash is not caused by another problem.

Warts

Adolescence is the peak time for warts to develop. They are more common among females than males. Warts are noncancerous skin growths caused by a virus that enters the body through a scrape or scratch. It takes two to three months for the wart to appear after the scratch. Warts usually go away on their own; a third disappear in six months and two thirds within two years.

The appearance of a wart depends on its location. Round, firm warts occur most frequently on the hands and fingers. Flat ones are found more often on the face, back of the hands, knees and wrists. Plantar warts occur at pressure points on the soles of the feet and cause pain on walking. They do not rise above the skin surface and may look like many black dots due to tiny amounts of clotted blood.

A number of methods exist to treat warts, such as cryotherapy (freezing with liquid nitrogen), acid plasters, medications applied to the wart (such as podophyllin), and surgical removal. Single, small warts on the hands, feet, neck, and arms can be treated at home with the over-the-counter products, but cutting a wart is never advised. A doctor should treat resistant warts and those that appear on the face.

Warts in the genital area are associated with sexually transmit-ted diseases (human papilloma virus, Chapter 21). They are flesh-colored, pink, or red, and may resemble cauliflowers or strawber-ries. They most often appear on the labia of the vagina, the penis, or scrotum but sometimes develop around the mouth. The appear-ance of any wart around the genitalia or the mouth requires medical attention and screening for other STDs.

Herpesvirus Infections

Herpesviruses are categorized as herpes type 1 and type 2. Type 1 infections typically occur in childhood and cause fever blisters or cold sores around the lips and mouth. Type 2 infections usually are sexually transmitted and cause painful blisters or ulcers in the genital and rectal areas.

The initial symptoms of both type 1 and 2 are pain, itching, or skin sensitivity, even before the blisters appear. The blisters may be either single or in clusters. Within a day of their appearance, the blisters break down to form a flat painful ulcer. In severe cases, there may be fever, swollen glands or lymph nodes, headache, and fatigue.

It is impossible to tell by physical examination alone if a herpes infection is caused by type 1 or 2. This requires a special culture of material swabbed from the blister or ulcer. Both types can be spread through sexual contact. Sexually active adolescents with new herpes outbreaks should assume that they became infected through sexual contact and should see a doctor both for treatment and examination for other STDs. The treatment for herpesvirus infections is described in Chapter 21.

Herpes zoster, better known as shingles, is a viral infection of the nerves beneath the skin's surface. It is much more common in older than younger people. It does occur in teenagers, though, especially at times of physical or emotional stress. Herpes zoster is caused by the chicken pox virus. After the rash of chicken pox clears, the virus enters an inactive state, or "goes to sleep" in a nerve. Years later, it may awaken, causing the rash of shingles.

Shingles begins with a tingling or burning sensation of the skin, followed within several days by the appearance of red, raised, painful bumps or blisters. The rash typically appears on one side of the chest, back, or face. It follows the path of the underlying, infected nerve on that side and does not cross to the nerve on the other side of the body. After five to ten days, the blisters crust over.

A doctor should always be seen if shingles is suspected. Most people recover without specific treatment, but the pain can be severe and can last several weeks. In addition to prescribing medication that helps the discomfort, the doctor will look for underlying illnesses that may have increased the likelihood of developing shingles. This is especially important in teenagers since shingles is relatively uncommon in the young.

Skin Reactions to Medication

Virtually any drug can cause a skin rash. Sometimes the rash is caused by an allergy. At other times, the medication may increase the skin's sensitivity to the sun, causing redness in sun-exposed areas. When the rash represents an allergy, the medication should be avoided in the future. When the rash represents increased sensitivity to the sun, exposure to the sun should be avoided while on the medication, but it is safe to take the medicine again in the future.

Drugs that commonly cause allergic reactions are penicillins (amoxicillin, ampicillin, Augmentin) and sulfas (Bactrim, Septra). Drugs that commonly cause sun sensitivity include tetracycline and minocycline.

Allergic skin reactions from drugs typically involve the back, chest, and abdomen but can spread to involve the face, hands, feet, and even the inside of the mouth and genitalia. The appearance of the rash may vary widely, from barely visible, to a sunburn-type redness, to red dots, to blisters.

If a teenager develops a rash while on medication, a doctor should be contacted immediately. If the doctor cannot be reached, it is always safer to stop the medication than to continue it. An allergic skin reaction is the body's way of saying that it cannot tolerate the medication. If the doctor feels that the rash is not caused by the medication, it can then be restarted.

Psoriasis

Psoriasis is a noncontagious skin disorder that often begins in adolescence and continues throughout adult life. Reddish patches appear on the scalp, elbows, knees, buttocks, and lower back. The patches, which can be teardrop size or several inches across, are covered by a white or silver scale. The cause of psoriasis is unknown. It affects females more than males and tends to run in families. If a parent or sibling has psoriasis, a teenager has a one in ten chance of developing it, which is ten times greater than the general population.

Emotional and physical stress may aggravate psoriasis. Puberty, menstruation, common colds, and school examinations all may precipitate flares. The readily visible skin patches and the flaking from scalp involvement are difficult at all ages, but perhaps especially during adolescence when personal appearance is so very important.

Psoriasis cannot be cured but can be controlled. Mild psoriasis often responds to prescription steroid creams and ointments applied to the skin and scalp. More severe cases may respond to ultraviolet light therapy administered by a dermatologist. *All* treatment requires close supervision by a physician who is familiar with the management of psoriasis and potential complications. In some instances, psoriasis can cause joint stiffness, pain, and swelling (psoriatic arthritis). The hands and feet tend to be involved more than the larger joints. Like the skin manifestations of psoriasis, the arthritis is not curable but it is controllable.

Sunburn

Despite increased public awareness about the dangers of overexposure to ultraviolet rays, the appeal of a tan is still strong among teenagers. One survey revealed that only 9 percent of teenagers use sunscreen consistently and 33 percent never use it.

The immediate reason to avoid sunburn is the pain, blistering, and peeling that will soon result. The long-term reason is the risk of skin cancer and early wrinkling. Before heading into the sun, teenagers should keep several recommendations in mind:

• Sunscreen lotions allow tanning but decrease the chance of burning. They are available in graduated concentrations of PABA (para-aminobenzoic acid) solutions; the higher the number, the more protection. Read the labels and use PABA numbers over 15, especially early in the exposure period. Creams containing zinc oxide or titanium dioxide block the sun's rays entirely and are often used on areas like the nose that are particularly sensitive to sunburn.

• Gradual exposure to the sun in small doses is safer than prolonged exposure over a few days. Avoid the sun midday, when its short ultraviolet rays are strongest. Begin with fifteen- to thirty-minute periods early in the morning or late in the afternoon and slowly build up to longer exposure times over the next few days. Give your skin a break from the sun from time to time by wearing a hat and clothing over a bathing suit.

• Do not be fooled by clouds, wind, and water at the beach. They make the day feel cool, but the sun's rays are still strong.

• Reapply sunscreen lotions frequently because swimming and perspiring wash them away.

• Some medications can increase the skin's sensitivity to the sun, including oral contraceptives, some antibiotics, sulfa drugs, and tranquilizers.

Even after a tan is achieved, it does not protect the skin from sun damage. Sunscreen use should be continued to prevent drying, wrinkling, thickening of the skin, and skin cancer later in life.

Hives

Hives (or urticaria) are itching, red bumps or blotches that appear suddenly and can spread quickly. They are caused by an allergic reaction either to something within the body (such as food or medication) or to something that has touched the skin's surface. Common causes of hives include shellfish, eggs, nuts, fresh berries, coffee, food additives, alcohol, medications, sunlight, cold weather, animal hair, pollen dust, mold, aerosol products, insect bites, and activities that produce perspiration.

Hives tend to last between a few hours to two days. Treatment involves first and foremost eliminating the cause. Itching can be relieved by cold compresses and antihistamines such as Benadryl (over-the-counter) or Atarax (by prescription). A doctor should always be consulted if hives persist or recur.

Tattoos

Tattoos carry many serious risks. The skin can be hypersensitive to the dye. Unattractive overgrowths of scar tissue, called keloids, can develop. Unsanitary methods of tattooing can lead to hepatitis and other serious infections. Attempts to remove tattoos by excision (cutting out) or dermabrasion (scraping the skin) often are unsuccessful. The decision to have a tattoo should never be made impulsively. It is a decision that leaves a permanent reminder and carries potential health hazards. (See body piercing, tattoos, and risk of HIV infection: Chapter 22.)

Moles and Changes in Pigmentation

Pigment is the material that gives the skin its color. The color of the skin may change in as small an area as a freckle or over large parts of the body.

Stretch marks (striae) frequently develop during the rapid growth phase of puberty. They are more common in females than males and usually occur on the breasts, abdomen, hips, buttocks, and thighs. The stretch marks look like thin, wrinkled stripes and may be purplish, pink, white, or skin tone. Striae tend to appear or become worse with rapid weight gain or loss, obesity, and pregnancy; they are seen, though, in many normal-weight teenagers following normal puberty. In most adolescents, the color of the striae fade over time and assume the same color as the surrounding skin.

Striae also occur in adolescents with chronic diseases who have been taking oral corticosteroids (prednisone) for long periods. Rarely, they are associated with a hormonal disorder called Cushing disease, in which the body produces excess amounts of corticosteroids (Chapter 33).

Moles are collections of pigment-producing cells that typically are brown, larger than a freckle, and may be either flat or raised. They can be present at birth or develop later in life. Moles that were flat during childhood may become raised during adolescence. Some may lose their dark color.

Malignant moles are called melanomas and are far less common during adolescence than later in life. Nevertheless, certain warning signs should be brought to a doctor's attention. These include size larger than half an inch, irregular borders, patchy coloring within the mole, loss of color within the mole, redness, bleeding, or pain.

Some moles may be precursors of future skin cancer, especially in families with a history of melanoma. These types of moles, called dysplastic nevi, often appear in childhood and increase in number during adolescence. *All* adolescents with moles and family history of melanoma *must* be followed closely by a dermatologist or other physician who is skilled at managing skin disorders.

Vitiligo is a rare condition characterized by the loss of normal pigment. Its cause is unknown. The faded patches appear slowly over bony parts of the body: knees, wrists, ankles. The areas rarely return to normal color. There is no single remedy, but ultraviolet light therapy combined with oral medication is effective in some cases. Special cosmetics are available to cover the depigmented skin. The areas are highly vulnerable to sunburn, so a sun block must always be applied before going outside. Vitiligo deserves medical attention because it can resemble other skin problems or can be associated with diseases elsewhere in the body, such as thyroid problems or diabetes.

Pityriasis alba causes pale pink or light brown areas with indistinct edges, often in the middle of the forehead and around the eyes and mouth. It also may appear on the neck, trunk, back, arms, legs, and scrotum. It first develops with two or three reddish spots that fade over several weeks and leave a whitish, powdery scale. Other than the change in color, the only symptom may be some itching.

Pityriasis alba usually appears between ages six and twelve, but 10 percent of the cases begin between thirteen and sixteen. It is most common among African-American children and teenagers.

The cause of pityriasis alba is unknown, and there is no clearly effective treatment. Most of the affected areas slowly disappear, but some may continue into adulthood.

Hair

For most adolescents, the appearance of the hair—its length, luster, color, and style—is one of their greatest concerns. If it is cut too short, how quickly will it grow back? If it falls out, what is wrong? What if too much hair grows in areas where it is unwanted?

How does the hair grow? The follicles in the skin, from which hairs grow, develop during fetal life. No new follicles develop after birth. Hair can thin if follicles die or if the hair shafts are broken off, but hair cannot thicken.

Hair grows in cycles. In its active, growing phase, hair increases in length about one tenth of an inch per day. It grows faster in warm weather than cold, and in females than males. But hair also has a resting phase when it stops growing and may fall out. Of the 100,000 hairs on the scalp, about 25 of 100 are shed every day. Most hairs, (80 to 90 percent) are growing right now. Between 10 and 15 percent are in a resting stage. The others are in transition.

HAIR LOSS

Any acute stress, illness, injury, or surgery can cause hair to stop growing for a while, usually six to ten weeks. When it begins growing again, the new hair will push the old, resting hair out. This hair loss will continue for one to three months and can cause teenagers considerable anxiety. Usually it is a sign that new, healthy hair is growing in.

Hair loss also may follow pregnancy, discontinuing oral contraceptives, crash dieting, malnutrition, anemia, and the use of certain medications. New hair growth resumes when the underlying problem ends.

Premature baldness may start in late adolescence for some males. The first sign can be thinning at the front and sides of the hairline. Most teenager boys with hair thinning have strong family histories of early baldness. Females rarely have premature baldness; if they do, they should consult a doctor.

Alopecia areata is patchy loss of scalp hair. The areas are well defined circles or ovals, and the loss is sudden. The skin underneath looks normal, but on microscopic examination, the hair shaft appears to have narrowed near the skin. Rarely, eyebrows, eyelashes, beard, and other body hair also may be lost.

The cause of alopecia areata is unclear, and its course is unpredictable. For many people, a full head of hair returns quickly. For others, it takes months or years. Still others remain partly bald. There are no clear-cut treatments, but a dermatologist should be consulted and accompanying medical conditions should be evaluated.

Hair loss also can be caused by tight braiding, twisting, pulling, hot combs, curlers, and overly vigorous brushing. The remedy depends on identifying and eliminating the damaging practice. Other causes of hair loss may be related to skin disorders like psoriasis or eczema, or to other underlying problems such as thyroid disease or malnutrition. It is always better to check with a doctor than to ignore hair loss during adolescence.

EXCESSIVE BODY HAIR

Excessive hair growth on the body can be just as disturbing to adolescents as hair loss from the scalp. *Hirsutism* is excessive hair on the face, chest, abdomen, or thighs in females who have no other male characteristics. *Virilism* is hirsutism with other male characteristics, such as deep voice, increased muscle mass, enlarged clitoris, or balding. There also may be a decrease in female characteristics, such as decreased breast development and irregular or absent menstrual periods. Virilism has a hormonal basis and is discussed in Chapter 33. *Lanugo* is an increase in fine, downy hair, usually on the back, shoulders, and upper arms. Lanugo most often accompanies anorexia nervosa (Chapter 7) and other conditions involving malnutrition and severe weight loss.

This section focuses on hirsutism. First, some basics: Hormones play an important role in hair growth and appearance. Androgens (male hormones) stimulate hair growth and increase its coarseness. Estrogens (female hormones) slow the rate of hair growth but may prolong the growing phase of the hair cycle.

Different ethnic and racial groups have different hair types and distributions. People from Mediterranean countries have darker, coarser, thicker hair, for example, than people from Nordic countries. Different families have different patterns of body and facial hair. Daughters tend to have patterns resembling those of their mothers or sisters. During puberty, it is normal to have rapid changes in body hair. It is normal for some hair to grow around the nipples of the breasts, on the lower abdomen, and on the inside of the thighs.

Hirsutism, when associated with other male characteristics or with menstrual irregularities, is not normal and a doctor must be seen when it occurs. Whenever body or facial hair causes anxiety or social discomfort, even if there are no other physical problems, a doctor's attention is warranted.

In most cases, there is no identifiable cause of hirsutism. Sometimes, it can be linked to a specific disorder, such as polycystic ovary syndrome (Chapter 17). Medications, both legal and illegal, can cause hirsutism. The most common illegal type is anabolic steroids, used by athletes to promote muscle development. Legal prescription drugs associated with hirsutism include diphenylhydantoin, or phenytoin (Dilantin), used for seizures, and minoxidil, used orally for high blood pressure and topically (Rogaine) for baldness.

The treatment of hirsutism varies depending on the cause and location. If the cause is identified, a doctor will try to treat the underlying problem usually by stopping the medication or correcting the hormonal problem. Temporary methods include cutting the hair, shaving, waxing, or bleaching. Electrolysis (removing each hair with an electric needle) is a longer-term method, but not always permanent. Electrolysis can be uncomfortable and cannot be used over large areas of the body.

Nails

Common conditions of the fingernails and toenails include the following:

Ingrown toenails develop when the top corner of the nail (usually on the large toe) becomes imbedded in the skin, causing pain, redness, and swelling. Ingrown toenails are caused by the shape of the nail, by cutting the nail too short, or by wearing tight shoes that squeeze the nail into the skin.

Ingrown toenails should be soaked in warm water, and then an antibiotic ointment should be applied. If there is no improvement, a doctor may prescribe an oral antibiotic. New tissue that grows and hardens around the area may need to be cauterized (burned) by a doctor with silver nitrate. Calloused skin around the ingrown nail may also need to be pared away.

When the nail and surrounding skin heal, the nail should be cut straight across and allowed to grow beyond the level of the skin. A recurrence of an ingrown toenail can be prevented if a bit of cotton is wedged under the corner of the nail, encouraging it to grow outward. Persistent ingrown toenails may require surgery to remove part of the nail.

Infection of the nail base is called paronychia. The skin around the nail becomes inflamed and tender or painful, and may be filled with pus. The nail should be soaked in warm water and an antibiotic ointment applied. If there is no improvement, a doctor may need to puncture the nail to drain the pus. An oral antibiotic also may be prescribed.

Thickened nails that are grooved, yellowish brown, and have reddened cuticles indicate a chronic infection, often caused by a fungus. A dermatologist should be seen. Part of the nail edge or plate may need to be removed, and an antifungal ointment or oral medication may be prescribed.

Nail biting is a common nervous habit. Teenagers who bite their nails are usually quite self-conscious about the appearance of their nails but do not know how to stop the habit. The answer is to focus less on the nails and to discover what is causing the anxiety that leads to nail biting. Talking with an empathic adult (parent, teacher, counselor, or therapist) and using relaxation techniques can help. Like most habits, nail biting cannot be stopped overnight. While working to diminish the underlying anxiety, a teenager also should try to avoid infection by keeping the fingers and nails clean.

Pale nails can be a sign of anemia (Chapter 35). This can be caused by blood loss through heavy menstruation or by inadequate iron in the diet. If anemia is the cause and it becomes severe, pale

nails will become brittle, flat, or concave, and ridges may develop
from base to tip.

Pitted or distorted nails can result from problems that affect other
parts of the body, such as psoriasis or vitamin deficiency. A doctor
should be consulted if the nail distortion persists longer than a
few months.

25

The Eyes, Ears, Nose, Mouth, and Throat

The Eyes

Eye problems can occur at any age, but certain symptoms and issues require special attention during adolescence. Schoolwork demands more reading. Blackboards and scoreboards require good distance vision. Sports participation should include protective eyewear to prevent injuries. Glasses worn throughout childhood may be pushed aside as concerns about appearance increase. Physical growth of the facial bones and the eye sockets can produce a change in visual acuity or clarity.

Most eye problems during adolescence are caused by growth-related changes or by irritations, infections, or injuries of the eye. Pain in or around the eyes, though, may signal trouble elsewhere, such as in the sinuses, facial muscles, skull, or brain. Some diseases of the eye are components of more widespread illnesses affecting distant parts of the body, such as the joints or intestines. Persistent problems related to the eyes *always* require medical attention. Even when there are no symptoms or problems, annual vision screening (often done through school) is recommended for all teenagers.

Before considering the causes and treatment of eye problems, some definitions of normal eye anatomy are useful:

The *conjunctiva* is a membrane that covers the white part of

311

the eye and the inside of the eyelids. It provides a clear mucus that lubricates the eyeball and keeps it clean.

The *sclera* is the white part of the eye. It is the outside coat that surrounds the eyeball.

The *pupil* is the opening in the front of the eye through which light enters. The pupil contracts (becomes smaller) in bright light and dilates (opens wider) in the dark.

The *iris* is the colored portion of the eye that surrounds the pupil. It absorbs strong light that could overpower the eye or blur vision.

The *cornea* is the transparent membrane, similar to a watch crystal, in front of the iris. The cornea allows light rays to enter the pupil.

The *lens,* located behind the pupil, bends the entering light rays so they focus on the retina.

The *retina,* the innermost layer of the eye, is the sensitive organ where light rays are focused and converted to electrical signals.

The *optic nerve* at the back of the retina collects the electrical signals and sends the visual information to the brain.

During an eye examination, the doctor looks at the appearance of the conjunctiva, sclera, pupil, iris, and cornea. The muscles that move the eye are checked by asking the adolescent to look far left, right, up, and down. Visual acuity or clarity is examined using an eye chart for distant vision and a reading card for near vision. A small light is shone into the eye to measure the contraction of the pupil. With an instrument called an ophthalmoscope, the doctor looks at the inside of the eye to examine the lens, retina, blood vessels, and optic nerve.

REFRACTIVE ERRORS

The most common eye problems during adolescence are caused by refractive errors. Refraction simply means the bending of incoming light rays. The eyes really do not see objects at all—they see the light that those objects reflect. That is why the eyes see nothing in darkness. Light rays from objects enter the pupil, are bent (or refracted) by the lens, and are changed into electrical signals by the retina. If the lens does not refract the light rays correctly so that they converge exactly at the retina, a blurred image occurs.

When teenagers have difficulty seeing the blackboard or the page in front of them, the problem usually is a refractive error. Types of refractive errors include the following:

Myopia is nearsightedness, or sharp near vision with blurred distance vision. It is the most common vision problem in teenagers. It usually begins during the rapid growth phase of puberty when the bones of the face surrounding the eyes mature.

Myopia occurs when light rays from distant objects converge before they reach the retina. Glasses or contacts with concave lenses correct myopia by bringing the rays together at the retina.

Teenagers with mild myopia may not recognize that they are having difficulty seeing objects at a distance. Some may complain of headache from squinting or eye fatigue. Many will express new difficulty seeing the movies or distant faces. Usually myopia stabilizes once puberty is completed. Myopia that continues to become worse during late adolescence and adulthood can be severe and requires close monitoring by an eye doctor.

Hyperopia is farsightedness, or sharp far vision with blurred near vision. It occurs when the incoming light rays reach the retina before they converge, placing the focal point behind the retina. Glasses or contacts with convex lenses will correct hyperopia.

Astigmatism is blurred vision at both near and far distances. It occurs when the lens does not refract properly and fails to bring light rays together at one point in the eye. Astigmatism typically begins in childhood. Glasses or contacts with cylindrical lenses can correct astigmatism.

Young children usually wear their glasses without much complaint. As they become older and more self-conscious about appearance, they may not comply as readily. Contact lenses or a fashionable pair of frames can be costly, but usually solve the problem. Contacts are available in many different forms, including hard lenses, soft lenses, disposable lenses, and tinted lenses that change eye color. For some eye disorders, contact lenses are preferable to regular glasses. Teenage athletes also find contacts better for sports like basketball, where breakage of eyeglasses is a risk.

If teenagers choose contact lenses, they must keep them clean to maximize comfort and prevent eye infections. Whether they opt for frames or contacts, adolescents need annual examinations because their vision may continue to change.

STRABISMUS

This condition is an asymmetry in the way the muscles that surround the eyes work. One eye may turn too far inward toward the nose (cross-eye) or outward toward the side (walleye). Each eye sees a different picture and sends a different message to the brain. The result can be double vision or a blurred image.

The imbalance may appear some or all of the time. It may occur when the eyes are at rest but not when they are in use and focusing. In some cases, strabismus is apparent only during an eye examination when one eye is covered and quickly uncovered. While covered, the deviant eye will drift out of place; on uncovering and focusing, it will snap back into center position. Strabismus occurs most often in young children. For some youngsters, wearing a patch over the stronger eye helps the deviating eye improve. If strabismus is not corrected early, vision in the weaker eye can be permanently impaired. If strabismus goes uncorrected until adolescence, the prevailing treatment is surgery on the eye muscles.

EYE TRAUMA

Teenagers are at greater risk for injuries of all types than younger children or adults. Eye trauma or injury is no exception. A corneal abrasion is the most common type of eye trauma. This is a scratch on the cornea, frequently caused by a contact lens or a makeup brush. If irritation persists, a doctor should be seen. A teenager who wears contact lenses should not put them back in until the scratch heals.

Another common eye injury is called a subconjunctival hemorrhage. It causes the white part of the eye to appear bloodshot and occurs when a small blood vessel under the conjunctiva ruptures. It can look quite frightening but usually is not serious, causes no pain, and disappears on its own within a few days.

Any significant injury to the eye should be evaluated by an ophthalmologist, especially if there is pain or any change in vision.

THE RED EYE

An eye or eyelid can become red for any number of reasons, some minor, others major. Any persistent red eye requires medical care. Some problems can threaten vision. It is always safer to use nothing in the eye than to guess at treatment without consulting a physician. Problems that can cause a red eye include the following:

Blepharitis is irritation of the eyelid. Its cause can be either within or outside the eye. The small glands in the eyelids may be secreting too much fluid. A form of dermatitis (skin inflammation) may cause scales and crusts to form on the eyelids. Nits (eggs of lice) on the eyelashes can irritate the lids. Dandruff from the scalp can irritate the eyes. A doctor can determine the cause of the irritation and recommend the appropriate treatment that both addresses the root cause and relieves the irritation.

Bacterial infections also cause blepharitis. The signs include a thick, yellow discharge or crust along the lids, thickened lids, loss of eyelashes, or a red swelling at the edge of the lid (a sty). A doctor should always be seen when a bacterial infection of the eye is suspected because prescription antibiotic ointments or drops usually are indicated.

A sty is a painful, swollen inflammation of a gland on the edge of the eyelid. Over several days, a sty grows from a small red spot to a pointed, pus-filled swelling that may rupture on its own. If the sty does not improve with warm water soaks and antibiotic ointment, a doctor can drain it to relieve the pain and speed its healing. Sties that recur should be evaluated for an underlying problem.

Conjunctivitis refers to any inflammation of the conjunctiva. It is often called pink eye and can be caused by an allergy, an injury from a foreign body, bacteria, or a virus. Less common causes include diseases that involve other parts of the body as well as the eye. For example, Reiter syndrome (Chapter 18) is a disease predominantly of adolescent males that involves inflammation of the eyes (conjunctivitis), joints (arthritis), and urinary tract (urethritis).

Periorbital cellulitis is a serious bacterial infection of the eye and surrounding tissues. It may begin with conjunctivitis, a sinus infection, or an ear infection. Whenever the eye and the skin around the eye become red, swollen, and painful, a doctor should be seen immediately. Periorbital cellulitis requires hospitalization and intravenous antibiotics to avoid serious complications.

Keratitis is an inflammation of the cornea. The symptoms include a red eye, moderate pain, some discharge, blurred vision, a cloudy cornea, and an abnormal sensitivity to light (photophobia). Keratitis can be caused by injury or infection. Depending on the cause, treatment may include eye drops, antibiotics by mouth, or, if there is no improvement, surgery. If untreated, keratitis can lead to scarring of the cornea and diminished vision.

Uveitis is an inflammation of the iris and/or the space in front of or behind the lens. The symptoms include pain, watery eyes, slightly blurred vision, small pupil size, and sensitivity to light. Uveitis requires immediate medical attention. It may be a complication of conjunctivitis or keratitis or may accompany injury to the cornea. In some instances, uveitis is a sign of more widespread disease, such as juvenile rheumatoid arthritis (Chapter 31) or colitis (Chapter 29).

The Ears

The ear is composed of three parts: the external, middle, and inner ear. The *external ear* includes the visible outer ear and the canal leading to the eardrum. The *middle ear* is made up of the eardrum or *tympanic membrane (TM)*, the small bones (ossicles) that conduct sound, and the space behind them. The *inner ear* is a complex system of tiny fluid-filled channels that control equilibrium (or balance) and a nerve that carries sound messages from the ear to the brain.

BLOCKED EAR CANAL

This condition may result from a buildup of earwax, a foreign object such as a piece of pencil eraser, or an infection. It is very important not to stick anything into the ear because the eardrum can easily be punctured.

Excess earwax (ceruminosis) may cause no symptoms, or there may be a sense of fullness, popping sounds, uneven hearing, or steady hearing loss. Earwax can be dissolved by over-the-counter ear drops such as Debrox or Cerumenex. If the block does not clear, a doctor may have to remove the wax and examine the ear canal for a foreign object or underlying infection.

Flushing the ear canal at home is not recommended because it can cause dizziness, nausea, or vomiting. If a foreign body is present, the flushing may force it deeper into the canal rather than washing it out.

OTITIS EXTERNA

"Swimmer's ear" is the common name for this inflammation or infection in the ear canal. Water that stays in the ear canal, as after swimming, can tip the acid balance of the canal to an alkaline one, allowing bacteria or fungi to thrive. Symptoms include discharge from the ear, swelling or redness of the ear canal, and pain, especially when moving the outer ear or opening the mouth.

Otitis externa has causes other than swimming. A foreign object (such as a pen or pencil) used to clean the ear can scratch the canal and cause otitis externa. Occasionally, a hair follicle in the canal can become infected. Eczema or seborrheic dermatitis (Chapter 24) can cause irritation of the ear canal.

Swimmer's ear is treated with prescription antibiotic ear drops. Once the infection clears, repeat episodes can be prevented with VōSoL ear drops, available by prescription, or by a homemade preparation of equal parts of rubbing alcohol and white household vinegar. A few drops of the mixture should be put in each ear soon after swimming. This treatment is recommended for teenagers who spend much time in the water, even if they have had only one episode of swimmer's ear.

Otitis externa usually responds quickly to prescription antibiotic ear drops. It should never be ignored, though, because persistent infection can damage the canal and spread to surrounding tissues and bone.

OTITIS MEDIA

Infection of the middle ear is referred to as otitis media. It is much more common in young children than in teenagers or adults. By adolescence, the eustachian tube, which connects the middle ear to the back of the throat, has grown and is less likely to become blocked and infected than in childhood. The lymph tissue also has shrunk by mid- to late adolescence so that the adenoids (lymph glands in the throat, behind the nose) no longer obstruct drainage of the middle ear.

Symptoms of otitis media include pain (often severe), fever, and sometimes a ringing sensation or decreased hearing. The treatment typically is a ten-to-fourteen-day course of antibiotics taken by mouth. If the infection does not clear, drainage and culture of the middle ear fluid may be required. Otitis media always requires medical attention and prompt treatment, both to alleviate the pain and to prevent serious complications.

SEROUS OTITIS MEDIA

This condition is caused by a collection of noninfected fluid in the middle ear. The usual symptoms are hearing loss and a sense of fullness, with no or minimal pain. Serous otitis media is much more common in young children than adolescents. After an infection such as the common cold, a thin yellow or clear fluid may collect in the ear. Over time, the fluid becomes thick and rubbery, resulting in the term "glue ear." This can cause marked hearing loss and destruction of the delicate tissues of the ear if left untreated. Another type of fluid that can collect in the middle ear is blood. This can happen after a blow to the ear or after scuba diving.

Treatment of serous otitis media varies, and no single approach is considered ideal. Fortunately, serous otitis media typically disappears on its own, without complications. Antibiotics alone or in combination with other medication help in some instances, but are ineffective if there is no infection of the fluid. Exercises such as gum chewing and balloon blowing may help the fluid drain. If it persists, a surgical procedure called a myringotomy may be recommended. The surgeon makes a small hole in the eardrum to allow the fluid to drain from the middle ear through the ear canal. A tiny myringotomy tube may be placed in the hole to keep it open. Eventually the tube falls out and the hole seals over. This procedure is performed very commonly in young children; it is used far less often in adolescents.

DEAFNESS

Deafness—either partial or complete—affects fifteen to twenty million Americans. Teenagers may not realize that their hearing is diminished. For some, undiagnosed hearing loss may be the cause of poor school performance. This is one reason why annual hearing checks are performed in many schools.

Temporary hearing loss is very common during adolescence. A teenager who has attended a rock concert may experience some hearing loss that can last from minutes to up to one week. Normal hearing will return if the ears are given a rest from loud noise. On the other hand, constant, repeated exposure to loud noise can cause permanent loss. Teenagers who play or sing with groups should rehearse with ear protectors or with amplifiers turned down. Permanent hearing loss can also result from listening frequently to a stereo system at a high volume. Teenagers who are exposed to a great deal of loud noise should have their hearing checked once or twice a year.

There are two types of hearing loss: conductive and sensorineural. *Conductive hearing loss* refers to impaired sound transmission through the ear canal or middle ear because of any of the problems described previously. *Sensorineural hearing loss* refers to disorders of the inner ear and the auditory nerve, which transmits sound messages to the brain. Sensorineural hearing loss frequently has a congenital cause—a problem before birth, when the mother was pregnant. The result is deafness or hearing loss at birth. Inherited disorders that run in families can cause progressive sensorineural hearing loss years after birth, often beginning in adolescence or adulthood. Other causes of sensorineural hearing loss that occur after birth include infections, trauma, medications, and tumors.

Conductive hearing loss typically has a better prognosis than sensorineural loss because the former responds to medication, surgery, or a hearing aid. The prognosis for sensorineural loss varies, depending on the cause, the age when it appeared, and how it was treated. Implants in the cochlea, the shell-shaped coil of the inner ear, improve hearing for some individuals. An adolescent with a significant sensorineural loss needs educational, social, and psychological support in addition to hearing aids that amplify sound.

The Nose and Sinuses

On the outside, the nose appears to be a simple protrusion in the middle of the face. On the inside, it is a complex organ necessary for breathing and smelling. Air flows through the nostrils into two nasal passages or tunnels, leading to the throat (pharynx), windpipe (trachea), and lungs. Odors are sensed when nerves in the mucous membranes of the nose detect chemicals in the air. The nerve fibers send impulses to two nearby parts of the brain called the olfactory bulbs (one is located just above each nasal passage). From here, impulses are sent to other parts of the brain, where they are recognized as particular odors.

The *sinuses* are air-filled cavities that surround the nose. The four pairs of sinuses are located in the front of the skull, and all connect to the nose. The largest pair (the maxillary sinuses) is located behind the cheekbones on either side of the nose. A small pair lies between the nose and eyes (the ethmoid sinuses), and a somewhat larger pair is behind those (the sphenoid sinuses). Another pair is located just above the eyes, behind the bones of the forehead (the frontal sinuses). The sinuses act as air-filled cushions that lighten the skull and protect the brain from impact injuries.

Nose and sinus problems produce many symptoms: a runny nose, sneezing, dizziness, headache, watery eyes, and pain in the face, eyes, or forehead. The causes may be allergies, viruses (most often the common cold), bacteria, smoke, climate, drafts of air, or drugs (marijuana, cocaine, or glue sniffing). Some of these problems require no medical attention or treatment. For example, the common cold will run its course in seven to ten days, regardless of treatment. Other problems, though, can be very serious. Sinus infections can cause high fever and pain, and can spread to the eyes or brain. Always seek medical care if the discharge from the nose is yellow or green; if high fever develops (over 101°F); if the area around the eyes becomes red and swollen; or if facial pain is severe or persistent. The most common nose and sinus troubles include the following:

RHINITIS

This condition is an inflammation of the nasal membranes that causes rhinorrhea, or runny nose. In adolescents, the usual causes are the common cold, allergies, excessive use of nose sprays or drops, side effects of certain drugs, withdrawal from narcotic substances, or an obstruction or foreign body in the nasal cavity.

An important—and not widely known—point: Repeated use of over-the-counter nasal sprays and drops containing decongestants should be avoided because they can cause dependence and rebound (a worsening of congestion when the medication wears off). If the sprays or drops are used repeatedly, the duration of relief will shorten and the rebound congestion will become worse. The more the sprays and drops are used, the more they are needed, creating a vicious cycle. Not all nasal sprays or drops cause problems, though. Preparations with corticosteroids alone (without decongestants) do not cause dependence or rebound and generally are safe in teenagers. They are used for allergic rhinitis, not for the common cold, and require a doctor's prescription.

Allergic rhinitis is often called hay fever, although the allergy need not be limited to hay or grass. House dust, mold, animal fur, and pollen from flowers, trees, and grass are common "allergens" (substances that cause allergic reactions). They typically follow the seasons: tree pollen in late summer and early autumn. Symptoms are all too familiar to sufferers: sneezing, runny nose, itchy eyes and nose, watery eyes. Allergic rhinitis often starts during adolescence. Teenage girls have allergic rhinitis more often than boys; there is no gender difference in younger children.

The best prevention is avoidance of substances that trigger allergic reactions. If the allergen is indoors—a dog, cat, house dust, or mold—the pet may need another home or housecleaning may need to be more frequent. Dusting with a dry cloth only moves dust around; a damp cloth is better. Removing carpets, drapes, stuffed animals, and feather pillows from the teenager's room may decrease symptoms. Air conditioners, air filters, and humidifiers can help. A dehumidifier can reduce mold in a damp basement. Bathrooms should be cleaned with cleansers that destroy molds.

Controlling or eliminating allergens in the environment is the first line of defense, but may be difficult or impossible to achieve. When symptoms flare, antihistamines and decongestants usually help. It may take some trial and error to see which works best and which has the fewest side effects (such as drowsiness). A phone call or visit to the doctor for advice is a good first step. For persistent symptoms, temporary use of an intranasal steroid or cromolyn (an anti-inflammatory medication) spray may be prescribed. Many children and teenagers with severe allergies improve with "allergy shots." These are injections, usually given weekly, that decrease sensitivity to a given set of allergens. The need for allergy shots usually diminishes by late adolescence.

Vasomotor rhinitis looks like allergic rhinitis, but it is not caused by an allergy to a particular substance. The symptoms (sneezing, runny nose, congestion) are precipitated instead by "nonallergic" conditions such as stress, menstruation, fatigue, air pollution, or extremes in outdoor temperature. The description of when the symptoms appear is less consistent than for allergic rhinitis, and the symptoms are less bothersome. Because no allergy is involved, antihistamines are not helpful. Treatment is usually unnecessary, but oral decongestants may relieve the symptoms. Excessive use of decongestant sprays or drops (as described earlier) should be avoided.

The common cold is a viral cause of runny nose. There are many different types of cold viruses. Treatment of a cold is no different for an adolescent than for anyone else. Staying home in bed is not necessary for most teenagers with colds. They can go to school if they feel well enough, but should remember that colds are highly contagious. Hand washing and covering coughs and sneezes can decrease the likelihood of spread. No matter what treatment is used, most colds persist for seven to ten days. Over-the-counter medicines can make symptoms more tolerable, but they are not a cure. If symptoms continue beyond ten days, or if the temperature reaches 101°F, a doctor should be contacted.

Other causes of rhinitis include withdrawal from certain illegal drugs and head trauma. Use of crack or repeated snorting of cocaine leads to inflammation of the nasal passages and constant runny nose. In cases of head trauma (a blow to the head, for example), a runny nose may result. Immediate medical attention should be sought in such instances.

SINUSITIS

Sinus infection, or sinusitis, is quite common among teenagers. Usually sinusitis is not serious. But if untreated, it can have very serious consequences: infection of the facial bones, the tissues around the eyes, or even the brain.

Infections spread easily from the nose to the sinuses because all sinuses are connected to the nose. The infection causes the lining of the sinus to swell, blocking the drainage of infected material. Symptoms of sinusitis vary from dull facial pain or headache to severe throbbing around the eyes or even the upper teeth. Other symptoms may include fever, lethargy, a yellow or green nasal discharge, or a tickling cough. Symptoms are worse in the morning after awakening because sinus and nasal secretions have collected overnight and further blocked the sinus cavities.

Sinusitis typically is caused by a bacterial infection and requires antibiotics prescribed by a physician. Pain relievers containing acetaminophen, like Tylenol, and oral decongestants help the symptoms but do not cure the underlying infection. The antibiotics often bring relief within two or three days but should be continued for ten to fourteen days to kill all the bacteria. If the symptoms do not improve, a physician should be contacted. Sometimes a different antibiotic continued for up to three weeks may prove effective. At other times, the physician may look for other, less common causes of sinusitis that require different treatment approaches.

RHINOPLASTY

Cosmetic surgery performed to change the shape or size of the nose is called rhinoplasty. It should not be performed until puberty and growth are completed and the facial bones have stopped growing. For most teenagers, this occurs by age sixteen to eighteen. A teenager who is concerned about the appearance of the nose should first talk with his or her doctor about the need for the procedure and referral to a surgeon. When rhinoplasty is done for cosmetic, nonmedical purposes, most health insurance policies will not cover it. The out-of-pocket costs can range from several hundred to several thousand dollars.

The Mouth

The most prevalent problems of the jaw, mouth, lips, and teeth during adolescence are described here:

Temporomandibular joint (TMJ) syndrome is a condition involving one or both sides of the jaw just in front of the ear. The symptoms include jaw pain, trouble chewing, a clicking or cracking sensation in the joint, trouble opening the mouth fully, or locking of the joint. TMJ syndrome also can cause symptoms less localized to the jaw, such as vague headache, toothache, or earache. TMJ syndrome affects adolescents more than any other age group because of the rapid growth of the facial bones during puberty. It can be caused by an asymmetry in the bite, a dislocation of the joint, or spasm of the muscles around the jaw. The symptoms of TMJ syndrome tend to become worse when emotional stress causes jaw clenching or teeth grinding.

The treatment of TMJ syndrome consists of resting the jaw. The adolescent should avoid foods requiring large bites or wide opening of the mouth. Heat and gentle massage to the area helps to relax the muscles. In some instances, a dentist may fit the teenager with an appliance to correct the jaw's misalignment or to prevent teeth grinding. Surgery is rarely necessary to correct dislocation of the jaw. In most cases, the jaw will shift back into place on its own. As the adolescent matures, TMJ syndrome improves and eventually disappears.

Cheilosis is painful cracking and redness at the corners of the mouth. Unlike chapped lips, which are caused by cold or dry climate, cheilosis is caused by an infection or, less frequently, by a vitamin deficiency. Over-the-counter creams that contain antibacterial medication (Polysporin) or antifungal medication (Lotrimin) may relieve pain and speed healing. If there is no improvement within two to three days, a health professional should be seen.

Fever blisters or cold sores ("herpes labialis") are painful clusters of small blisters on the lips or in the mouth. They may appear at times of physical or emotional stress, such as during an illness, menstruation, or final examinations. At first, the area may be painful without any apparent sore. Within a day or two, one or more painful blisters appear. Over the next six to ten days, the blisters crust over and disappear.

Herpes labialis is caused by Herpes simplex virus (HSV) type 1 or, less often, type 2. Most adolescents with herpes labialis acquired the infection during childhood via nonsexual transmission. Among sexually active adolescents, however, HSV infection is epidemic and can cause either mouth or genital lesions (blisters). A doctor should be consulted for a first outbreak of herpes labialis, both to make the diagnosis and recommend treatment. For the first episode, a medication called acyclovir, taken either orally in tablet form or applied to the lips as a cream, can shorten the duration of symptoms. Acyclovir has not been shown to be effective in subsequent outbreaks, although some individuals still find that it decreases the pain. Other topical creams or ointments may be recommended by the physician to numb temporarily the area around the sores.

Canker sores ("aphthous ulcers") are small, white sores that appear on the inside of the mouth, the gums, or tongue. They are particularly sensitive to acidic foods such as orange juice. Canker sores can be caused by local injury, dental braces, or biting the inside of the mouth. At other times, there may be no apparent cause. Canker sores typically heal by themselves within ten days regardless of treatment. Over-the-counter medications (like Orabase) applied directly to the sore can relieve the pain temporarily. If the pain is severe, a doctor or dentist can apply silver nitrate to the sore, creating a type of scab or crust. Canker sores generally are harmless and do not require medical treatment. In rare instances, though, recurrent canker sores may be associated with serious underlying disease such as inflammatory bowel disease (Chapter

29). A doctor should always be told of canker sores when they are a frequent, recurring problem.

Dental problems are best prevented by regular dental checkups and daily flossing and brushing. Adolescence is the prime time for dental cavities. Good oral hygiene is important during these years to control plaque, which can lead to tooth damage, cavities, and gum problems. Keeping high-sugar foods (candy, soda) at a minimum and using fluoride toothpastes also help prevent cavities.

Facial bones grow and change through puberty, and alignment of the teeth and jaw may shift. A dentist may recommend that the older child or young adolescent see an orthodontist, who can help determine if and when correction is indicated. The appliances used to correct the alignment of the teeth or jaw include braces, headgear, retainers, and expanders. Some of this treatment may be covered by dental insurance policies; much is not. Adolescents should understand that the treatment is expensive and requires consistent use of the appliances and regular dental visits. They should be informed, at the first visit, what to expect and what will be expected of them.

Another dental problem that appears commonly during adolescence is impaction of the wisdom teeth. When these large, hindmost teeth crowd other teeth, or cannot break through the gum surface, the dentist will recommend extraction. The removal usually can be done in the office using local anesthesia.

Halitosis, or bad breath, is a major concern of teenagers. It usually is caused by inadequate hygiene of the gums and teeth. Flossing will remove plaque and loosen tiny food particles from between the teeth that may decay and cause halitosis. Flossing, brushing, and using mouthwash at least twice a day eliminate halitosis for most teenagers. If it persists, a dentist should be consulted.

The Throat

Sore throat is ubiquitous during adolescence. The medical term is *pharyngitis,* an inflammation of the mucus membrane of the throat, or pharynx. The most common cause of sore throat is a cold virus, which runs its course in seven to ten days. Other viruses that cause sore throat in teenagers include Epstein-Barr virus (infectious mononucleosis, Chapter 34) and influenza virus. The typical treatment for all of these viral infections is acetaminophen (Tylenol) and gargling with warm salt water or mouthwash (like Chloraseptic).

At times, the cause of sore throat may be noninfectious, such as throat irritation from smoking cigarettes or marijuana, dehydration, shouting, or dry air. Sore throats from these causes typically are not severe and are not accompanied by fever, but they can recur frequently. Whenever a sore throat is severe, prolonged, recurrent, or associated with fever, a doctor should be contacted. Causes of sore throat that commonly affect teenagers and require medical attention include the following:

Strep throat is an infection caused by bacteria called streptococci. The symptoms of strep throat include severe soreness, difficulty swallowing, and fever. Strep throat can look the same as a viral throat infection. The diagnosis requires a laboratory test. The back of the throat is swabbed and the material is sent to the laboratory for culture. Because cultures require forty-eight hours, kits have been developed for use in the doctor's office to speed the diagnosis. Strep throat responds well to penicillin or other antibiotics such as erythromycin. If strep throat is suspected, a doctor should be contacted immediately because late or no treatment can lead to rheumatic fever (Chapter 34) or a kidney problem called glomerulonephritis (Chapter 30).

Mycoplasma is another bacterial infection that causes sore throat and is more common during adolescence than at any other age. Mycoplasma also can cause ear infections or pneumonia. The symptoms of mycoplasm infection include fever, achiness, sore throat, earache, headache, and a persistent dry, hacking cough. The symptoms improve with antibiotics such as erythromycin, though the cough may linger for several weeks.

Sexually transmitted diseases can cause sore throat through oral–genital contact. The most common is gonococcal pharyngitis. The gonorrhea bacteria infects the throat, resulting in pain, redness, pus, swollen glands, and fever. Some individuals may harbor gonorrhea in the throat but have no symptoms. Whenever and wherever gonorrhea is present, regardless of symptoms, antibiotic treatment is imperative for the individual and for all sexual partners. Other sexually transmitted diseases that can cause sore throat are chlamydia, herpes, and syphilis. These infections are discussed in Chapter 21.

Tonsillitis, or infection of the tonsils, causes sore throat, difficulty swallowing, and fever. Most sore throats do not involve the tonsils and, therefore, are called pharyngitis. In tonsillitis, the cause may be either viral or bacterial, and a culture is needed to make a final diagnosis. Tonsillitis usually is managed in the same way as pharyngitis. A medical emergency arises when the tonsils are so swollen that they block the airway, when the infection spreads outside the tonsil (peritonsillar cellulitis), or when pus collects around the tonsil (peritonsillar abscess). These conditions require emergency medical treatment, usually with hospitalization, intravenous antibiotics, and sometimes surgery to drain the infection. The signs of these serious conditions include severe sore throat, fever, trouble swallowing even saliva, trouble breathing, and neck swelling. *These conditions require an immediate visit to a doctor or emergency room.*

In early adolescence, a teenager's tonsils may appear large even when not infected because all lymph glands, including the tonsils, have grown very rapidly during late childhood. Size alone is not a reason to remove them. Tonsils are not removed routinely, as they were a generation ago.

A tonsillectomy (surgical removal of tonsils) is usually performed only when the tonsils are so large that they interfere with breathing or when strep throats are so frequent that they endanger the teenager's health and function. This usually means at least four strep throats, proven by culture, over the course of one year. Even then, many physicians opt to treat early with antibiotics and avoid surgery. As the teenager matures, the tonsils shrink and the infections become far less frequent.

26

The Breast and Chest

The first part of this chapter discusses conditions of the breast. Most of these conditions pertain to females, though gynecomastia, or breast enlargement, is a common concern of adolescent males. The second part of the chapter discusses the many causes of chest pain in adolescents. Additional information specific to the lungs and heart can be found in Chapters 27 and 28.

The Breast

The first visible sign that puberty in girls has begun is breast budding. This often occurs between ages eight and thirteen, shortly before the growth spurt.

Breast development marks a new threshold for a young woman. She may be comfortable and delighted with her changing body, or she may be self-conscious or worried about the size and shape of her breasts. Increased public awareness of breast cancer has produced anxiety for many teenage girls. Any perceived abnormality may be incorrectly interpreted by the teenager as breast cancer. During adolescence, breast cancer is exceedingly rare, but other breast problems are very common. It is important that the adolescent discuss her concerns with a health professional. She should learn how to examine her breasts because a good habit established during adolescence may be lifesaving later in adulthood. A nurse or doctor can show her how to examine her breasts, or she can obtain a pamphlet from the American Cancer Society or the National Cancer Institute (see Resources at the end of the book).

ASYMMETRICAL BREASTS

It is not unusual for one breast to develop earlier or faster than the other. One breast may seem more tender, firmer, or better defined than the other. The asymmetry is most pronounced when the breasts are growing rapidly. In most girls, the slower-developing breast eventually matures to resemble the other. Until then, a padded bra cup can make outward appearance more symmetrical.

In a very small percentage of women, there is an absence of breast tissue or the nipple on one or both sides. This can be surgically corrected once puberty is completed. Between 1 and 2 percent of women have extra nipples, usually located just below the breast or on the upper abdomen. This too can be corrected surgically.

UNDERDEVELOPED BREASTS

Fashion dictates more than hemlines or fabrics. It also defines desirable body shape. When fashion promotes a full figure, adolescents with small breasts may worry about their development or may feel less attractive. When the flat-chest look is in, adolescents who develop earlier than peers or who have large breasts may feel self-conscious.

Breast size has nothing to do with sexuality, femininity, childbearing, or breast-feeding. For many teenagers, concerns about underdeveloped breasts diminish with increasing maturity and stabilization of body image. If the concern persists into young adulthood, surgical enlargement of the breasts can be considered. Many problems have been reported with the use of silicone implants. A young woman should talk with an experienced surgeon and should ask about all potential short-term and long-term complications. Nonsurgical techniques to increase breast size, such as creams, pumps, and massage, do not work. Exercise can increase the size of the chest muscles around the breast but does not increase the breast tissue itself. Hormonal medications such as oral contraceptives can result in some increase in breast tissue.

Teenagers should recognize that a condition that causes significant weight loss will cause a decrease in breast size. The concern should focus on the cause of the weight loss rather than on the breast.

ENLARGED BREASTS

This can happen when the developing breast tissue is unusually sensitive to estrogen. Large breasts can lead to shoulder and neck pain, skin inflammation beneath the breasts, difficulty exercising, unkind comments from peers, and extreme self-consciousness. Breast size may decrease somewhat once puberty is completed but rarely enough to affect the physical symptoms. If enlargement is physically or psychologically debilitating, some breast tissue may be removed surgically, regardless of age or pubertal stage. The adolescent should be fully informed about the procedure, likely outcome, and future precautions. She should know where and how large the scar will be. There may be altered sensation, such as numbness, in the area around the scar. If the surgery is done before puberty is completed, a second procedure may be necessary to remove additional breast tissue. If the surgery involves moving the nipples, breast-feeding later in life may be affected. The ability to become pregnant or to deliver a baby is *not* affected in any way by breast surgery.

DISCHARGE FROM THE BREAST

Galactorrhea is the medical term for secretion of breast milk. It is normal to secrete milk after giving birth, during nursing, or occasionally following miscarriage or abortion.

Galactorrhea is associated with elevated levels of prolactin, a hormone secreted by the pituitary gland. Medications, including oral contraceptives and several psychiatric medications, can cause galactorrhea. Excessive stimulation of the breast can increase prolactin levels, resulting in galactorrhea. When amenorrhea (absence of menstrual periods) accompanies the galactorrhea, the cause may be a small tumor of the pituitary gland (Chapter 17). Galactorrhea always requires medical attention.

BREAST PAIN

Most breast pain is a harmless part of the normal menstrual cycle. It begins several days before and disappears toward the end of the menstrual period. It can be eased with heat, a firmly supportive bra, or anti-inflammatory medications such as ibuprofen. If the discomfort is extreme, hormonal therapy (such as oral contraceptives) may help. Breast pain and tenderness that is not associated with the menstrual period should always be discussed with a physician.

BREAST MASSES (LUMPS, TUMORS, CYSTS)

Breast cancer is *very rare* in adolescence. Far less than 1 percent of all breast lumps in teenagers are malignant, or cancerous. The vast majority of breast cancer (98 percent) affects women over age twenty-five.

Most breast masses in teenagers are benign (noncancerous), solid tumors called *fibroadenomas.* These lumps usually are smooth, rubbery, firm, and movable to the touch. They can grow slowly, disappear entirely, or remain the same size. Fibroadenomas may be detected at any time after puberty begins but are more frequent late rather than early in adolescence.

Fluid-filled cysts also cause breast lumps but less often in adolescents than in older women. In fibrocystic breast disease (FCBD), several small cysts throughout the breasts may come and go over time. FCBD is far more common among women in their thirties and forties than among adolescents. The signs of FCBD include small, firm, movable, tender lumps scattered throughout the breasts. The tenderness and size of the lumps tend to increase before and decrease after the menstrual period.

WHAT TO DO ABOUT BREAST MASSES

First and foremost: do not panic. The vast majority of breast lumps in teenagers are harmless and will disappear without any treatment. If a lump persists beyond one month, a doctor should be consulted. In teenagers—but not in older women—the doctor may decide to follow the lump for a few months. This is because breast cancer is so rare during adolescence and neither fibroadenomas nor cysts cause damage or threaten health.

Some women find that FCBD improves if they avoid foods containing caffeine (coffee, tea, cola). If FCBD persists and causes recurrent pain or discomfort, the doctor may recommend oral contraceptives to suppress the body's hormone production, which causes changes in the breast tissue.

The pubertal stage in which a lump appears is important. The breast bud of early puberty can feel like a lump and absolutely should *not* be removed because the breast then will not develop. If left alone, the breast bud will grow and the lumplike character will disappear.

If a lump appears later in adolescence, the doctor may recommend an office procedure called aspiration. A needle is inserted into the lump and, if it is a cyst, the fluid is withdrawn. If there is no fluid on aspiration, the doctor may recommend the removal of a small amount of tissue for diagnosis (biopsy). This same-day surgical procedure involves a small incision and may be done with either local or general anesthesia. The reason for the biopsy is to be absolutely certain that the lump is benign.

Mammography (X-ray of the breast) generally is not useful during adolescence. The young breast is very dense, obscuring the difference on the X-ray film between the lump and the surrounding tissue. During adulthood, the fat content on the breast increases, giving the breast a less dense appearance on the film. Mammography then becomes a very important screening test for breast cancer.

All the preceding comments regarding breast masses pertain to teenagers, not to adults. Breast cancer is rare in adolescents and common in adult women. One in ten adult women develops breast cancer. While mammography is not helpful in teenagers, it is very important in adult women. Many lumps in adolescents can be observed for months without aspiration or biopsy; few lumps in adults should be observed that long. Any adult woman with a breast lump should see her doctor early—as soon as she detects the lump.

GYNECOMASTIA

As discussed in Chapter 2, gynecomastia, or enlargement of the male breast, occurs in 60 percent of normal adolescent boys and typically disappears as puberty progresses. If it persists beyond two years, surgical removal of the breast tissue is an option.

In obese adolescents, fatty tissue may look like breast enlargement. This "pseudogynecomastia" will decrease with weight loss but not with progression of puberty alone. Surgery is discouraged for pseudogynecomastia because, without weight loss, the fat will reaccumulate.

Rarely, gynecomastia during adolescence is caused by an underlying medical problem. In these cases, though, there are signs in addition to breast enlargement. An inherited disease called Klinefelter syndrome (Chapter 33), for example, results in delayed puberty and small testes as well as gynecomastia. Thyroid and liver disorders can trigger gynecomastia. Certain drugs may cause gynecomastia, such as antidepressants, steroids, insulin, amphetamines, narcotics, and marijuana.

Chest Pain

Young people aged ten to twenty-one make 650,000 annual visits to doctors' offices or clinics because of chest pain. Fortunately, chest pain in adolescence seldom signals a major medical problem. But it can be frightening, especially if there is a family history of heart disease.

Although chest pain in teenagers is common and usually not serious, it raises a complex medical question because of its many possible causes. In addition to the heart, which is rarely the source, chest pain can originate in the bones and muscles of the thorax (the chest cage), the lungs, or the esophagus (the tube leading from the mouth to the stomach). Even the organs located high in the abdomen (the liver, spleen, and stomach) can be the site of chest pain.

The most common causes of chest pain in teenagers include the following:

MUSCULOSKELETAL CAUSES

Pain originating in the muscles and bones of the thorax is rarely serious. The four most common types are:

• A sudden, sharp, knife-like pain that lasts only seconds or minutes. Most often, it is on the left side of the front of the chest and is intensified by taking a deep breath. This type of pain is not serious and needs no treatment.

• An aching or throbbing pain that lasts days to weeks. The muscles in the chest wall can be strained by coughing, heavy lifting, or exercise. Deep breathing, twisting, and raising the arms make the pain worse. The muscle will feel tender when touched. This type of pain can be quite bothersome but is not at all dangerous. It generally improves with acetaminophen (Tylenol), aspirin, or ibuprofen and resting the sore muscle area.

• A sharp, sticking pain that lasts days to weeks. A blow to the chest or a bad coughing spell can cause a rib fracture or muscle bruise. The injured site is tender to the touch and the pain gets much worse with deep breathing or coughing. A rib fracture usually requires no treatment, but it *hurts*. An Ace bandage around the chest, along with aspirin or ibuprofen, can help relieve the pain.

• A constant, aching pain and tenderness along the breastbone that last days to months. This is called costochondritis, and is an inflammation of the cartilage (the elastic gristle) that connects the ribs to the breastbone. The inflammation sometimes causes swelling or a lump, usually along the edge of the breastbone. The pain and swelling may be in a single or several spots. The pain may be mild to severe, may begin suddenly or gradually, and may spread to the shoulder or arm. Breathing and movement—even sneezing—may increase the pain. A heating pad, aspirin, or ibuprofen help relieve the pain.

ANXIETY

Chest pain frequently accompanies anxiety or stress. The pain may be described as almost anything—tightness, heaviness, aching, or stabbing pain. It has no relation to physical movement or exercise. When it starts and how long it lasts are unpredictable. Anxiety or panic attacks (Chapter 13) typically cause chest pain, rapid heart-beat, shortness of breath, and light-headedness. These attacks are very frightening but are not physically dangerous. Effective modes of treatment are available.

PAIN FROM THE LUNGS

Chest pain that comes from the lungs is more diffuse than musculo-skeletal pain and is more likely to be associated with other symptoms. There are a number of causes:

Pleuritis, or pleurisy, is caused by an inflammation of the *pleura,* the lining around the lungs. The pain is stabbing and increases with inspiration, or breathing in. Pleuritis often is accompanied by fever, cough, sore throat, or achiness. Viral infection is frequently the cause, but other infections and many noninfectious diseases can also cause pleuritis. A doctor should be seen whenever pleuritis is suspected.

Pneumonia is an infection of the lungs. Its symptoms include fever, cough, shortness of breath, and chest pain (Chapter 27).

Spontaneous pneumothorax produces acute, severe stabbing pain on one side of the chest, with varying degrees of shortness of breath. It is caused when the small air sacs of the lung rupture, leaking air into the space between the lungs and the thorax. As the air pressure in the space increases, it forces collapse of the lung. Spontaneous pneumothorax typically happens in healthy ado-lescent and young adult males who have no history of previous lung problems. It is very important to see a doctor immediately if a pneumothorax is suspected. A small pneumothorax will not interfere with breathing or oxygen delivery to the blood and may require no specific treatment. Close observation and frequent chest X-rays are very important, though, because a small pneumothorax can enlarge, resulting in a life-threatening problem. If this happens, a chest tube will be inserted into the space between the lung and the thorax. As the collected air is drawn off, the lung reexpands.

Once a pneumothorax has healed, there is no need to limit exercise. Activities that involve rapid changes in pressure, such as scuba diving or flying in small aircraft, should be avoided. Teenagers who have had one spontaneous pneumothorax are at risk for a second. Repeated episodes are an indication for correction, especially if the episodes involve both sides. The correction usually is done surgically by tacking the lung to the thorax so that the lung is unable to collapse. Nonsurgical correction also can be effective. Medications are placed into the space around the lung through a chest tube. The medication causes inflammation followed by scarring of the space so that the lung becomes permanently fused to the thorax. Decisions about corrective methods usually are made jointly with the teenager's physician and a consulting chest surgeon.

A pulmonary embolus is a blood clot in the lung (Chapter 27). It is a small piece of a larger blood clot, usually in the leg, that has broken off and traveled through the bloodstream to lodge in the lung. The symptoms include sudden shortness of breath, acute chest pain, and usually thigh or calf pain and swelling. While it is quite rare in teenagers, risk factors include oral contraceptives, cigarette smoking, obesity, and immobilization, such as after an injury or fracture.

A pulmonary embolus is a very serious, life-threatening condition. If it is suspected, the adolescent should seek immediate medical care. The treatment involves hospitalization and intravenous medication to dissolve the clot. Following the hospital stay, oral medication to prevent a clot from reforming is continued for several months.

CARDIAC CAUSES

The heart rarely causes chest pain in teenagers, but possible problems are discussed below.

Pericarditis is an inflammation of the pericardium, or lining around the heart. The inflammation causes sharp pain in the center or left side of the chest that is aggravated by lying flat in bed and deep breathing. The pain is diminished by sitting up and leaning forward. Usually pericarditis is caused by a virus and disappears without treatment. There are many causes, though, that do require very specific treatment and can be life-threatening if left untreated. A doctor, therefore, should always be seen when pericarditis is suspected (Chapter 28).

Mitral valve prolapse (MVP) is a very common, but seldom serious, problem in teenagers. The mitral valve controls the flow of blood from the upper left chamber (the atrium) to the lower left chamber (the ventricle) of the heart. In MVP, the valve is slightly thickened and billows (or "prolapses") upward into the left atrium when the heart contracts. This billowing produces a heart murmur that can be heard with a stethoscope. MVP usually causes no symptoms and is found incidentally on a routine physical examination. When symptoms do appear, the most likely are vague pain under the breastbone and palpitations, or the sensation that the heart is beating irregularly (Chapter 28).

EVALUATING CHEST PAIN

Whenever chest pain is severe or persistent, see a doctor. Usually a diagnosis can be made by a medical history and physical examination alone. Sometimes it may be necessary to do a chest X-ray or an electrocardiogram (ECG or EKG), which is a recording of the heart's electrical impulses. If the doctor suspects MVP, an echocardiogram may be done. An echocardiogram uses sound waves to assess the heart's structure and blood flow. Other laboratory tests to examine the heart are discussed in Chapter 28.

27

The Lungs

The respiratory system incudes the two lungs and the airways leading to them from the nose and mouth (Figure 27.1). The *trachea* is the main airway leading from the throat into the chest. The *bronchi* branch off the trachea like tree limbs and, in turn, lead to smaller airways called *bronchioles.* Eventually the air reaches the *alveoli,* which are tiny air sacs within the lungs, arranged in a honeycomb pattern. *Pulmonary arteries* supply blood to the lungs, and *pulmonary veins* carry blood away from the lungs. Like the bronchi, they branch into increasingly smaller vessels, ending in capillaries.

The major diseases affecting the trachea, bronchi, and lungs will be discussed in this chapter. Though it would be easier for readers if this information were organized by symptoms—cough, fever, or shortness of breath—almost all lung diseases can cause any or all of these symptoms. This chapter, therefore, is organized by specific disorders rather than symptoms.

Bronchitis

Bronchitis is an inflammation of the trachea and/or bronchi. It can be caused by an infection or an irritant such as cigarette smoke. A healthy teenager is more likely to develop bronchitis if precipitating factors are present: an infection of the nose or throat (a head cold, for example), sinusitis (an infection of the sinuses around the nose),

337

The Lungs

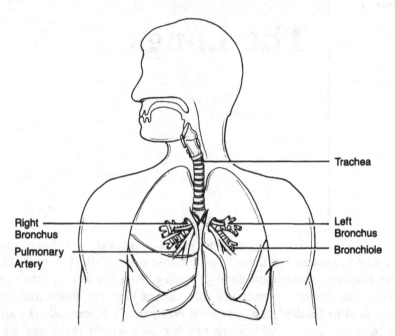

Figure 27.1

air pollution, cigarette smoke, noxious fumes (such as sulfuric acid, ammonia, chlorine, sulfur dioxide), or allergies. These factors can damage the cells that line the trachea and bronchi, resulting in inflammation and accumulation of mucus.

The earliest symptom of bronchitis usually is a dry, hacking cough, often associated with a common cold. Within a few days, the cough begins to produce mucus. Other symptoms may include pain around the breastbone (often from persistent coughing), fever, and shortness of breath. The cough tends to outlast other symptoms, lingering for several weeks in some instances.

Bronchitis typically disappears within one to four weeks. If the irritation is persistent, the bronchitis can become a chronic, ongoing condition. This is especially true in cigarette smokers whose airways have become so inflamed that they cannot clear mucus normally. The typical symptom is a "smoker's cough" that produces thick mucus in the morning.

Bronchitis that clears within a few weeks or even a few months does not cause permanent damage to the lungs. Chronic bronchitis, though, with excessive mucus, may be a sign that a destructive process is involving the bronchi and bronchioles. This destruction, called bronchiectasis, is uncommon in adolescents, but a doctor should always be seen when a cough persists beyond two weeks.

TREATMENT OF BRONCHITIS

Several basic rules apply when bronchitis develops. Avoid irritants like cigarette smoke and dry air. A humidifier in the bedroom at night can help. If the bronchitis is caused by an infection rather than allergies, avoid antihistamines because they may dry the lung's secretions and make it difficult to cough up mucus.

A chest X-ray is not needed to diagnose bronchitis. The doctor will make the diagnosis based on the symptoms and physical examination. If the bronchitis is caused by a bacterial infection, the cough will produce mucus that appears yellow, gray, or green. If the cause is a viral infection, there is little or no mucus and it is clear or white. Bronchitis caused by a bacterial infection is treated with prescription antibiotics such as amoxicillin, erythromycin, or tetracycline taken orally for seven to ten days. Bronchitis caused by a viral infection will not improve with antibiotics and does not require any specific medication.

The symptoms of both bacterial and viral bronchitis can be relieved by drugs that either inhibit coughing ("antitussives") or promote the expelling or coughing up of mucus ("expectorants"). Many over-the-counter medicines contain both antitussives and expectorants. These medications generally are safe but may cause drowsiness. They do not "cure" the bronchitis and should never be used longer than one to two weeks without a doctor's knowledge. Antitussives are most useful before bedtime to suppress nighttime coughing.

Pneumonia

Pneumonia is an infection of the lung tissue. It differs from bronchitis and is more serious. Patients with pneumonia are sicker—they have fever, often have a headache and chills, may have chest pain when taking deep breaths, are often short of breath, and usually have a cough. An X-ray will be abnormal with pneumonia but normal with bronchitis.

The most common cause of pneumonia is a virus. Viral pneumonia typically starts with coldlike symptoms (runny nose, sore throat, achiness) that progress to a cough and fever. There is no specific treatment for viral pneumonia other than rest and over-the-counter medications to relieve its symptoms.

Bacterial pneumonia is less common and more severe than viral pneumonia. Bacterial pneumonia often comes on suddenly with fever, chills, chest pain, a hacking cough, and shortness of breath. Initially the cough may be dry, but eventually it produces discolored mucus that may be blood-streaked. Bacterial pneumonia always requires specific treatment with appropriate antibiotics.

The vast majority of teenagers with pneumonia recover completely within one to two weeks. If complications do develop, they can take four forms:

• *Pleural effusion* is a collection of fluid in the space around the lung. The fluid can impair the expansion of the lung, making the shortness of breath or the chest pain worse. It usually clears on its own.

• *Empyema* is a collection of infected pus around the lung. If left untreated, it can cause scarring and permanent lung damage. Empyema requires hospitalization and drainage either by a needle or by a tube that remains in the chest for days to weeks.

• *Lung abscess* is a collection of pus in a cavity within the lung. This is rare in teenagers, but it requires weeks of antibiotics, often drainage, and sometimes surgery.

• *Spread of infection through the bloodstream* always requires hospitalization and intravenous antibiotics.

Pneumonia is a serious but curable infection. *Always* see a doctor when it is suspected. Early diagnosis and treatment lead to rapid improvement of symptoms and minimize the likelihood that complications will develop.

Environmental Irritants

Indoors and out, the air is full of agents that can irritate the lungs—smoke, pollens, gases, pesticides, perfumes, pollutants, house dust. Everyone breathes these irritants, but teenagers are more sensitive to them than most adults. Adolescent lungs and respiratory muscles are still growing. At the same time, puberty puts extra demands on the lungs because the whole body is calling for oxygen and energy as it grows. As a result, teenagers may be especially susceptible to irritants in the air they breathe.

Just how the adolescent lungs respond to outside irritants depends on several factors: genetics, the amount of exposure to irritants, and the type of irritant. If there is a family history of allergies, for example, a teenager has an increased chance of asthma or allergic response to dust, pollen, and a host of other irritants. Where you live is also a major factor. Problems are more common in industrial areas with factories, smelters, and high air levels of heavy metals, or in areas of heavy agriculture, mining, and forestry. The indoor environment also plays a role—teenagers whose homes have gas stoves, who live with tobacco smokers, and who have pets have more respiratory problems.

Avoiding active smoking (tobacco, marijuana, crack) is essential for any teenager with respiratory problems; so is avoiding exposure to the passive smoke of others, industrial smoke, or household pollutants. When lung problems arise, it is important to identify and eliminate the irritant. Sometimes the cause may be obvious but, in other instances, a doctor may need to conduct a series of tests to discover the source of the problem.

Asthma

Asthma is best described by its symptoms—difficulty in breathing, wheezing, and gasping for air. Medically defined, asthma is airway obstruction that happens periodically when the bronchi become inflamed and clogged with mucus. Between attacks, most adolescents with asthma have no or few symptoms.

Asthma is the most common chronic lung condition of teenagers. Millions of children and adolescents have asthma, making it a frequent cause of school absence. For unclear reasons, both its prevalence and severity have increased in the past decade. If asthma is suspected, medical care should be sought early, before the next attack. Treatment is highly effective and can prevent suffering and even death.

Many factors can cause asthma flares—air pollution, cold air, mold, mildew, dust, animal hair, smoke, pollen, food or medication allergies, respiratory infections, emotional stress, and exercise. Many adolescents with asthma have a parent or sibling with asthma or allergies.

SYMPTOMS

Asthma attacks occur when stimulants irritate the airways and cause them to constrict or narrow. The resulting symptoms include wheezing (especially at night), shortness of breath, pain or tightness in the chest, a hacking cough, and a choking sensation. The coughing can be so bad that the adolescent gags, vomits, or complains of abdominal pain. The shortness of breath can begin very suddenly or can increase gradually as the teenager tires from the work of trying to breathe.

Symptoms vary widely in frequency, severity, and duration. They may last minutes to days. Some teenagers have one episode a year, while others wheeze almost daily. At its worst, asthma is a life-threatening condition that causes intense anxiety and a suffocating sensation.

When seeing a physician about asthma, it is important to spell out the specific symptoms, when they occur, and how often. The doctor will ask about previous emergency room visits, hospitalizations, and medications for asthma. Situations within the home—cigarette smoke, animals, emotional stress—may exacerbate the teenager's asthma. The goal of the history taking is to prevent asthma attacks by identifying and correcting as many precipitating factors as possible.

EMERGENCY SIGNS

The following signs call for emergency care:

- inability to speak in full sentences because of shortness of breath,
- difficulty breathing when lying down,
- use of neck or stomach muscles to breathe instead of the usual chest muscles,
- increasing sleepiness as the breathing becomes worse,
- *no* wheezing with severe shortness of breath.

Wheezing is one of the most obvious signs of asthma. If the teenager feels increasingly short of breath but stops wheezing, it can mean that air flow to and from the lungs is blocked. This is a life-threatening condition that must be treated immediately.

When a patient is taken to a physician or an emergency room for an acute asthma attack, several tests may be performed to measure respiratory distress. An instrument called a spirometer measures the lungs' capacity to fill and empty. A "peak flow meter" is a small, hand-held instrument that measures how fast air is expelled from the lungs. A blood test or a small gauge worn on the finger (called a pulse oximeter) may be used to measure the amount of oxygen in the blood. A chest X-ray may be done to look for problems that can make asthma worse, such as pneumonia. If the attack is severe, though, treatment will begin before any tests are done.

MANAGING ASTHMA

There is no magic cure for asthma, but it can be controlled. Avoiding factors that trigger asthma is a basic rule of thumb. Most adolescents with asthma improve when dust is minimized, particularly in their bedrooms. This means giving away stuffed animals; using synthetic rather than feather pillows; enclosing mattresses in plastic covers; replacing draperies or miniblinds with pull-down shades; eliminating high-pile carpets, upholstered furniture, and houseplants. It may also mean finding another home for a beloved furry pet.

Vacuuming frequently, dusting with a damp cloth, damp-mopping uncarpeted floors, and using antimildew products to clean bathrooms are all helpful measures. If the bedroom is on the ground floor, basement dampness or mold from leaves around the outside of the house may contribute to asthma. Installing air conditioners, electronic air filters, and dehumidifiers can help, but filters should be cleaned regularly.

Asthma can be treated with medication on a daily basis or as needed at home and school. The most common form of treatment is a small, hand-held inhaler that delivers preset doses of medication. *All* asthma medication should be used with a doctor's knowledge and instruction. It is wrong to think that more is better. Overuse of asthma medication can cause life-threatening problems, such as irregular heartbeat or seizures. If an asthma attack requires using inhalers more frequently than four times a day, the adolescent should call a doctor or go to an emergency room. Deaths from asthma occur when an adolescent either waits too long for treatment or overuses medications in an attempt to control the symptoms.

If a doctor recommends an inhaler, it is important to learn how to use it properly. The inhaler should be held in front of the open mouth, squeezed, and the released puff of medication should be inhaled deeply. Lips should not be sealed around the mouthpiece during inhalation because that delivers the medication to the roof of the mouth rather than into the trachea.

A variety of asthma medications are available for home use. If a doctor prescribes one type and the teenager finds that it is not effective or has side effects, it is important to call the doctor and explain the details. Another type of medication may be more appropriate.

Asthma medications, with some trade names in parentheses, come in the following forms:

• Inhaled bronchodilators (Ventolin, Proventil, Alupent) are metered-dose medications, dispensed by hand-held inhalers. They relax the muscles of the airways, allowing the airways to open up. These medications can be used up to four times a day, one or two puffs at a time. They work quickly and can be very helpful during an asthma attack. Care must be taken not to use them excessively during an attack. Overuse of bronchodilators can cause jitteriness, headache, and rapid or irregular heartbeat.

• Inhaled cromolyn sodium (Intal), also dispensed by a hand-held inhaler, takes several weeks to reach a maximum effect. It is not helpful during an acute asthma attack. It suppresses the allergic or inflammatory reactions that are associated with asthma and is used on a daily basis regardless of asthma symptoms.

• Inhaled corticosteroids (Vanceril, Beclovent, AeroBid, Azmacort) are anti-inflammatory medications dispensed by metered-dose inhalers. Unlike oral corticosteroids taken in pill or liquid form, inhaled corticosteroids have very low rates of absorption into the bloodstream. Inhaled corticosteroids work by decreasing the inflammation and swelling of the lining of the airways. They help to prevent asthma attacks but are of little help in the midst of an attack.

• Oral corticosteroids (prednisone) are taken in pill or liquid form once or twice a day when all other medications are not adequately controlling the asthma. Prednisone typically is prescribed in a tapered dose, meaning a decrease in dose every few days until it can be stopped completely without a flare in the asthma. Prednisone may be started at home to break an acute attack or it may be started after an attack has been brought under control in an emergency room or hospital. Administration of this drug is stopped as soon as possible (usually within a week) because prolonged use interferes with the body's ability to make its own corticosteroids.

Side effects of prolonged use include interference with growth, weight gain, osteoporosis (thinning of bone), and susceptibility to infection.

• Oral theophylline (Slo-Bid, Slo-Phyllin, Theo-Dur, Uniphyl) is used for long-term treatment of moderate to severe asthma. It is taken daily as pills, liquid, or "sprinkles" on soft food such as applesauce. It works by relaxing the muscles of the airways and the blood vessels in the lungs. Theophylline has many side effects that become worse as the dose increases. These include nausea, abdominal pain, vomiting, jitteriness, agitation, irritability, headache, and rapid or irregular heartbeat. Severe overdosage of theophylline can cause seizures (convulsions) or life-threatening arrhythmias (irregular heartbeats). This rarely happens if the medication is taken as prescribed. The dose should *never* be increased without talking with a doctor first, even if the asthma symptoms are becoming worse.

Some medications (such as erythromycin), when taken with theophylline, can increase the level of theophylline in the bloodstream. Because of the many side effects associated with theophylline, it is no longer prescribed as the first drug to treat asthma. It may be useful, though, when inhaled medications are insufficient.

EMERGENCY TREATMENT OF ASTHMA

Adolescents who require emergency room care or hospitalization for asthma usually are given several different medications simultaneously. The adolescent will be asked to breathe a "nebulized" mist that contains a bronchodilator such as Ventolin, oxygen, and humidified air. If the attack is severe, corticosteroids and theophylline may be given intravenously.

An adolescent with a very severe attack that does not respond to medication may require "intubation." A tube, inserted through the mouth and into the lungs, is connected to a ventilator, a machine that takes over the work of breathing. Intubation gives the teenager a chance to rest while the airways open up. The tube usually can be removed within a few days or even hours. The vast majority of adolescents with asthma never need intubation.

LIVING WITH ASTHMA

Asthma can be a major challenge for busy teenagers. They dislike the daily details—keeping their rooms dust-free, remembering to pack an inhaler in the bookbag, using it during school hours. Yet those routine precautions are the keys to controlling asthma and preventing emergencies.

Compliance—following doctor's orders—is a problem for many adolescents. The reasons include confusion about the treatment plan, side effects of the medication, rebellion ("I don't want to deal with it right now"), denial that the problem is that serious, or fear that the symptoms will spin out of control. All of these reasons should be discussed with the doctor. Asthma is managed most successfully when a teenager learns how to judge the severity of an attack and what to do about it. Armed with knowledge and a plan, the teenager becomes more confident, begins to relax, and feels in control.

Many teenagers worry that asthma will inhibit their participation in sports. Asthma does *not* rule out athletics, as a few Olympic medalists with asthma well know. Exercise should be a regular part of every teenager's life. The key is to work with a doctor on controlling symptoms and to select activities that are tolerated. Some sports, like swimming, may be better handled than others, like basketball or tennis, which require considerable stop-and-start running.

In exercise-induced asthma, symptoms usually appear five to ten minutes after the exercise begins and disappear fifteen to thirty minutes after it ends. A bronchodilator, inhaled ten to twenty minutes *before* exercising, prevents or diminishes the symptoms for many teenagers. Millions of young athletes, in consultation with their doctors, manage their asthma successfully.

Cystic Fibrosis

Cystic fibrosis is a hereditary disease that involves the lungs and several other organs of the body. It is most common among whites (about 1 in 2,500), but it affects African-Americans (1 in 17,000) and Asians (1 in 90,000) as well. The gene for cystic fibrosis is present in 4 to 5 percent of whites, but very few of these individuals have any signs of the disease. Children who are born with two genes for cystic fibrosis—one from the father and one from the mother—have the disease, but the symptoms range from very mild to very severe. Males with cystic fibrosis generally fare better than females, especially during puberty.

Cystic fibrosis carried a dire prognosis until recently. In the 1960s, children with cystic fibrosis died at an average age of seven years. By the 1980s, medical science had pushed the average life expectancy to the late twenties. Cure, through gene therapy, is becoming a possibility that only a few years ago seemed unattainable. Prognosis, or outcome, now depends largely on early diagnosis and aggressive treatment.

Cystic fibrosis damages the lungs by producing abnormally thick mucus that clogs the airways and causes infections. Over time, the lung tissue scars and breathing becomes increasingly difficult. Mucus also collects in the intestines, interfering with the absorption of nutrients and with normal bowel function. Infants with cystic fibrosis may develop a mucus obstruction which prevents the intestine from propelling its contents toward the rectum. Older children and adolescents more typically experience frequent stools or diarrhea. Delayed growth and inadequate weight gain are hallmarks of cystic fibrosis because of the poor absorption of calories and essential nutrients. The pancreas, liver, and gallbladder all may be damaged by the abnormal mucus that accumulates.

The reproductive system is also affected by cystic fibrosis. About 85 percent of males with the disease are sterile. Most females with cystic fibrosis are able to have children, but they may have polyps of the cervix or thickened vaginal/cervical secretions that decrease fertility.

Genetic analysis now allows screening of individuals for the cystic fibrosis gene before they consider childbearing. It also allows in utero diagnosis of the fetus. This testing is not recommended routinely for all couples because of the low prevalence of the gene in the population at large. It is an important option, though, for families with a history of cystic fibrosis.

SYMPTOMS

Cystic fibrosis is an inborn disease, present from the moment of conception. The diagnosis is made during infancy or childhood in 90 percent of individuals with the disease. Ten percent have relatively mild symptoms that remain undiagnosed until adolescence or adulthood. Teenagers with undiagnosed cystic fibrosis may have the following problems: frequent pneumonia or sinus infections, chronic cough, delayed puberty, poor weight gain, or persistent diarrhea.

DIAGNOSTIC TESTS

A "sweat test" is a readily available screening test for cystic fibrosis. A small sample of perspiration is collected on filter paper and measured for its content of chloride. A second test, on a sample taken on another day, should be done if the test is positive. Genetic analysis is the most definitive way to diagnose—or exclude—cystic fibrosis. If it is confirmed, other tests (chest X-rays, breathing tests, blood samples, and cultures from the respiratory tract) will be done to monitor the course of the disease.

TREATMENT

The treatment of cystic fibrosis involves many combined methods. The regimen may be complex and may require frequent adjustment. It is important to work with physicians who are experienced in treating the disease and who are comfortable caring for adolescents.

Depending on the individual situation, treatment generally involves oral or aerosol antibiotics (often taken daily) to fight lung infection, bronchodilators to keep airways open, oral medications to enhance absorption of nutrients from the intestines, and chest physiotherapy to help break up mucus. During chest physiotherapy, the adolescent lies on one side and then the other while a friend or family member "thumps" the back with cupped hands. This helps the mucus dislodge and encourages the adolescent to cough it up.

Nutritional counseling and dietary supplements are particularly important for teenagers with cystic fibrosis. High-calorie, high-protein foods and vitamin supplements are necessary, particularly as the disease progresses. Extra salt is recommended when the teenager is perspiring from exercise, hot weather, or fever. Fluid intake also should be increased at these times because dehydration thickens the mucus and increases the risk of infection.

Frequent hospitalizations are common as cystic fibrosis progresses, but home management has become much more feasible in recent years. Teenagers and their parents can learn to administer intravenous medications at home, which not only is less expensive, but also spares the adolescent exposure to hospital infections. To keep weight stable, some teenagers with cystic fibrosis use nighttime feeding tubes inserted through the nose into the stomach. Another type of feeding tube can be inserted directly through the skin overlying the stomach and concealed under clothing. Home treatment gives an adolescent a greater sense of control over the disease and reduces the anxiety that often accompanies hospitalization.

In emergencies, such as severe shortness of breath or pneumonia that does not respond to home antibiotics, admission to a hospital is vital. These situations may require intravenous fluids, several different intravenous antibiotics, oxygen therapy, frequent chest physiotherapy, and more aggressive nutritional supplementation than has been done at home. The hospitalization also may provide a time for the adolescent, family, and doctors to regroup and adjust the home management plan.

Cystic fibrosis places enormous stress on an adolescent and the entire family. Teenagers resent the limitations imposed by the disease—both everyday annoyances and the possible future implications. They worry not only about the progress of the disease, but also about their ability to have children, to plan for college and career, to live independently.

Many adolescents with cystic fibrosis are physically smaller, thinner, and less developed than their same-age peers. They may be self-conscious about looking different or maturing later. All adolescents with cystic fibrosis—whether the diagnosis is new or old—benefit from a team approach to their care. This involves doctors, nurses, social workers, and counselors who understand the many issues of both the disease and adolescence. Many hospitals throughout the country have teams of health professionals who specialize in cystic fibrosis.

Adolescents with cystic fibrosis and their families face many challenges in the day-to-day management of the disease and in its emotional ramifications. A key ingredient is giving these teenagers the opportunity and tools to help them make decisions and assume responsibility for routine health care.

Tuberculosis

Tuberculosis was a very common disease in the United States prior to the 1950s. Better public health measures, along with a wide array of medications effective against tuberculosis, led to a steady decline in the disease from the 1960s into the 1980s. In 1985, the trend reversed and the incidence began to climb. Strains of drug-resistant tuberculosis began to emerge in the early 1990s.

Children and adolescents living in crowded areas are at greater risk for this highly contagious disease than they were a decade ago.

Individuals at highest risk are children and adolescents who live in the same household with a person who has untreated tuberculosis.

Tuberculosis is caused by very small bacteria, called mycobacteria, that are transmitted through airborne particles. When a person with active tuberculosis coughs, the bacteria are propelled into the air, where they can be inhaled by others.

Routine tuberculosis testing is an essential part of health screening. The tests for tuberculosis are called the Tine test and the PPD test. The Tine test is a four-pronged prick of the skin on the inner surface of the lower arm. The PPD test is a small injection under the skin of the lower arm. If, after forty-eight to seventy-two hours, the prick spots or injected area becomes swollen and raised, the test is positive. This does *not* mean that the individual has active tuberculosis. It means that the young person has been infected with tuberculosis at some time in the past. The vast majority of people with positive skin tests do not have active disease, are healthy, and are not contagious. To confirm that there is no active disease, a chest X-ray should always be done if the skin test is positive. Adolescents with positive skin tests are at increased risk for activation of the quiet, or latent, infection. To decrease the risk of activation—even when the X-ray is negative—a medication called isoniazid, or INH, may be recommended for six to twelve months. The medication is taken in pill form once a day.

Children and adolescents who are exposed to someone with active tuberculosis should see a doctor immediately for a skin test. If the test is positive, the adolescent will be treated with isoniazid. If the test is negative, many physicians will still prescribe the medication because it may take several weeks or months for the skin test to become positive. If the later skin test is still negative, the medication can be stopped.

Certain medical conditions place an individual at increased risk of tuberculosis. They include other lung diseases, diabetes mellitus, prolonged use of corticosteroids, malignancy, HIV infection or AIDS, kidney disease, poor nutrition, and marked weight loss.

There are two types of active tuberculosis: primary and reactivation. Primary tuberculosis occurs with a new infection. It usually causes no symptoms, but there may be a mild cough, low fever, or fatigue. These symptoms disappear within one to two weeks, and the tuberculosis enters a dormant phase. The skin test may not become positive for up to two months following the infection.

In reactivation tuberculosis (also called postprimary or secondary), the infection "wakes up" and progresses to pneumonia or bronchitis. The mycobacteria can spread through the bloodstream to other parts of the body. Symptoms of reactivation tuberculosis include fever, night sweats, cough with mucus or blood, and weight loss. The diagnosis is made by chest X-ray, skin test, and microscopic stains and cultures of the mucus. The greatest risk of reactivation is in the year following initial infection, but it can occur at *any* time, especially at times of physical stress like puberty.

Tuberculosis can be cured if medication is taken as prescribed. Active infection is treated with two or more medications taken daily for six months to a year. It is important for teenage patients to establish a regular schedule for the medication because compliance is critical to cure. Within one to two weeks of beginning the medications, most patients are no longer contagious. But they are not cured at this point and will become ill if they discontinue the medications before completing the full six- to twelve-month course.

Medications commonly prescribed for tuberculosis include isoniazid, rifampin, ethambutol, streptomycin, and pyrazinamide. All can have side effects, and monitoring by a physician is important. A chest X-ray will be done every few months during the first year of treatment, particularly if the adolescent is still progressing through puberty. Close family and friends may want to discuss a plan of preventive treatment with a doctor.

Blood Clots in the Lungs

A blood clot in the lung (a pulmonary embolus) is rare during adolescence. It happens when a small piece of a larger blood clot in the leg or pelvis breaks off and travels through the bloodstream to lodge in the lung. This is a life-threatening condition that requires emergency care and hospitalization.

The major risk factors for pulmonary embolus during adolescence are oral contraceptive use and cigarette smoking. Even among girls who smoke and use the pill, though, the risk of a blood clot remains very small. The risk of death from a blood clot among fifteen-to-twenty-four-year-old women who use the pill and smoke is less than 10 per 100,000 women. The risk for the same age group who use the pill but do *not* smoke is nearly 0 per 100,000. As women get older, especially beyond age thirty-five, the risk of a blood clot among pill users—both smokers and nonsmokers—increases dramatically.

Even though the risk is small, adolescents who smoke and use the pill should recognize the signs of a blood clot in the leg (thrombophlebitis) or lung (pulmonary embolus). These include calf or thigh pain, leg redness and swelling, chest pain, shortness of breath, coughing up blood, increased or irregular heartbeat, lightheadedness, and fainting. If these symptoms develop, a teenager should seek medical care immediately.

Young people with sickle cell disease, blood clotting problems, circulatory disorders, or prolonged bedrest (such as after a fracture of the pelvis or leg) are also at somewhat higher risk of a pulmonary embolus.

The diagnosis of thrombophlebitis is confirmed by an intravenous dye study or an ultrasound study of the leg. The diagnosis of pulmonary embolus is confirmed by either a scan or a dye study of the lung that shows areas of decreased blood flow. The treatment begins in the hospital with an intravenous medication called heparin to thin the blood. Once the adolescent is stable, the heparin is stopped and treatment continues at home for several months with an oral blood thinner called warfarin (Coumadin).

Teenagers who have had blood clots should not smoke and should not take oral contraceptives.

28

The Heart and Blood Vessels

Adolescence is a significant time for the cardiovascular system. The heart and blood vessels grow rapidly during these years and must meet the demands of a maturing, active body. In addition, many habits established in adolescence determine cardiovascular health in adulthood.

The heart (Figure 28.1) is a muscle and, like all muscles, increases in mass during puberty. As the heart gets larger and stronger, the amount of blood pumped with each heartbeat increases. This greater work efficiency means that the heart does not have to beat as fast to provide blood to the rest of the body. Consequently, the heart rate, or number of heart muscle contractions per minute, is slower in teenagers than in young children.

The stronger force of each heart contraction creates a higher blood pressure inside the arteries (vessels that carry blood from the heart). Blood pressure normally increases in both females and males during adolescence, but more so in males. If the increase in pressure is too much, high blood pressure, or hypertension, results.

As the heart grows and changes, the teenager makes decisions about tobacco use, diet, and exercise that affect both its current function and future health. Over time, these decisions may become habits that are associated with adult heart disease from atherosclerosis, or narrowing of the arteries. A few risk factors, such as family history of early heart disease, cannot be changed. Many others can be avoided or altered. The time to begin is *now*—don't smoke, exercise regularly, and watch your diet and weight.

353

THE HEART

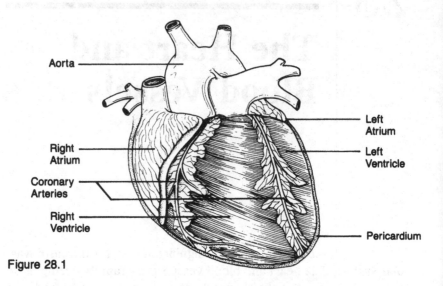

Aorta

Left
Atrium

Right
Atrium

Left
Ventricle

Coronary
Arteries

Right
Ventricle

Pericardium

Figure 28.1

This chapter reviews the major risk factors for adult heart disease and what to do about them. It also discusses the heart conditions commonly seen during adolescence: congenital heart disease, murmurs, infections of the heart, and irregular heartbeats.

Adult Heart Disease

Heart disease is not a sudden, single episode, but an ongoing process. Studies have shown that the process begins in childhood and adolescence. To understand the factors that contribute to this process, some definitions are useful:

Atherosclerosis, sometimes called hardening of the arteries, results from a buildup of plaque on the inner lining of the arteries. The plaque is a deposit of fats (called lipids), cells, and blood-clotting factors. As the plaque accumulates, it narrows and stiffens the arteries so that less blood flows into the surrounding tissues.

Coronary artery disease (CAD), or coronary heart disease (CHD), is the narrowing of the small blood vessels called coronary arteries that supply oxygen-rich blood to the heart muscle itself. The most common cause of CHD is atherosclerotic plaque inside the coronary arteries. This process can begin in childhood and adolescence but rarely causes problems until the thirties or later in life.

Angina is chest pain caused by inadequate blood flow through the coronary arteries. Just as a leg muscle will cramp during exercise if it does not get enough oxygen through the blood, the heart muscle also sends a distress signal: pain in the chest. Angina rarely is the cause of chest pain in teenagers (see the section entitled Chest Pain, in Chapter 26).

Myocardial infarction, or heart attack, occurs when one or more coronary arteries are so narrowed that the blood flowing through them cannot meet the oxygen demands of the heart. When this happens, a portion of the heart muscle may die and eventually scar. This part of the heart cannot pump blood or conduct the electrical signals of the heart. Myocardial infarction is exceedingly rare in teenagers. The likelihood of myocardial infarction increases with advancing adult age and is strongly correlated with risk factors for CHD.

Despite a twenty-year decline in its mortality rate, CHD remains the leading cause of death in the United States. About 1.25 million Americans suffer heart attacks each year, and 500,000 die yearly of CHD. Seven million have symptoms of CHD, accounting for ten million doctors' visits and two million hospitalizations. Many adult patients have children who are at risk for future adult heart disease.

During childhood, streaks of fat may appear in the *aorta,* the large artery leading from the heart. By adolescence, fatty streaks may develop in the coronary arteries. Studies of young soldiers (average age twenty-two) killed in the Korean and Vietnam wars showed that three fourths had plaque in their aortas and coronary arteries.

Two risk factors for CHD, sex and family history, cannot be altered. Males are at greater risk than females. Individuals of either sex are at increased risk if they have a parent or sibling who had CHD, heart attack, or sudden death from heart disease by age fifty-five. Other risk factors, though, can be changed. They include cigarette smoking, sedentary life-style, obesity, high cholesterol levels, hypertension, and diabetes mellitus (Chapter 33).

Tobacco use is the leading preventable cause of death in the United States. Public awareness of its dangers has led to a decline in use among adults. More than thirty million Americans have stopped smoking cigarettes in the last three decades. Unfortunately, the initiation of smoking during the teenage years has shown no decline over the past decade (Chapter 12). Cigarette smoking poses a risk for CHD on its own, but it also aggravates other risk factors. For example, smoking can increase the levels of "bad" cholesterol, decrease the levels of "good" cholesterol, and increase blood pressure.

A sedentary life-style is another risk factor that can begin—or change—during adolescence. Regular exercise dilates (opens up) the arteries, increases "good" cholesterol, decreases blood pressure, keeps the heart muscle efficient, and helps fight obesity. The ideal frequency and duration of the exercise varies depending on the activity, but a reasonable goal is thirty to sixty minutes at least three times weekly. Aerobic exercises, such as walking, jogging, dancing, swimming, and bicycling, provide more cardiovascular benefit than resistance-type exercises such as weight lifting. The benefits of regular physical exercise go beyond cardiovascular fitness or muscle development. Exercise promotes a sense of well-being, enhances self-image, and provides a structured time for social interaction (Chapter 4).

The incidence of obesity among American children and teenagers has risen alarmingly (Chapter 6). Obesity in adults is associated with CHD and with other risk factors such as hyperlipidemia (high cholesterol levels) and high blood pressure. Obesity in adolescence is correlated with obesity in adulthood, and at least one study has shown that obesity in adolescence is directly associated with CHD in adulthood. Many treatment programs for adolescent obesity have been studied. The most effective incorporate both a decrease in caloric intake and an increase in exercise.

Hyperlipidemia

Cholesterol and triglycerides are lipids, or fats, that are carried through the bloodstream by special protein particles. The lipid–protein package is called a lipoprotein. There are three types of lipoproteins:

• VLDL (very low density lipoprotein) carries mainly triglycerides; there is little association between VLDL and CHD.
• LDL (low density lipoprotein) carries mainly cholesterol; LDL is strongly linked with CHD and is sometimes called "bad"

cholesterol because the higher its level, the higher the risk of atherosclerosis and CHD.
• HDL (high density lipoprotein) also carries mainly cholesterol, but HDL is called "good" cholesterol because the higher its level, the lower the risk of CHD.

Many factors affect the circulation of lipoproteins and the levels of cholesterol and triglycerides. Genetic abnormalities may cause an increase in these levels, but diet is also important. Saturated fats and cholesterol can raise lipid levels when consumed regularly and excessively. When lipid levels are high, it is called hyperlipidemia.

WHY SHOULD TEENAGERS WORRY ABOUT CHOLESTEROL?

Many large studies of adults show that the blood cholesterol level is a very strong predictor of CHD. Studies of adults also show that lowering the blood cholesterol level is associated with stabilization, or slower progression, of atherosclerosis. Some research even suggests that atherosclerosis may decrease with control of cholesterol.

No studies have directly shown that lowering blood cholesterol levels in children and teenagers decreases the risk of adult heart disease. However, there is extensive indirect evidence:

• American children and teenagers have higher blood cholesterol levels and higher dietary intake of saturated fats and cholesterol than their peers in other countries, just as American adults have higher rates of CHD.
• Cholesterol levels are associated with atherosclerotic lesions (streaks of fat and plaque in the arteries) in teenagers and young adults.
• Young people with high cholesterol levels often have a family history of CHD.
• High cholesterol levels in childhood and adolescence tend to remain high in adulthood. Adult hypercholesterolemia (high cholesterol levels) clearly is associated with adult CHD.

WHAT CAUSES HIGH BLOOD CHOLESTEROL?

Genetics offers some answers. Inheritance of a single gene can produce very high cholesterol and/or triglyceride levels. In some families, the high levels may appear early in childhood; in many, the levels may be normal until young adulthood.

Inheritance of several genes ("polygenic") can also predispose a young person to high cholesterol, but the levels usually are not as high as the single-gene type of hyperlipidemia. Most children, teenagers, and families with high cholesterol fall into the polygenic category. Diet, exercise, weight, cigarette smoking, and alcohol are very important in the management of this type of hyperlipidemia.

The types and amounts of food that adolescents eat have a definite effect on cholesterol and triglycerides. The link is clear when the diet of young people in various countries is compared to their cholesterol levels. Children in the Philippines and Italy, for example, where 10 percent of the average diet is saturated fat, have lower cholesterol levels than children in the Netherlands and Finland, where 15 to 17 percent of the average diet is saturated fat.

Factors other than genetics and diet also effect lipid levels. Obesity increases both cholesterol and triglycerides. Cigarette smoking increases "bad" cholesterol and lowers "good" cholesterol. Less common causes of hypercholesterolemia include an underactive thyroid gland (hypothyroidism); some medications such as oral contraceptives, diuretics (for high blood pressure), corticosteroids, anticonvulsants, Accutane (for acne), and phenobarbital (for epilepsy); alcohol use; some forms of liver and kidney disease; illegal steroids used by athletes to build muscles; diabetes mellitus; pregnancy; and anorexia nervosa.

CHOLESTEROL CHECKS—WHO? WHEN? WHERE?

With so much public attention on cholesterol in recent years, many families are confused by these questions. The National Cholesterol Education Program (NCEP) recommends that all adults over age twenty have their cholesterol levels checked. It is not recommended, though, for all children and teenagers. Cholesterol should be measured in any child or adolescent who has:

• another risk factor for CHD, such as hypertension, diabetes mellitus, obesity, or cigarette smoking.

• a parent or grandparent who had heart problems diagnosed before age fifty-five (these problems include heart attack, stroke, angina (p. 355), sudden cardiac death, or heart surgery for blocked coronary arteries); or

• a parent with high blood cholesterol.

Cholesterol screening should be done as part of a health care visit. The first cholesterol screening does not require fasting ahead of time. If the test is normal, it need not be repeated for five years. If the test shows a high cholesterol level, a second test should be done after a twelve-hour fast (nothing to eat or drink except water).

WHAT IS A NORMAL CHOLESTEROL LEVEL?

There are three parts to the measurement of cholesterol: total cholesterol, LDL cholesterol, and HDL cholesterol. The total cholesterol level includes LDL cholesterol, HDL cholesterol, and other fats in the blood. The total and the LDL cholesterol measurements are categorized as acceptable, borderline, or high. The following definitions are for children and adolescents:

Acceptable means that the total cholesterol is below 170 mg/dL (milligrams of cholesterol per deciliter of blood serum) and the LDL cholesterol is below 110 mg/dL.

Borderline is a total cholesterol of 170 to 199 mg/dL and an LDL of 110 to 129 mg/dL.

High is a total cholesterol at or above 200 mg/dL and an LDL at or above 130 mg/dL.

If a teenager's level is borderline or high, the recommendations in the following section will apply.

HOW TO LOWER CHOLESTEROL LEVELS

The 1992 report of the NCEP took a two-pronged approach to the treatment of high cholesterol: for the population at large and for the individual.

The population approach aims at lowering the cholesterol levels of *all* Americans by widespread changes in nutrition and eating patterns. These recommendations apply to everyone over age two years:

• Eat a wide variety of foods.
• Get enough calories to support growth and development and to reach or maintain a desirable body weight for age, height, and sex.
• Keep saturated fats below 10 percent of total calories, total fat below 30 percent of total calories, and dietary cholesterol below 300 mg/day.

Many food labels list the grams of fat contained in an average serving. To calculate how many grams of fat per day you should eat, first estimate your ideal caloric intake. Let's assume that you should eat 2,300 calories daily. No more than 30 percent of this, or 690 calories, should come from fat. Since each gram of fat contains nine calories, you should eat no more than 77 grams (690 ÷ 9) of fat daily.

The NCEP recommends that schools, health professionals, government agencies, the food industry, and the mass media promote the population approach to lowering cholesterol levels for all Americans. The individual approach, on the other hand, is aimed at identifying and treating children and teenagers who have high cholesterol now or are at risk of developing it as adults. For these young people, the NCEP recommends a two-step diet to reduce the amount of saturated fat and cholesterol that they eat.

The Step-One Diet is suggested for those whose cholesterol levels fall in the borderline range. It involves the same daily intake as recommended for the whole population, but it calls for detailed instructions by a professional trained in nutrition. Table 5.2 in Chapter 5 lists foods that are low in fat and cholesterol.

The Step-Two Diet is suggested for those whose cholesterol levels fall in the high range and for those whose borderline levels do not improve after three months on the Step-One Diet. Step-Two requires a reduction in saturated fat intake to less than 7 percent of calories and in cholesterol intake to less than 200 mg/day. Step-Two should be undertaken only in consultation with a qualified dietitian or nutritionist to assure a proper balance of nutrients, vitamins, and minerals (Chapter 5, Table 5.1).

Medication may be recommended for children aged ten and older whose cholesterol levels have not improved after six to twelve months of Step-One and Step-Two diets. The NCEP recommends drug therapy if: (1) the LDL remains at or above 190 mg/dL, or (2) the LDL remains at or above 160 mg/dL *AND* there are other risk factors for CHD.

The home environment plays a key role in helping an adolescent with high cholesterol follow dietary recommendations. A healthy, low-fat eating pattern for the entire family removes the focus from the teenager and diminishes struggles over who can eat what. A positive, balanced attitude toward eating is far more successful than a tally of every calorie or gram consumed. Some recommendations include:

• Provide meals that are low in fats and cholesterol; allow healthy snacks to offset hunger and alleviate feelings of dietary deprivation.

• Break the habit of unnecessary eating when not hungry; eliminate reminders to "clean your plate."

• Try to make meals and snacks consistent in size and time of day.

• Plan ways in advance to cope with parties, restaurants, or meals at friends' homes.

• Accept that slip-ups happen, but quickly get back to a low-fat eating pattern.

High Blood Pressure (Hypertension)

Blood pressure is the force that drives the blood from the heart and through the arteries to every part of the body. Blood pressure varies throughout the day, depending on physical activity, stress, and body position. It is higher when you are exercising than sleeping, anxious than relaxed, lying down than standing up. These transient ups and downs are normal.

Most teenagers have had their blood pressure measured during a medical examination. A cuff, wrapped around the arm above the elbow, is attached to a pump and a meter filled with mercury. As the pump is squeezed, the cuff fills with air and tightens around the upper arm. When the pressure in the cuff exceeds the pressure forcing blood through the arteries of the arm (the blood pressure), blood flow to the arm will cease. As the air is released from the cuff, the blood flow will return. Using a stethoscope placed over the artery on the inside of the elbow, the nurse or doctor can hear the beats when the blood flow returns. At this point, the pressure in the cuff (and measured in the mercury meter) is called the *systolic* blood pressure. This is the highest pressure and reflects the heart's contraction. Eventually, as the cuff deflates more, the nurse or doctor will no longer hear the beating sound. The pressure on the meter at this point is the *diastolic* blood pressure. This is the lowest pressure and reflects the heart's relaxed, noncontracting phase.

Hypertension is defined as the level of systolic or diastolic blood pressure at which there is an unacceptable risk of cardiovascular problems. This is a statistical definition that corresponds to one's age, sex, and physical maturity.

Most people with high blood pressure have no symptoms. Because of this, the blood pressure should be measured annually from early childhood throughout life. It should be done in a quiet setting, and the readings should be correlated with standardized tables for age, sex, height, and weight. The physician will use the tables to translate the reading into a percentile. The blood pressure is "normal" if it falls below the ninetieth percentile, "high normal" if it falls between the ninetieth and ninety-fifth percentile, and "high" if it is above the ninety-fifth percentile. Hypertension is the same as high blood pressure. A diagnosis of hypertension should never be made on the basis of one reading. It requires three separate readings, taken on different days, that are all above the ninety-fifth percentile.

Hypertension has two classifications: primary and secondary. Primary, or essential, hypertension has no identifiable cause, but usually is associated with a family history of high blood pressure. Over 90 percent of teenagers with high blood pressure have primary hypertension. Secondary hypertension has an identifiable cause, usually from a vascular (blood vessel), kidney, or hormonal problem. The younger the adolescent, the more likely it is that the hypertension is secondary.

Adolescents with secondary hypertension are more likely to have symptoms than adolescents with primary hypertension. The symptoms vary widely, depending on the underlying cause. In both primary and secondary hypertension, symptoms tend to appear as the blood pressure climbs higher. Symptoms can include headache, chest pain, shortness of breath, rapid heartbeat, light-headedness, flushing, change in vision, fluid retention (which appears as swelling of the feet, hands, or face), or palpitations. Palpitations are a sensation that the heart is beating too fast, flip-flopping, skipping beats, or adding beats. They can last seconds to hours.

Untreated hypertension, regardless of cause, is dangerous. In the short term, very high blood pressure can cause seizures, stroke, or coma. Over many years, hypertension can cause CHD, heart failure, kidney failure, eye damage, stroke, and damage to the blood vessels in the abdomen or legs.

WHAT CAUSES HIGH BLOOD PRESSURE?

The list of possible causes of hypertension is long and complicated. *All teenagers with high blood pressure must see a doctor for evaluation and treatment.* Primary hypertension is not curable but is controllable with diet or medication. Many types of secondary hypertension are curable if treated early. All types can be controlled given the many types of antihypertensive medications that are now available.

Some possible causes of secondary hypertension include the following:

• recurrent childhood urinary tract infections that can scar the kidneys and lead to high blood pressure (pyelonephritis, Chapter 30);
• other causes of chronic kidney disease (Chapter 30);
• narrowing of the artery that supplies blood to one of the kidneys (renal artery stenosis);
• congenital heart disease (discussed below);
• thyroid disorders (Chapter 33);
• disorders of the adrenal glands (the small glands in the abdomen that produce corticosteroids, Chapter 33);
• medications, including oral contraceptives, some asthma medications, corticosteroids (such as prednisone);
• illegal drugs (crack, cocaine, amphetamines, anabolic steroids);
• pregnancy.

HOW IS HIGH BLOOD PRESSURE TREATED?

Before treating hypertension in teenagers, it is important to be sure that the diagnosis is correct. Remember: A single high blood pressure reading does *not* mean hypertension; the diagnosis requires at least three high readings on separate days. An incorrect label of hypertension creates unnecessary anxiety for the teenager and family. The teenager may lose or avoid certain job opportunities, have difficulty obtaining health insurance, or take unwarranted medications that could have negative side effects.

When diagnosed correctly, the treatment of hypertension depends on its cause and severity. A very high blood pressure reading requires immediate treatment. Searching for the cause will be delayed until the blood pressure is under better control. Most adolescents with hypertension do not have severe elevations, and evaluation and treatment may proceed simultaneously.

General recommendations for controlling hypertension include the following:

• If overweight, restrict caloric intake;
• Restrict salt intake;
• Exercise;
• Do not use tobacco.

Caloric restriction is *not* recommended for hypertensive teenagers who are of normal weight. It is very important, though, for those who are overweight. Weight reduction in overweight and obese teenagers is associated with a fall in blood pressure during adolescence and a decreased likelihood of hypertension later in adulthood.

Most individuals with hypertension, regardless of weight or age, should restrict their salt intake. Salt, or sodium chloride, causes fluid retention, which increases blood pressure. Fresh foods can be prepared with a small amount of salt, but the salt shaker should not be used at the table. Packaged and frozen foods usually have salt added. It is best to check their labels for sodium content. Most teenagers with hypertension should try to limit their sodium intake to 2,500 mg daily. Foods that are high in sodium include most sauces and soups; condiments such as mustard, catsup, relish; and snack foods such as salted chips, pretzels, and popcorn; and breakfast and lunch meats. Favorite foods of American teenagers—fast foods and pizza—also tend to be high in sodium. Before going to a restaurant, plan ahead and eat sensibly. If one meal is high in sodium, cut back on sodium in subsequent meals.

Exercise is important for all adolescents, especially those with hypertension. Aerobic exercises such as running, swimming, bicycling, or using a treadmill can actually help lower blood pressure over time. Isometric exercises, such as weight lifting or wrestling, are more controversial because they may increase blood pressure during the activity. Adolescents with hypertension who do isometric exercises should be supervised with frequent blood pressure checks and should begin gradually and work up slowly.

If the blood pressure does not come under control with diet and exercise, a physician may prescribe medication. There are many different types of antihypertensive medications, and the choice must be tailored to the individual teenager. A medication that works well for a parent or grandparent may be absolutely wrong for a teenager. Family members should not share their blood pressure medications or change their doses without talking with their doctors. Antihypertensive medications are safe when used appropriately, but they can cause side effects and even organ damage when taken incorrectly. Hypertension may not be curable, but it is controllable. Once it is brought under control, it imposes no risk to the adolescent.

Congenital Heart Disease

Most congenital heart defects—meaning those present since birth—are discovered before age ten. A few may not become apparent until the rapid growth phase of puberty. Whether the diagnosis is old or new, teenagers with congenital heart disease are faced with conflicting prospects. On the positive side, surgical repair has improved survival and function for many adolescents with congenital heart disease. Some of the advances in surgical techniques and medications are still so new, though, that lifelong predictions cannot be made. For some teenagers, treatment may have delayed the progression of symptoms from childhood to adolescence. For others, the treatment may have allowed survival but could not fully correct the problem. These teenagers may experience poor growth, delayed puberty, and chronic fatigue or breathlessness.

In addition to the medical problems, congenital heart conditions may affect the teenager's self-image, socialization, evolving autonomy, and future plans. Sports and recreational activities may be limited, leaving the teenager isolated from same-aged peer groups. As children with congenital heart disease mature in adolescence, they begin to ask questions about relationships, marriage, and childbearing. The risk of having a child with the same heart problem ranges from 1 to 7 percent for men and 3 to 16 percent for women with congenital heart disease. Adolescents need help in interpreting their risks and in making important life decisions. This help begins with the family and physicians, but other members of the health care team—social workers, psychologists, nurses—may become increasingly important as the teenager struggles with these complex issues.

Adolescents with congenital heart disease need continuous, regular health care that promotes a smooth transition from pediatric to adult-centered care. The best overall care comes from health professionals who understand both the adolescent's specific heart problem and the developmental issues common to all teenagers.

Heart problems typically diagnosed in childhood are not discussed here. The following descriptions apply to a few selected congenital heart defects that may not be diagnosed until adolescence or that may progress during puberty.

AORTIC VALVE DISEASE

The aortic valve is located between the lower left chamber of the heart (the left ventricle) and the main artery leading from the heart (the aorta). Normally this valve consists of three cusps that resemble rounded leaves. The cusps open when the heart contracts, allowing blood to flow forward from the ventricle into the aorta. When the valve closes, the heart relaxes and blood is prevented from flowing backward from the aorta into the ventricle.

If the cusps thicken, the aortic valve cannot open as fully as it should and the forward blood flow is impaired. This is *aortic regurgitation.*

A common congenital heart problem that may not be recognized until adolescence is *bicuspid aortic valve,* in which there are two instead of three cusps. The bicuspid valve may function normally or may thicken over time, causing aortic stenosis and/or regurgitation.

Symptoms of aortic valve disease include light-headedness, fainting, chest pain, and shortness of breath. On physical examination, the doctor will hear a distinctive heart murmur through the stethoscope. If an abnormal aortic valve is suspected, the doctor will order an echocardiogram, a type of ultrasound study. This is a painless test that uses sound waves to assess the heart's anatomy and blood flow. An electrocardiogram (ECG) will also be done to record the heart's electrical activity. A cardiologist (heart specialist) will usually be consulted to help advise the teenager with aortic valve disease about treatment, exercise, and sports participation.

A serious potential complication of aortic valve disease is infection of the valve by bacteria in the bloodstream. Antibiotics, such as penicillin, usually are prescribed before procedures that can cause bacteria to enter the blood (discussed below).

The treatment of aortic valve disease depends on the abnormality and the severity. A bicuspid aortic valve that functions normally requires no treatment other than antibiotic prophylaxis (preventive measures) and close follow-up. Aortic stenosis or regurgitation significant enough to cause symptoms usually requires surgery. If the problem is stenosis, "balloon valvuloplasty" may relieve the obstruction. A thin tube, called a catheter, is inserted into an artery in the groin or arm and threaded up to the heart until it crosses the aortic valve. A small balloon at the tip of the catheter is then inflated to widen the valve. Severe aortic regurgitation usually requires open heart surgery with replacement of the aortic valve.

ATRIAL SEPTAL DEFECT (ASD)

This congenital defect is a hole in the heart between the two upper chambers, the left and right atrium. An ASD usually causes no symptoms in childhood and may be missed on routine physical examination. The defect may first become apparent during puberty when growth places extra demands on the heart. The diagnosis can usually be confirmed by echocardiogram.

The effects of ASD vary from one individual to another, but they usually become worse over time, leading to exercise intolerance and irregular heart rhythms during young adulthood. When ASD is diagnosed, correction generally is recommended. Surgery has been the main method of correction for forty years, but a newer method involves patching the hole through a cardiac catheter (see above).

COARCTATION OF THE AORTA

In this condition the aorta, the main artery leading from the heart, is severely narrowed. It is usually diagnosed in childhood but may not become apparent until adolescence. The typical signs are high blood pressure measured in the arms, much stronger pulses in the arms than legs, and a murmur. The diagnosis is confirmed by echocardiogram or magnetic resonance imaging (MRI), a technique for seeing internal organs without the radiation of an X-ray.

Coarctation of the aorta in a teenager usually is treated surgically, with excision or widening of the narrowed area. In some patients, the balloon catheter is used to dilate, or widen, the aorta, but the long-term results of this method are unclear. After surgical repair of the coarctation, high blood pressure is common and should be treated.

ASYMMETRIC SEPTAL HYPERTROPHY (ASH)

This is an inherited disorder in which the wall separating the two lower chambers of the heart (right and left ventricles) thickens. In severe cases, it blocks the flow of blood out of the heart. ASH usually goes undetected until adolescence. All teenagers with a family member who has ASH should see a doctor for evaluation. Even if there are no symptoms, there is a risk of heart problems, especially during exercise. When symptoms do appear, they may include exercise intolerance, chest pain, light-headedness, or irregular heartbeat. An echocardiogram confirms a diagnosis of ASH.

ASH is a leading cause of sudden death in adolescent athletes. If the obstruction or symptoms are severe, surgery can reduce the thickness of the wall and improve blood flow.

Heart Murmurs

Cardiac murmurs are sounds caused by the flow of blood through the heart. Most are heard only with a stethoscope, but a few are audible to the individual or to others standing nearby. The discovery of a heart murmur by a physician can surprise and upset a teenager. Remember that murmurs are very common in adolescence and that the great majority are harmless. Between 20 and 40 percent of teenagers have murmurs discovered during routine or sports examinations. Most murmurs are not associated with heart disease and should not restrict physical activity.

Harmless murmurs are called benign, innocent, or functional. These terms all mean the same thing: The murmur is simply the sound that the blood makes as it flows through a normal heart. The sound can come from several sources:

- the flow of blood out of the heart when it contracts;
- the flow of blood through the veins leading into the heart;
- the very rapid flow of blood out of the heart when the body is stressed, as in fever.

MITRAL VALVE PROLAPSE (MVP)

This condition causes one of the most common murmurs to appear during adolescence. The mitral valve controls blood flow from the left atrium (upper left chamber) to the left ventricle (lower left chamber). If the valve is thicker than normal, it can billow, or "prolapse," upward into the atrium when it closes, causing a clicking sound. If the valve opens as it billows, blood flows backward from the ventricle into the atrium (mitral regurgitation), causing a murmur. Some people have both a click and a murmur, while some have just one or the other.

MVP is seldom a serious problem in teenagers and usually causes no symptoms. It is often found during a routine physical examination. If symptoms do appear, they tend to be vague pain under the breastbone, palpitations, fatigue, light-headedness, fainting, or anxiety. If a teenager has symptoms and a physical examination does not reveal MVP, the doctor may order an echocardiogram, which is an excellent test for MVP.

As many as 20 percent of teenagers have MVP. It is two to three times more common in females than in males. The vast majority of adolescents with MVP have no complications and are not at increased risk for adult heart disease. They can participate in all activities, including competitive sports. MVP does not place a woman at risk during pregnancy or delivery, and there is no significant evidence that oral contraceptives place a woman with MVP at risk. The only medical recommendation for adolescents with MVP is to take antibiotics before certain dental and surgical procedures to prevent infection of the heart valve (discussed below).

Infections of the Heart

Infections of the heart are unusual. They generally take three forms:

• *Endocarditis* is infection of the heart valves or the inside lining of the heart;
• *Myocarditis* is infection of the heart muscle;
• *Pericarditis* is infection of the fluid-filled sac surrounding the heart.

ENDOCARDITIS

The most common type of endocarditis is "subacute bacterial endocarditis," or SBE. It is called "subacute" because it comes on gradually, over days or weeks. Bacterial infection of the heart valve or lining can occur under two conditions. One is a structural abnormality of the heart, as in congenital heart disease. The second is intravenous drug use in which infected material is injected into the bloodstream and lodges in the heart.

Fever is always a symptom of SBE. Other signs may include a new or changed heart murmur, pain or tenderness in the upper left abdominal area caused by an enlarged spleen, and joint aching or swelling. Rare symptoms are tender, discolored nodules, or bumps, under the skin of the fingers or toes or splinterlike marks under the nails.

The complications of SBE are serious. The infection can spread through the bloodstream to other organs, such as the brain, lungs, and kidneys. The infection can damage the heart and cause heart failure. Death can result from untreated SBE. It is a *very serious* illness that requires immediate medical attention.

SBE should be suspected if a teenager has a persistent fever and any one of the following:

- congenital heart disease,
- mitral valve prolapse,
- history of rheumatic fever (discussed below),
- intravenous drug use.

The diagnosis of SBE is made by a blood sample cultured in a laboratory. An adolescent with suspected SBE will be hospitalized before the diagnosis is confirmed by laboratory culture. It is not unusual that three or four blood samples may be required to make the diagnosis.

Treatment of SBE involves four to eight weeks of antibiotics, depending on the type of infection. Adolescents who are at risk for SBE because they have heart abnormalities or a previous history of endocarditis can help prevent SBE by taking antibiotics before and after dental and some surgical procedures.

RHEUMATIC FEVER

Over the last quarter century, the incidence of acute rheumatic fever declined dramatically. Unfortunately, the number of cases has begun to increase recently.

Rheumatic fever follows a streptococcal bacterial infection of the throat (see Strep throat, in Chapter 25) that has not been treated with antibiotics. Strep throat, even if untreated, usually clears on its own and does not cause later problems. Sometimes, though, the body's reaction to the infection causes a delayed set of symptoms, beginning one to six weeks after the sore throat. These signs and symptoms make up some of the criteria for diagnosing rheumatic fever. They include a positive throat culture for strep, swelling of the joints, a characteristic rash, inflammation of the heart, and nodules under the skin. Less convincing criteria include fever and joint aching without swelling.

Uncontrolled movements of the arms and legs, called *chorea* or St. Vitus' dance, are an important, and often delayed, sign of rheumatic fever. It may follow strep throat by as long as six months and affects females more often than males. Chorea begins with restlessness, irritability, or excitability. These changes are followed by involuntary, uncoordinated movements, an awkward walk, garbled speech, or trouble with handwriting. Chorea usually disappears on its own within three to four months.

The most serious sign of rheumatic fever is carditis (inflammation of the heart) because it can result in permanent damage to the heart valves. The symptoms of carditis include rapid or irregular heart rate, shortness of breath, chest pain, swelling of the feet or legs, and light-headedness.

Rheumatic fever always requires treatment with an antibiotic. After the initial treatment, monthly injections of a long-acting penicillin or daily doses of oral antibiotics are recommended for at least five years in adolescents without carditis and for life in those with carditis. This is done to prevent recurrences of acute rheumatic fever.

The fever and joint pain of acute rheumatic fever respond well to aspirin or ibuprofen. Adolescents with carditis will also be given oral corticosteroids (prednisone) to decrease the inflammation. As the inflammation fades, the prednisone and aspirin will be tapered off gradually.

Teenagers with rheumatic fever need to recognize the seriousness of the disease and the importance of following doctors' orders to prevent future recurrence and permanent heart damage.

Arrhythmias

Heart rate varies widely in teenagers. Serious arrhythmias—irregularities in the heart rate or rhythm—are uncommon in adolescents. When arrhythmia does occur in a teenager, the heart is usually structurally normal. This is very different from arrhythmias in older adults, which generally indicate some underlying heart disease. Even in the young, though, arrhythmias warrant a doctor's attention. When the heart beats irregularly, it may not pump blood efficiently. It is this abnormal pumping that causes the palpitations, chest pain, breathlessness, or light-headedness of arrhythmias. A very rare complication of an arrhythmia is cardiac arrest. This occurs when the electrical impulses in the heart are either absent or so disorganized that they fail to stimulate contraction of the heart muscle. If the heart is not stimulated to contract, death will occur within minutes.

Arrhythmias during adolescence may be uncommon, but they

can be serious. Teenagers who are concerned about their symptoms should talk to their doctors immediately.

WHICH TEENAGERS ARE AT RISK?

Adolescents at risk for serious arrhythmias often have a family history of irregular heart rhythms, sudden death, or neuromuscular disorders, such as muscular dystrophy. Teenagers who have had cardiac surgery are also at increased risk.

If a serious irregular rhythm is discovered, an adolescent should be evaluated for underlying heart disease. A doctor usually will begin with an electrocardiogram (ECG), which records the heart's electrical impulses over seconds or minutes. The ECG will miss an irregularity that does not happen to appear during that precise, short time. Long-term, or Holter, ECG monitoring can be used to provide a record over several days. Electrodes are taped to the chest and connected to a small box that the teenager wears on a belt. The Holter monitor records the heart rhythm constantly and notes the exact times of all irregular beats. Another type of monitor records only when the adolescent has symptoms and instructs the monitor to begin recording. It will therefore miss arrhythmias that occur when the adolescent is asleep or preoccupied with other activities.

When there is strong evidence of serious arrhythmias, electrophysiologic studies are done. These involve threading a cardiac catheter from a blood vessel in the groin or arm into the heart. The heart is stimulated electrically, through the catheter, and its electrical response is measured.

COMMON ARRHYTHMIAS

Irregular rhythms often found in adolescents fall into three categories:

Ventricular extrasystoles are extra beats of the lower chamber of the heart. Other terms for the same irregularity are premature ventricular contractions (PVCs) or ventricular premature beats (VPBs). If an adolescent has no other symptoms and a normal physical examination, no treatment or restrictions are required. If lightheadedness, dizziness, or fainting occur, the teenager should have a full evaluation by a cardiologist.

Bradycardia is a slow heart rate. Heart rates vary widely in teenagers, making it difficult to set a definitive lower limit. Heart rate depends on the teenager's age, sexual maturity, activity level, and body temperature. A resting heart rate of fifty beats per minute is acceptable for Jack, a sexually mature eighteen-year-old soccer player. But the same rate might warrant medical evaluation in Bob, a sedentary twelve-year-old who is just entering puberty.

Tachycardia is a rapid heart rate. Just as the lower limit of the heart rate varies among individuals, so does the upper limit. Sarah, a healthy twelve-year-old who has not yet begun puberty, has a normal resting heart rate of 110 beats per minute. This same heart rate might not be normal in her seventeen-year-old sister, who has completed puberty and is an athlete.

Arrhythmias can be dangerous. There are many different types, and their evaluation is complicated. Many forms of treatment—medications, pacemakers, surgery—are available for serious arrhythmias. In the vast majority of teenagers, arrhythmias are not dangerous and do not need treatment. But, if there are symptoms, they should always be brought to the attention of a doctor.

29

The Digestive System

Abdominal complaints are very common during adolescence. Most of these problems originate in the digestive, or *gastrointestinal,* system (Figure 29.1), which includes the esophagus (the tube connecting the mouth and stomach), stomach, small intestine, large intestine, rectum, liver, gallbladder, and pancreas.

The first four sections of this chapter address common digestive symptoms—abdominal pain, diarrhea, constipation, and rectal problems. Liver disease is discussed separately in the last section because it may cause vague, overlapping symptoms. Specific diseases are described within each section. For example, ulcer disease is discussed under abdominal pain. A cautionary note about this organization: Diseases do not follow instructions. An ulcer *usually* causes pain, but not always. It may begin with nausea or vomiting. Milk intolerance *usually* causes diarrhea, but not always. It may appear as cramping or bloating. Whenever symptoms are unclear or persistent, talk with a doctor. Do not attempt to make a diagnosis or begin treatment alone.

Abdominal Pain

Severe abdominal pain that begins suddenly or becomes worse steadily can signal a medical emergency. It always demands an immediate call to the doctor or visit to the emergency room.

Most abdominal pain does not represent a medical crisis. It can

The Digestive System

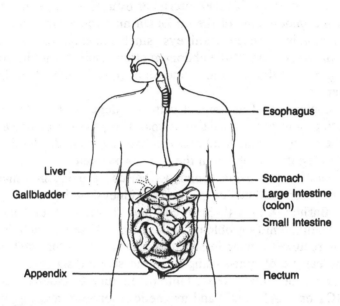

Figure 29.1

have many causes, some physical and some emotional. Pain that is caused by a physical problem is called organic pain. Pain that is caused by emotional distress is called functional pain. Organic pain can have functional consequences, such as poor school attendance or irritability. Similarly, functional pain can have organic consequences, such as weight loss or poor growth.

Organic and functional abdominal pain have different characteristics. Organic pain tends to localize to one place, interferes with normal activities, may disrupt sleep, and often is relieved by medications such as acetaminophen or antacids. Functional pain tends to vary in location and frequency, does not disrupt sleep, and is not relieved by medication. A teenager with organic pain usually is able to pinpoint something particular—like a certain food, activity, or position—that brings on the pain. A teenager with functional pain may have difficulty identifying any specific trigger.

Whether organic or functional, pain is real. It hurts. It should not be ignored or minimized. Emotional distress should be taken as seriously as any physical cause. Counseling, stress reduction techniques, and other psychological measures can be very effective in relieving functional pain and understanding the cause.

The list of physical causes of abdominal pain is long and complex. Pain in the lower abdomen, below the belly button, may result from a problem in the bladder, uterus or ovaries, or large intestine. Pain in the middle part of the abdomen may represent a problem in the abdominal muscles, kidneys, small intestine, or pancreas. Pain in the upper part of the abdomen often originates in the stomach, first part of the small intestine (duodenum), gallbladder, liver, or spleen.

The evaluation of abdominal pain will depend on its location, description, and associated symptoms. The physical examination helps the doctor decide if laboratory tests are needed. Blood tests can help identify a problem in the liver or pancreas. Ultrasonography, a painless test using sound waves, can provide information about the liver, gallbladder, pancreas, kidneys, and gynecological organs. Barium X-rays ("upper GI" and "lower GI," or "barium enema") help identify problems in the inside of the stomach, intestines, or rectum. Similar information about the rectum and large intestine can be obtained using a lighted scope ("sigmoidoscope" or "colonoscope") that is passed into the rectum. Computed tomography (CT or "CAT scan") and magnetic resonance imaging (MRI) provide information about the abdominal cavity and the general size and shape of the abdominal organs.

Appendicitis. The appendix is a three-to-four-inch projection of the large intestine. If the appendix becomes inflamed (appendicitis), it must be removed surgically before it ruptures. The incidence of appendicitis peaks in early adolescence and is more frequent among males than females. The earliest symptom is often generalized abdominal pain that begins gradually. As the pain becomes worse, it begins to localize around the belly button and then to the lower right side of the abdomen. It can become so intense that the teenager does not want to move, stand, or straighten the legs. Fever, nausea, vomiting, and constipation frequently accompany the pain. On examination, the doctor finds tensing of the abdominal muscles and tenderness in the lower right side. The white blood cell count usually is high, indicating inflammation or infection. The treatment for appendicitis is surgical removal of the appendix.

Gastritis and peptic ulcers. Two sets of forces—active and passive—are at work in the stomach and duodenum (the first part of the small intestine). To break down and digest food, there must be active production of acid, enzymes, and bile. A constant, passive force is required to protect the stomach and duodenum from these compounds. This protection comes from the mucosa (the lining of the stomach and intestine). The mucosa has a mucus coating and is richly supplied with oxygen and nutrients from the bloodstream. Normally, the active and protective forces are in balance. When they are not, problems arise.

Gastritis is inflammation of the lining of the stomach. The symptoms include a gnawing or burning pain in the upper mid-abdomen, nausea, a frequent sensation of hunger, belching, a sour taste in the mouth, and "heartburn" (a burning sensation under the breastbone). The symptoms improve temporarily with milk, small amounts of food, and antacids such as Maalox or Mylanta. Severe gastritis can cause bleeding of the stomach. Vomited blood resembles coffee grounds because of the effect of the stomach acid on the blood. Blood from the stomach will make the stool appear black or tarlike. *Bleeding is an emergency—call the doctor or go to the emergency room immediately.*

The causes of gastritis include certain medications (like aspirin or ibuprofen), alcohol, a bacteria called *Helicobacter pylori,* and physical stress. It is less clear if and how emotional stress contributes to gastritis. Once present, it can make the gastritis worse, but emotional stress probably is an uncommon sole cause of gastritis.

The diagnosis of gastritis is usually made on the basis of the teenager's history of symptoms rather than by physical examination. A doctor may order an "upper gastrointestinal series" (UGI) or "endoscopy." For the UGI, the teenager drinks a cup of chalky liquid called barium that coats the stomach. X-rays of the stomach and duodenum are then taken. Irregularities in the barium coating will show up on the X-ray.

Endoscopy is an outpatient procedure that involves passing a tube (called an endoscope) from the mouth, through the esophagus, and into the stomach and duodenum. The tube contains a light and magnifying scope through which the doctor examines the mucosa. Small, painless "bites," or biopsies, of the mucosa can be taken through the scope. These samples are examined under a laboratory microscope or cultured for bacteria.

The treatment of gastritis depends partly on the cause, but all treatments try to minimize the acidity of the stomach. Antacids help but need to be taken frequently. Some can cause diarrhea (like Maalox or Mylanta), while others (like Amphojel) can cause constipation. Teenagers generally prefer "H_2 blockers," which are pills taken once or twice daily that block acid production by the stomach. Examples of H_2 blockers include cimetidine (Tagamet), ranitidine (Zantac), and famotidine (Pepcid).

Antibiotics are required to treat gastritis if *Helicobacter pylori* bacteria are found by endoscopy. Most adolescents with gastritis come to endoscopy only after a trial of H_2 blockers has proven ineffective or when their symptoms recur.

Teenagers with symptoms of gastritis should avoid alcohol, coffee, aspirin, and anti-inflammatory drugs. It also helps to eat small, frequent meals. A bland diet is not necessary, but very spicy foods can make symptoms worse. If belching and heartburn persist, it helps to stay upright for one to two hours after eating and to elevate the head of the bed at night by placing blocks, bricks, or books under the mattress.

Ulcer or "peptic ulcer," is an inflamed sore or small crater in the stomach or duodenum. Three fourths of peptic ulcers occur in the duodenum and one fourth in the stomach. They are more common in males than in females.

The symptoms of peptic ulcer disease resemble those of gastritis but are usually more severe. The abdominal pain can be intermittent or constant, stabbing or burning. The pain does not seem to come from an exact place, and teenagers with peptic ulcers often find that their distress is vague and difficult to describe. Peptic ulcers have no clear-cut triggers, such as certain types or amounts of food, but often produce greatest discomfort when the stomach is empty.

Over half of adolescents with ulcer disease will experience a recurrence when they stop their medication. Factors associated with recurrence include a family history of peptic ulcer disease and infection with *Helicobacter pylori*. Complications are more common with peptic ulcer disease than gastritis. All complications, though, are far more common in adults than adolescents and with recurrent than with first ulcers. Life-threatening bleeding occurs in less than 5 percent of first ulcers. Perforation (when the ulcer erodes a hole through the stomach or duodenum) occurs even less often. Scarring, which can obstruct the flow of food, is very rare in teenagers but does occur in adults with a long history of recurrent peptic ulcer disease.

Diagnosis of peptic ulcer disease is made either by endoscopy or UGI. Endoscopy is the preferred method if the adolescent has vomited blood. A bleeding ulcer requires immediate medical attention and usually hospitalization. It is a curable problem that can be fatal if untreated.

The treatment for peptic ulcers is similar to, but longer than, that for gastritis. Ulcers generally heal in one to three months with either antacids or H_2 blockers. As with gastritis, H_2 blockers are easier to take and better tolerated than antacids. It is very important that the teenager take the medicine as prescribed for the full course (usually four to eight weeks). The symptoms may disappear within a few days of treatment, but full healing requires much longer. Antibiotics are required for *Helicobacter pylori,* as discussed above.

Other medications that may be used to treat ulcers are sucralfate, omeprazole, and misoprostol. Sucralfate binds to the ulcer crater and protects it from further damage. Omeprazole blocks the secretion of acid in the stomach. Long-term studies about its safety in adolescents are limited, and it is used only in severe ulcer disease that has not responded to other therapy. Misoprostol both blocks acid secretion and protects the mucosa. It too has not been studied in teenagers. It absolutely must not be used in females of childbearing age who are having unprotected sexual intercourse because it can cause miscarriage.

Little is known about the usefulness of psychological counseling in either treating ulcer disease or decreasing the chance of recurrence. The weight of the evidence suggests that it is of limited help. Once established, ulcer disease requires a medical regimen and close medical follow-up. Counseling can, however, help the adolescent comply with the regimen and understand both the serious and treatable nature of the problem.

Gallbladder Problems. The gallbladder is a hollow, pear-shaped organ located below the liver in the upper right side of the abdomen. It stores and concentrates bile, a fluid that is produced in the liver and contains chemicals necessary for digestion.

Pain from the gallbladder may be caused by inflammation (cholecystitis) or stones (cholelithiasis). Cholecystitis is uncommon in adolescents. Occasionally, it can appear in teenagers who have a family history of gallbladder problems and in those with recent dieting, pregnancy, or oral contraceptive use. It also can be precipitated by certain diseases in which red blood cells are broken down (such as sickle cell disease). The breakdown products form gallstones, which can inflame the gallbladder. Most gallstones are not caused by red blood cell problems but rather by imbalances in the composition of the bile. The stones can vary in size from as small as gravel to as large as a lemon.

Cholecystitis and cholelithiasis often coexist. The signs and symptoms of gallbladder problems include pain, nausea, and bloating. The pain can be in the upper right side or in the upper mid-abdomen, just below the rib cage. The symptoms become worse after eating fatty foods. If the inflammation is severe, symptoms will escalate to include fever and vomiting. Serious complications can develop, such as obstruction of the bile duct leading from the gallbladder to the small intestine, infection, or perforation (tearing) of the gallbladder wall.

Diagnosis of gallbladder disease is made by a history of symptoms, physical examination, blood tests, and special scans or ultrasound of the gallbladder. Once the acute pain disappears, surgery may be recommended, especially if there are gallstones. An alternative to surgery for gallstones is "lithotripsy," which uses shock waves under general anesthesia to shatter the gallstones.

Pancreatitis. The pancreas is a gland in the middle of the abdomen that secretes enzymes necessary for digestion. It also makes insulin, a hormone that controls the level of sugar in the bloodstream. Pain from the pancreas usually is caused by inflammation, called pancreatitis.

Pancreatitis can be caused by viral infections (such as mumps, mononucleosis, or hepatitis), alcohol use, medications (such as oral contraceptives or corticosteroids), or abdominal injury. Less common causes include pregnancy, diabetes mellitus, peptic ulcer disease, cystic fibrosis, and other disorders.

The primary symptom of pancreatitis is pain in the middle of the abdomen and back. It may be mild, or it may come on suddenly and increase in severity within a few hours. It can occur once or recur over time. Other symptoms may include nausea, vomiting, and fever.

The diagnosis of pancreatitis is made by the history, physical examination, and blood tests to measure enzymes produced by the pancreas. If pancreatitis is present, the level of those enzymes (amylase and lipase) will be higher than normal. An ultrasound or CT scan of the pancreas may also be used to confirm the diagnosis.

Treatment of pancreatitis usually requires hospitalization, with intravenous fluids and a tube passed through the mouth to the stomach to keep it empty of secretions. The goal is to avoid stimulating the pancreas with food until it can rest and recover.

Diarrhea

Diarrhea is the passing of loose or liquid stools three or more times daily. It causes the loss of important body water, nutrients, and electrolytes like potassium, sodium, and chloride. Diarrhea can last a few days or can be chronic, with episodes periodically over many years.

Intestinal infections, resulting in diarrhea, can be caused by viruses, bacteria, fungi, or parasites. *Viral gastroenteritis,* sometimes called a "stomach flu," causes nausea, vomiting, diarrhea, and low-grade fever (below 100°). The symptoms usually disappear without treatment within a few days. It is important to prevent dehydration by drinking extra fluids such as tea, Gatorade, or flat sodas. Milk and citric juices should be avoided.

Food poisoning also causes nausea, vomiting, and diarrhea, but no fever. The symptoms can appear within an hour after a meal or up to a day later. Food poisoning usually results from bacteria, such as *Staphylococcus aureus,* which grow in spoiled foods. Poorly refrigerated foods are often the culprits, particularly salads made with mayonnaise or eggs, custards and cream fillings, and poultry stuffing. Symptoms usually improve within one to two days without treatment. It is best not to use antidiarrheal medicines such as Kaopectate, Imodium, or Lomotil because they can prolong the diarrhea by slowing the passage of the bacterial toxins through the intestine.

One of the most common intestinal infections is called "traveler's diarrhea" because it occurs while visiting parts of the world where the food or water may be contaminated with bacteria different—and more toxic—than bacteria at home. With no treatment, traveler's diarrhea ends within a week. Antibiotics, such as Bactrim, often are recommended because they can shorten the duration of the diarrhea.

Salmonella **and** *Shigella* are bacteria that cause infections as either isolated cases or epidemics. Both cause bloody diarrhea, fever, vomiting, nausea, and cramping. Both are diagnosed by stool culture. *Salmonella* typically clears within five days without treatment. *Shigella* is treated with antibiotics.

Giardia is a parasite that invades the small intestine; the resulting infection, giardiasis, causes diarrhea, bloating, and flatulence (gas). A diagnosis is made by microscopic examination of a stool specimen. An antibiotic called metronidazole (Flagyl) is used to treat giardiasis.

Frequent or prolonged use of antibiotics can cause a severe form of diarrhea, signaled by bloody stool, fever, and abdominal pain. The normal, healthy intestine contains bacteria that aid food digestion. Excessive antibiotics kill the normal bacteria and allow overgrowth of a bacteria called *Clostridium difficile,* which causes the diarrhea and other symptoms. Treatment requires discontinuing the first antibiotic and beginning another (metronidazole or vancomycin) that destroys the *Clostridium difficile.*

Irritable bowel syndrome (IBS), also called spastic colitis, is less common in teenagers than adults. Its hallmark is diarrhea or loose stool alternating with constipation. In most people, one or the other predominates and is more bothersome. Associated symptoms include abdominal cramping, bloating, gas, and passage of mucus. The symptoms become worse during periods of stress and are relieved with bowel movement. IBS does not cause blood in the stool, weight loss, or poor absorption of food and nutrients. It is uncomfortable and bothersome, but it is not dangerous or progressive.

IBS has no known cause, and neither blood tests nor barium X-rays show any abnormalities. The diagnosis is based primarily on the history of the symptoms and excluding other possible diagnoses, such as giardiasis or milk intolerance (discussed below).

A diet high in fiber often helps relieve the symptoms and regulates bowel movements. The food highest in fiber content is bran, and the easiest way to eat it is as a breakfast cereal (such as All-Bran or Fiber One). Increased fiber intake only works if fluid intake also is increased. This is because the fiber draws fluid into the stool, increasing its bulk and easing its passage. If symptoms persist after dietary changes, over-the-counter bulking medications such as Metamucil may help. The dose should be adjusted until the adolescent is having one or two bowel movements each day. Bloating and gas may increase temporarily with both fiber and bulking agents. It helps to avoid sodas, chewing gum, and artificial sweeteners.

Milk intolerance is also called lactose intolerance or lactase deficiency. Lactase is an enzyme necessary for the digestion of lactose, the sugar in milk. If there is insufficient lactase in the intestine, the lactose is not digested properly and the normal bacteria in the intestine convert it to gases and fatty acids. The resulting symptoms are bloating, gas, abdominal pain, and diarrhea. Sometimes, the teenager can clearly link the symptoms to drinking milk. Many foods, though, contain hidden milk products. The teenager may need to keep a careful dietary record to discover which foods lead to symptoms. Lactase deficiency typically begins to cause symptoms in late childhood or adolescence.

Diagnosis is made primarily by a history of symptoms linked to milk intake. Other diagnostic measures are available for more obscure cases, but usually are unnecessary. Treatment involves reducing or eliminating milk and milk products in the diet, drinking lactose-free milk, adding lactase to milk, or taking lactase tablets (sold over-the-counter) with meals.

Malabsorption disorders occur when the bowel is unable to absorb food and nutrients normally. The symptoms of malabsorption include malodorous, bulky, light-colored stools; abdominal bloating; weight loss or poor weight gain; delayed growth; and fatigue. There are many causes of malabsorption, including an intolerance to certain food (such as milk), a deficiency of pancreatic enzymes necessary for the digestion of food (as in cystic fibrosis), or a defect in the absorbing surface of the intestine (as in celiac disease).

Celiac disease in children, called nontropical sprue in adults, causes a typical malabsorption disorder. It is more common in females than males and probably is inherited. It is characterized by an abnormality in the absorbing surface of the small intestine and an intolerance to gluten, a protein found in wheat. Eighty percent of people with celiac disease improve when they eliminate gluten from the diet. The diagnosis is based on a history of malabsorption related to wheat ingestion and on a biopsy of the small intestine done through an endoscope (p. 377).

Inflammatory bowel disease (IBD). IBD is a serious cause of persistent diarrhea. About 2.5 million Americans have IBD, and nearly a third are first diagnosed during adolescence. It tends to run in families and is more common in whites than other racial groups. The prevalence is especially high among the Jewish population in North America.

The term IBD includes two similar but distinct diseases: *ulcerative colitis* and *Crohn disease* (also called regional enteritis or granulomatous ileocolitis). The symptoms of the two diseases are similar, but each involves a different part of the digestive system.

Ulcerative colitis is an inflammation of the inside lining of the colon, the five-to-seven-foot-long large intestine that connects the small intestine to the rectum. Crohn disease is an inflammation of the entire intestinal wall and can affect any part of the intestinal tract from the mouth to the anus.

The symptoms of IBD include diarrhea that may be bloody, rectal bleeding, recurrent fever, loss of appetite and weight, poor growth, delayed puberty, a plateau in sexual development once puberty has begun, anemia, and fatigue. In Crohn disease, symptoms such as heartburn, nausea, and vomiting suggest involvement of the upper intestinal tract.

The failure to grow and develop is caused by inadequate food intake and, to a lesser degree, malabsorption of essential nutrients. Teenagers with IBD find it difficult to consume enough food to support the growth spurt of puberty. They avoid eating because it triggers diarrhea and cramping. Many feel bloated or "full" well before ingesting adequate calories and nutrients.

IBD can affect parts of the body other than the digestive tract, but such involvement is far more common in Crohn disease than in ulcerative colitis. The symptoms include joint aching or swelling; skin rashes, ulcers, or painful red nodules; eye inflammation; and liver or kidney inflammation. Crohn disease often causes painful tears around the rectum (fissures) and tracts that burrow through tissues and connect one part of the bowel to another (fistulae).

A long-term complication of ulcerative colitis is cancer of the colon. The risk of cancer increases 1 to 2 percent per year in individuals who have had ulcerative colitis for over ten years. Up to ten years, there is no increased risk of cancer. The risk of malignancy in Crohn disease is far less than in ulcerative colitis. It is probably not much higher than the general population without IBD.

The diagnosis of IBD is based on a combination of findings from the history, physical examination, and endoscopy or barium X-rays. The adolescent with mild IBD may have few symptoms and a normal physical examination. In more severe disease, the teenager may have a very tender abdomen, especially in the right lower side where the inflammation is often at its worst. The doctor may notice hemorrhoids or small tags of skin around the rectum, both of which are abnormal in teenagers though common in healthy adults.

No specific blood test is available to diagnose IBD or to distinguish Crohn disease from ulcerative colitis. The final diagnosis will depend on the results of barium studies and sigmoidoscopy or colonoscopy. In sigmoidoscopy, a lighted scope is passed into the rectum and left side of the colon. In colonoscopy, the scope is passed into the rectum and through the entire colon, or large intestine. Biopsies can be taken during either procedure. The pattern of bowel involvement and the microscopic appearance of the biopsy tissue differentiate Crohn disease from ulcerative colitis.

There are no medications that cure IBD, but there are many that help control it. The goal of treatment is to decrease inflammation in the intestines. The drugs used to do this include sulfasalazine (Azulfidine), salicylates, and corticosteroids (prednisone). Every attempt is made to limit the use of corticosteroids because they carry risks, such as interference with growth, thinning of the bones (osteoporosis), and susceptibility to infection. Sometimes other medications may be added to allow a decrease in the dose of corticosteroids.

Surgery is reserved for the most severe cases of IBD. The role of surgery is different in ulcerative colitis than in Crohn disease. Ulcerative colitis involves, at most, the large intestine and the last segment of the small intestine (the terminal ileum). Removing the entire colon (a total colectomy) cures ulcerative colitis and removes all risk of future colon cancer.

Because most teenagers have not had the disease for more than ten years and because the surgery carries both medical and psychological risks, surgery generally is avoided if possible during adolescence. If a total colectomy is done, a loop of small intestine is pulled to the skin surface, allowing bowel movements into a disposable bag that is sealed over the area. Most adolescents with ulcerative colitis who require surgery have a subtotal colectomy in which the rectum is left in place. The colon is removed and the ileum is connected to the rectum. This procedure can be done if there is no disease in the rectum. A risk is that disease or cancer will develop later in the rectum. Close follow-up, and sometimes later surgery, are necessary.

Surgery in Crohn disease, unlike ulcerative colitis, is not curative because Crohn disease can involve the entire intestinal tract. It is not possible to remove all areas at risk. Surgery is done only when a segment of the intestine is so inflamed that medications have proven ineffective. Unfortunately, even after surgery, recurrences are very common and about three quarters of adolescents will require another surgical procedure within five years.

Adolescents with IBD grow and develop fully if adequate nutrition is maintained. Most teenagers with IBD are able to eat normally. Some may need to adjust their diets with nutritional supplements to maintain weight and promote growth. A few will require periods of bowel rest when they receive very simplified, elemental nutrition through a tube that is placed through the mouth and into the small intestine. Others may need longer periods of bowel rest with all nutrition given intravenously. Whichever route is necessary, nutrition to support growth and sexual maturation is always possible. The feeding regimen may begin in the hospital but, with the help of visiting nurses and parents, usually can continue at home.

IBD can make adolescence an especially trying time. Frequent bowel movements during a school day may be embarrassing. The feeling of having no control of symptoms is difficult at a stage in life when increasing autonomy is the norm. Looking different because of delayed growth or side effects of medication causes great pain for teenagers who, as part of social development, compare themselves to their peers. Parental anxiety about the child's health may complicate the separation that begins during adolescence. Many of the problems are common to all chronic illnesses of adolescence; some are quite specific for IBD. It helps to talk with other adolescents and young adults with IBD. Many communities have IBD support groups. It also helps to work with a multidisciplinary team of health professionals (physicians, nurses, social workers, psychologists) who are comfortable with the issues of both IBD and adolescence. Many community hospitals and most academic medical centers can provide help and guidance.

Constipation

Constipation is the infrequent, difficult, and sometimes painful passing of firm bowel movements. Small children may develop chronic constipation by trying to withhold bowel movements which, they know from past experience, can be painful. Over the years, this voluntary withholding can become involuntary, producing chronic constipation by adolescence. The consequences include abdominal discomfort, soiled underwear, and bleeding from the rectum.

Other common causes of chronic constipation include insufficient fiber in the diet, low fluid intake, and physical inactivity. Medications such as iron, antidepressants, narcotics, bismuth (Pepto-Bismol), and aluminum-containing antacids (Amphojel) can aggravate constipation. Diseases associated with constipation include hypothyroidism (underactive thyroid), anorexia nervosa, and depression. Rarely, chronic constipation is caused by an abnormality in the nerves that supply a segment of the colon (Hirschsprung disease), resulting in poor propulsion of the stool to the rectum.

Constipation that is not part of a chronic pattern often is precipitated by changes in the usual routine, such as travel, vacations, summer camp, or entering college. A sudden change in bowel pattern, though, can signal serious disorders. If the constipation is associated with other symptoms, such as abdominal pain, nausea, vomiting, or fever, medical care should always be sought.

Most constipation improves with several changes in diet and daily routine:

• Drink at least eight glasses of fluid daily and even more after exercise or in hot weather.
• Increase fiber intake through bran cereals or breads, fruits, and leafy vegetables.
• Establish a regular time for bowel movements, usually within thirty to forty-five minutes of a meal. Morning is preferable but not always feasible on school days. After dinner is more convenient for most adolescents. Sit on the toilet for about twenty minutes and make periodic attempts to move the bowels. A suppository inserted into the rectum ten minutes beforehand can make elimination easier and less painful.
• If these measures are insufficient, the next step is to try a bulk laxative, such as Metamucil, which increases stool volume and shortens the travel time through the colon. It should be taken every day rather than periodically as with other laxatives. It works best when taken with at least eight ounces of water and should *never* be taken dry. Two to three weeks are required to see its full effect.
• If bulk laxatives are unsuccessful, short term use of other laxatives may be necessary. Mineral oil (Kondremul), stool softeners (Colace), milk of magnesia, or magnesium citrate are the best choices. Long-term use of laxatives that stimulate the bowel to contract (such as Ex-Lax) can damage the intestine, leading to dependency on laxatives.

Constipation often is considered a "minor" problem that does not need medical evaluation. Usually it is temporary and responds to simple changes. Whenever it is persistent or causes worry, it warrants discussion with a doctor.

Rectal Problems

Pain, discharge, tears, bleeding, or itching in the rectal area are symptoms that require diagnosis and treatment and should not be ignored.

"Proctitis" refers to inflammation of the rectum. It may cause pain on bowel movement, blood-streaked stools, or rectal mucus or pus. The most common cause is a sexually transmitted disease (STD), such as gonorrhea or chlamydia (Chapter 21). Other causes include bacterial infections and inflammatory bowel disease (discussed above).

Rectal tears, fissures, or hemorrhoids that cause pain or blood streaks during bowel movements are usually the result of constipation, anal intercourse, or pregnancy. While the underlying cause is diagnosed and treated, symptoms can be relieved by warm baths, topical creams (such as Anusol, Xylocaine, or Nupercainal), and the measures to reduce constipation previously described.

Itching in the rectal area is called pruritus ani and can be caused by irritation from poor hygiene, yeast infections, pinworm, tight clothing, STDs, or allergies to soap or bubble baths. The underlying cause should be identified whenever possible and eliminated. Pruritus ani often is "idiopathic," meaning no cause can be found. The symptoms then can be controlled by attention to hygiene and the use of topical steroid creams.

Liver Problems

The liver, the body's largest gland, is located in the upper right side of the abdomen. It has many functions, including protein and carbohydrate (sugar) metabolism, digestion, the breakdown of medications and hormones produced by the body, and the production of proteins that are essential for blood clotting. Diseases of the liver can be caused by infections, alcohol use, medications, diseases beginning in other parts of the body (such as diabetes or cystic fibrosis), cancer, inherited disorders, starvation (as in anorexia nervosa), and abnormalities of the blood vessels supplying the liver.

In the earliest stages, most liver diseases cause an abnormality in the "liver function tests" (LFTs) but no symptoms. LFTs require a single tube of blood and are part of many routine blood test panels. If the liver disease becomes worse, symptoms begin to appear. These vary depending on the cause, but may include right-sided abdominal pain or tenderness, jaundice (a yellowing of the skin and eyes), tea-colored urine, light-colored stool, nausea or vomiting, and enlargement of the abdomen. In very severe liver disease, there may be internal bleeding, progressive mental confusion, and coma. It is impossible to survive if the liver fails completely. Liver transplantation then can be lifesaving.

It is impossible to cover all liver diseases in this section. The five that follow either are common during adolescence (such as hepatitis) or are uncommon but tend to appear during adolescence (such as Wilson disease).

Hepatitis is a viral infection that inflames the liver. Many different viruses can be responsible, including hepatitis A, B, C, D, and E viruses, the Epstein-Barr virus (EBV) that causes infectious mononucleosis, and cytomegalovirus (CMV). EBV is discussed in Chapter 34. Of the five hepatitis viruses, A and B are the most common.

Hepatitis A is transmitted through food and water and from person to person through stool, oral secretions, and sexual contact. Symptoms appear fifteen to fifty days after infection and include fever, fatigue, nausea, vomiting, pain in the upper right abdomen, loss of appetite, and jaundice. In many cases, symptoms are very mild or even absent. When present, they usually disappear on their own within a few weeks, though it may take up to two months for the LFTs to return to normal. Chronic liver damage is extremely rare following hepatitis A, and chronic infection does not happen. Hepatitis A is diagnosed by a blood test that measures antibodies to the hepatitis A virus.

Hepatitis A is contagious during the two weeks before and after symptoms appear. All people who live in the same household or have had sexual contact with the infected person should receive an injection of immune globulin as soon as possible to decrease their chance of infection. The injection has no protective effect if given more than two weeks after exposure.

Adolescents who are exposed to hepatitis A in school are not considered at risk and should not receive immune globulin. Adolescents with hepatitis A should not return to school until the jaundice clears or for at least one week after the illness begins. Careful bathroom hygiene and hand washing are very important in preventing the spread of the disease.

Hepatitis B virus infection is associated with a broad spectrum of manifestations, including nausea, lethargy, jaundice, and abdominal pain. In most individuals, there are no symptoms and the only evidence of past infection is the presence of antibodies in the blood. There is a 45-to-160-day delay between exposure to someone with hepatitis B and the onset of symptoms. It can take up to four months for LFTs to return to normal. Unlike hepatitis A, hepatitis B can progress to a chronic form called chronic active hepatitis in which liver inflammation, infection, and contagiousness persist for life. Chronic carriers of the hepatitis B virus are at high risk of developing liver cancer or cirrhosis, a disease in which scar tissue replaces liver cells and obstructs the flow of blood through the liver.

Hepatitis B virus is spread through sexual contact, intravenous drug use, and contact with infected blood, and from mother to fetus. The infection is diagnosed by a blood test that measures both hepatitis B antigen (a marker of the virus) and hepatitis B antibody (the body's normal response to the virus). Chronic active hepatitis is diagnosed by a liver biopsy in which a needle is passed through the skin and into the liver. The small piece of tissue collected through the needle is examined under a microscope.

Hepatitis B infection can be prevented by a vaccine that is now recommended for all children and adolescents. The vaccine is a series of three injections given over the course of six months. Individuals who are exposed to hepatitis B via a household member should receive the vaccine. Sexual partners should receive both the vaccine and an injection of hepatitis B-specific immune globulin within two weeks of exposure.

Toxin-induced liver damage. "Toxins" refers to alcohol, illegal drugs, medications, or environmental pollutants that damage body tissues. In adults, the most common hepatic (liver) toxin is alcohol. Liver disease secondary to alcohol use is far less common in teenagers because they have not yet had years of drinking. Nevertheless, short-term heavy use can cause fatty infiltration of the liver (called alcoholic fatty liver) and inflammation of the liver (alcoholic hepatitis). In alcoholic fatty liver, the liver becomes enlarged and the LFTs are abnormal. If the drinking stops, the liver may return to normal. Alcoholic hepatitis is more serious than alcoholic fatty liver and over many years can progress to alcoholic cirrhosis and even death.

Certain drugs—both legal and illegal—can cause severe liver damage. Drugs that are potentially toxic to the liver include anesthetic agents, psychiatric medications, seizure medications, analgesics (painkillers), hormonal medications, antibiotics, some vitamins, and illegal drugs such as cocaine. The only treatment in most cases is to stop the offending drug.

Acetaminophen (Tylenol) is probably the most common cause of drug-induced liver disease in teenagers. Acetaminophen is very safe when taken in recommended doses. When an overdose is taken, as in a suicide attempt, the result can be permanent damage to liver cells. Within several hours of the ingestion, the teenager may develop nausea and vomiting. The LFT values begin to increase within forty-eight hours, and liver failure can follow within three to five days. Early treatment is imperative and lifesaving. If the level of acetaminophen in the blood is high, an oral medication called acetylcysteine (Mucomyst) will be given to try to prevent liver damage. It must be given within twenty-four hours of the ingestion to be effective.

Aspirin is another important cause of liver damage in children and teenagers. Like acetaminophen, it can cause direct damage. It also can cause indirect damage through an association with viral illnesses. In the 1970s, it became apparent that aspirin use in children who had influenza or chicken pox increased their risk of Reye syndrome. This disease begins within a week of the viral illness with severe vomiting, irritability, and fatigue. Most patients then begin to improve, and their liver function returns to normal. Some children, though, progress to seizures, coma, and even death.

Most causes of Reye syndrome are in children aged six to eight years, although it occurs in adolescents as well. Reye syndrome is rare, but its severity has led to the recommendation that aspirin should not be used for viral illnesses in children and teenagers.

Inherited disorders of the liver. There are many inherited diseases that affect the liver. Some are very mild and cause elevated LFTs with no symptoms. Others are quite severe, resulting in progressive liver failure. Some are apparent from birth, while others may first appear during adolescence or young adulthood.

Gilbert disease is an inherited disorder affecting 2 to 6 percent of the population. It is caused by an abnormality in the liver's metabolism of bilirubin, a breakdown product of red blood cells. The LFTs are normal except for a high bilirubin level. Dieting, fasting, and weight loss all may increase the bilirubin level up to threefold in adolescents with Gilbert disease. This disease causes no symptoms, is not progressive, and requires no treatment.

Wilson disease is a more serious inherited disease that typically becomes apparent during adolescence. It is caused by an abnormality in copper metabolism, resulting in the accumulation of copper in the liver, eyes, brain, and kidneys. The first signs of the disease usually are liver enlargement or symptoms resembling hepatitis. Some teenagers develop psychiatric or neurologic problems. These are usually subtle, such as mild changes in speech, school performance, or mood.

Wilson disease should be considered in all teenagers with unexplained liver disease. The diagnosis is made by blood test, eye examination, and liver biopsy. Untreated Wilson disease ultimately is fatal. Early diagnosis and proper treatment with a medication called D-penicillamine results in an excellent outcome for most young people with the disease.

30

The Urinary Bladder and Kidneys

The kidneys, bladder, and urinary tubes (Figure 30.1) function together to remove waste products and water from the body. The *kidneys* are a pair of organs in the mid-back of the abdomen, one on each side of the spine. Each kidney is connected to a small tube called the *ureter* that carries the urine to the *bladder*. The bladder stores the urine, which continually drains from the kidneys through the ureters. As the bladder fills with urine, its walls expand like a balloon. A ring of muscles around the neck of the bladder, called the *urethral sphincter*, acts as a door to keep the urine within the bladder. When the bladder becomes full, it sends a message to the spinal cord and the urge to urinate results. The urethral sphincter relaxes and opens, the muscles of the bladder wall contract, and the urine is expelled through a tube called the *urethra*.

During adolescence, a disorder of the urinary tract may be the continuation of a childhood condition or may signal a new problem. Some urinary conditions cause straightforward symptoms. For example, bladder infections typically cause pain on urination and cloudy or bloody urine. Other urinary problems, though, cause vague symptoms such as nausea, backache, or fever. The following symptoms suggest that the cause may be in the urinary tract:

- pain in the mid-back or flank (the side of the body from the lowest rib to the hip);
- pain radiating from the abdomen or back to the groin (where

393

The Urinary System

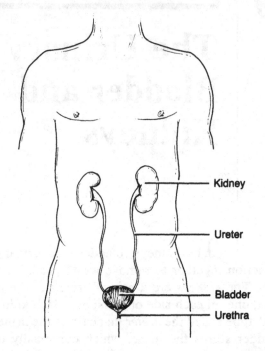

Kidney

Ureter

Bladder

Urethra

Figure 30.1

the thigh and abdomen meet), scrotum, or labia (the outside of the vagina);
- pain in the lower pelvis (the ring of bones in the hip area);
- blood in the urine;
- pain on urination;
- frequency, urgency, or hesitancy in urinating;
- incontinence (involuntary urination or the inability to withhold urine).

These symptoms should always receive medical attention. The doctor will begin the evaluation with a thorough history and physical examination. In females, this may include a pelvic examination (Chapter 3) to determine if the problem is originating in the vagina, uterus, or ovaries.

Depending on the suspected location of the problem, the following laboratory tests or procedures may be done:

Urinalysis involves a urine sample that the teenager provides by voiding into a jar. The urine is then checked for protein, sugar, and blood by a dipstick that changes colors if these substances are present in abnormal amounts. The urine also is examined under a microscope for cells and bacteria.

Urine culture involves a "clean catch" urine sample. The teenager is asked to wash the penis or vagina thoroughly with an antiseptic soap before urinating into a sterile jar. The sample is sent to the laboratory, where it is tested for bacteria. Normally, the urine is sterile.

Blood tests for two compounds called blood urea nitrogen (BUN) and creatinine are done to measure kidney function. These compounds normally are present in the blood in very small quantities. If the kidneys are not functioning properly, the BUN and creatinine levels increase.

Cystoscopy is an outpatient procedure that is performed by passing a very thin, lighted tube through the urethra into the bladder. The lining of the bladder can be examined and a biopsy (removal of a small sample of tissue) can be done of any abnormal areas.

Voiding cystourethrogram (VCUG) is an outpatient procedure in which a small catheter, or tube, is placed through the urethra into the bladder. The bladder is then filled with water and its filling capacity and emptying function are measured.

Intravenous pyelogram or urogram (IVP or IVU) is an X-ray test in which a dye is injected into an arm vein. The dye travels though the bloodstream and shows up on the X-ray as it is excreted through the kidneys, ureters, bladder, and urethra.

Renal ultrasound is a painless test that provides a picture of the size and shape of the kidneys using sound waves. "Renal" means the same as "kidney."

Renal scan is done by injecting a tiny, harmless amount of radioactive tracer into an arm vein. The tracer travels through the bloodstream and is picked up and excreted by the kidneys. A scanning device, run over the outside of the body, detects the tracer and gives a picture of the kidneys.

Kidney biopsy is a procedure in which a hollow needle is inserted through the skin of the back into one kidney. A small sample of kidney tissue is removed through the needle and examined under the microscope. The biopsy requires sedation, local anesthesia, and an overnight hospital stay.

Urinary Tract Infections

Cystitis is a bladder infection. It affects females much more commonly than males because a female's urethra is shorter and closer to the rectum, where bacteria normally grow. Between 10 and 20 percent of women experience at least one episode of cystitis. Factors that increase a female's risk of cystitis include sexual intercourse, use of a diaphragm for contraception, poor hygiene of the vaginal–urethral–anal area, pregnancy, and anatomic abnormalities of the urinary tract. Males with cystitis are far more likely to have anatomic abnormalities than are females.

The symptoms of cystitis include frequency, urgency, hesitancy, pain on urinating, lower abdominal pain, and blood in the urine. A diagnosis is made by a urinalysis that shows many white blood cells and a urine culture that grows bacteria.

The medical evaluation of cystitis depends on gender and the frequency of infection. Even one bout of cystitis in a male warrants evaluation because of the likelihood of finding an anatomic problem. Cystitis in females usually is not evaluated unless the infections recur frequently. The tests for males and females may include an IVP, a voiding cystourethrogram, and cystoscopy.

Cystitis is treated with antibiotics. About 85 percent of females with cystitis are cured of the infection by a single oral dose or single injection of antibiotics. All males—and females who do not improve with single-dose therapy—are treated with oral antibiotics for seven to ten days. A urine culture should be repeated after treatment is completed to be sure the infection is cured.

Females with recurrent cystitis should take precautions to avoid the risk factors previously mentioned. Sexually active females should urinate before and after intercourse to keep the bladder empty. If these preventive measures are ineffective, a six-month course of low-dose antibiotics may be prescribed to prevent recurrences.

Mothers of today's teenagers may have been treated for cystitis years ago by "urethral dilation," or stretching of the urethra. This method is ineffective and is no longer used to prevent cystitis.

Pyelonephritis is an infection of one or both kidneys. It is more serious than cystitis and causes a more severe illness. The symptoms of pyelonephritis include pain in the mid-back or flank, fever, chills, nausea, vomiting, and cloudy urine. The diagnosis is made by a history of these symptoms in the presence of a urine culture that grows bacteria. Pyelonephritis is treated with antibiotics for fourteen days. If the teenager is not too ill and is able to keep pills down, the antibiotics may be taken orally. Many adolescents with pyelonephritis require several days of hospitalization for intravenous antibiotics. Once the fever is down and nausea ceases, they may go home to complete the full course of antibiotics orally. After treatment is completed, a urine culture must be repeated to be certain that the infection is cured.

Enuresis (Bedwetting)

Enuresis, or involuntary wetting, is stressful for both adolescents and their families. It typically happens at night, during periods of heavy sleep. Teenagers with enuresis may feel embarrassed, guilty, and confused about how to overcome a problem that usually occurs when they are asleep and unaware. Concealing enuresis, or deciding just to tolerate it, is always a mistake. Talk to your doctor about it; there are many new, effective methods of treatment.

The prevalence of enuresis decreases throughout childhood and adolescence. Up to 20 percent of five-year-olds have enuresis. The rate falls to less than 10 percent at age ten and less than 2 percent at age eighteen. Over three quarters of these teenagers have enuresis only at night, while a quarter have episodes both day and night. Enuresis is more common in males than females and in teenagers with a parent who had enuresis.

The majority of teenagers have no identifiable physical or psychological cause for the enuresis. Conditions that are associated with it include spinal cord problems, frequent urinary tract infections, and diabetes mellitus. Some teenagers with daytime and nighttime wetting have diabetes insipidus, a disorder in which the kidneys cannot hold on to water. These teenagers have a lifelong history of drinking great quantities of fluid to keep up with the losses through the kidneys. It now is thought that some children and teenagers with nocturnal enuresis have a very mild form of this disorder in which the normal nighttime increase in the hormone responsible for water retention does not occur. This hormone, called antidiuretic hormone, or vasopressin, can be given as a nasal spray medication called DDAVP. When taken at bedtime, DDAVP can help control enuresis with few side effects. Once the enuresis is controlled, the DDAVP should be tapered off gradually.

Several other therapies usually are tried before DDAVP. All should begin by addressing the feelings and responses of the adolescent and family. All family members should recognize that enuresis affects hundreds of thousands of teenagers, not just their teenager. Guilt and blame are understandable reactions but serve no part in its treatment. Teenagers should take an active part in dealing with the problem—changing the sheets, for example—and parents should diminish their involvement. This helps diffuse the angry feelings and focuses on changing the behavior.

A method that helps many teenagers is an alarm with a moisture-sensing clip that attaches to the underwear and a beeping device worn like a wristwatch. When the sensor detects a small amount of moisture, it activates the wrist alarm. As the teenager awakens, the urethral sphincter closes, allowing time to go immediately to the bathroom. Over several weeks, the teenager learns to wake up with the urge to urinate, before the alarm goes off. Some will be able to suppress the urge through the night; others will learn to get up quickly and go to the bathroom.

An exercise method may help adolescents with small bladders who urinate frequently day and night. The exercise requires holding back the urine as long as possible when the urge to urinate arises. Over time, this can help increase the bladder's holding capacity and muscle tone. Some adolescents find it helpful to measure the amount of urine as a way of assessing their progress. The exercise should be done in conjunction with other therapies because it usually does not control enuresis on its own.

Medications other than DDAVP can help diminish the frequency of enuresis, but none are completely effective. Imipramine (Tofranil) helps over a quarter of adolescents with enuresis, but side effects such as anxiety, light-headedness, and abdominal discomfort are common. Another drug called Ditropan is taken three times daily and decreases bladder contraction. It is more helpful for adolescents who urinate frequently during the day than for those with nocturnal enuresis.

In many cases, enuresis disappears on its own with time. Sometimes, though, it continues into adulthood. Don't wait for a spontaneous cure; discuss treatment options with a physician.

Kidney Stones

Kidney stones are far more common in adults than in teenagers or children. Factors that predispose adolescents to stone formation include a family history of kidney stones, recurrent urinary tract infections during childhood, bladder dysfunction, abnormalities in kidney shape, and prolonged immobilization. Teenagers with these factors may be at even greater risk of kidney stones if their diets are high in certain substances, such as calcium from large quantities of milk products or antacids and oxalate from tea, cranberry juice, and spinach.

The kidneys normally collect wastes and dilute them with water. If the urine is too concentrated, either because of excessive waste or insufficient water, crystals will form. Very small clusters or crystals, or "stones," can pass through the urinary tract without any problem. Larger stones can cause irritation, bleeding into the urine, obstruction of the flow of urine, and pain.

The pain of kidney stones varies from a dull ache in the mid-back or flank on one side to an excruciating pain in the back or abdomen that radiates down to the groin. The pain may—or may not—become worse with urination.

A preliminary diagnosis of kidney stones is based on the history of the symptoms and urinalysis. Small stones, or "gravel," sometimes can be found by collecting the urine and pouring it through a fine cloth sieve. The gravel then can be sent to the laboratory to determine its components. If a kidney stone is suspected or collected, an IVP usually is done to examine the structure of the urinary tract and the location of the stone or stones.

Treatment depends on the type and size of the stone and the underlying cause. Small stones often will pass spontaneously though the urinary tract. Larger stones that do not move and cause discomfort or obstruction may require a procedure called lithotripsy, which shatters the stone with shock waves. The tiny, broken-up particles then can pass freely through the urinary tract. Lithotripsy is done under general anesthesia but does not require an incision. Surgery has become an uncommon method of treating kidney stones.

Teenagers with a history of kidney stones should increase their fluid intake to help keep the urine diluted. They may also need special nutritional counseling or medications that prevent stone formation. Regular medical care throughout adolescence and adulthood decreases the chance of future recurrences.

Protein in the Urine

Protein is not normally found in the urine, but there are times when it does appear without any harmful effects. These temporary appearances of "proteinuria" tend to coincide with strenuous exercise, a fever, dehydration, or extreme hot or cold weather. Another common cause is called postural proteinuria because the protein appears after standing and disappears after a night's sleep. It is not associated with kidney disease and carries no risk for the adolescent.

In up to 5 percent of adolescents, proteinuria is found on routine urinalysis. The majority have normal physical examinations. Microscopic examination of the urine reveals no abnormal cells. Their kidney function measured by simple blood tests (BUN and creatinine) are normal. Up to half of these teenagers may continue to have small amounts of proteinuria into adulthood, but they are not more likely than adolescents without proteinuria to develop kidney disease.

Some adolescents excrete greater quantities of protein. The urinalysis dipstick provides a rough estimate, which, if high, should be quantified exactly by measuring the protein in a twenty-four-hour collection of urine. Potentially serious underlying causes must be considered if the proteinuria is significant. Kidney infections and kidney stones can cause proteinuria. There may be a problem ("nephritis") in the small tubules that collect urine within the kidney. Proteinuria can signal chronic diseases such as diabetes mellitus, high blood pressure, or sickle cell anemia. It can be caused by infections outside the kidneys such as syphilis or hepatitis. It is a common complication of pregnancy that requires very close prenatal care. Certain medications and illegal drugs can cause proteinuria.

An important cause of significant proteinuria in children and teenagers is called *idiopathic nephrotic syndrome*. It typically begins after a minor viral illness with swelling around the eyes or in the feet and hands. As the kidneys leak more protein into the urine, the fluid retention (edema) becomes worse. There may be abdominal distention from fluid in the belly or difficulty breathing from fluid in the chest. The diagnosis may be suspected from the symptoms, physical examination, and urinalysis, but must be confirmed by a kidney biopsy.

Corticosteroids such as prednisone are used to treat idiopathic nephrotic syndrome. Most adolescents respond to corticosteroids and, over time, the disease disappears completely. The minority of adolescents who do not respond to corticosteroids have a poorer outcome and may face eventual kidney failure.

Glomerulonephritis, another cause of proteinuria, is an inflammation of the tiny blood vessels clustered throughout the kidney. It can be a complication of an autoimmune disease such as lupus (Chapter 31) or can follow an infection elsewhere in the body. "Poststreptococcal glomerulonephritis" appears within two weeks of a strep throat (Chapter 25) or skin infection. The signs and symptoms include blood in the urine, swelling of the face or feet, decreased urine output, fatigue, fever, back or abdominal pain, and high blood pressure. The diagnosis is made by the history, physical examination, urinalysis, and blood tests. The treatment involves an antibiotic for ten days to kill the bacteria. Other members of the household should have throat cultures done and should take antibiotics if they are positive for strep. Over 90 percent of adolescents with poststreptococcal glomerulonephritis recover completely.

Blood in the Urine

Blood in the urine, or *hematuria,* can make the urine appear brown, amber, red, or pink. If the blood originates in the kidney, the color is likely to be brownish. If it comes from the lower urinary tract (the bladder or urethra), it may be pink or red and may contain small blood clots. More often, the urine looks normal but blood is detected with a dipstick and by examining the urine under a microscope.

False hematuria frequently occurs in females due to vaginal bleeding, especially during the menstrual period. It is called false because the bleeding does not originate in the urinary tract. Certain foods and medications can also produce false hematuria by reacting with the urine dipstick. The clue here is that no red blood cells are seen with the microscope.

True hematuria has many possible causes. The most common in teenagers are cystitis, urethritis (Chapter 18), back and abdominal injuries, and strenuous exercise—especially running. In exercise-induced hematuria, the urinalysis is normal before the exercise but reveals blood for several hours or even days after the exercise. It generally does not indicate kidney disease and carries no risk for the teenager. Other less common causes of hematuria include kidney stones, sickle cell disease (Chapter 35), glomerulonephritis (discussed above), blood clotting disorders (Chapter 35), and—very rarely in teenagers—tumors of the kidney or bladder.

Several inherited kidney diseases can cause hematuria. Some, called benign hematuria, are *not* associated with kidney failure and cause no symptoms. Another, called Alport syndrome, is associated with kidney failure, deafness, and vision problems.

IgA nephropathy, or Berger disease, begins with hematuria during adolescence or young adulthood and is six times more common in males than females. "IgA" refers to a type of antibody that is produced by the body in response to an outside antigen such as a virus or toxin. The antibody and the antigen bind together and become trapped in the kidneys, causing inflammation. The resulting hematuria and proteinuria may come and go, often following colds or minor viral illnesses. Sometimes the flares are associated with pain, but usually there are no symptoms.

IgA nephropathy is diagnosed by a kidney biopsy. The disease has no known cause or cure. Despite the bouts of hematuria, two thirds of affected adolescents have normal kidney function. A third develop scarring of the kidney and are at risk for progressive kidney failure.

Kidney Failure

When the kidneys fail, the body is unable to excrete its waste products. Acute renal failure means that kidney function has declined suddenly over days or weeks. Chronic renal failure means that it has declined gradually over months or years. The most important laboratory indicators of kidney failure are increasing blood levels of BUN and creatinine. The signs and symptoms include poor growth, fatigue, anemia, loss of appetite, nausea, and vomiting.

Renal failure is treated with either dialysis or kidney transplant. Dialysis is the process of removing wastes from the bloodstream by an artificial kidney machine. Without treatment, renal failure eventually leads to electrolyte imbalances that may produce irregular heart rhythms or seizures. Increasing mental confusion and eventually coma and death are inevitable in progressive renal failure.

The causes of acute renal failure are divided into three groups: decreased blood flow to the kidneys, problems in the kidneys themselves, and obstruction or blockage of the urine flow from the kidneys. Some causes of decreased blood flow are hemorrhage from somewhere else in the body and overwhelming infections of the blood. Problems within the kidneys that can lead to acute renal failure include glomerulonephritis and certain medications. Examples of obstruction include kidney stones and tumors that block both ureters.

The most common causes of chronic renal failure in adolescents are inherited kidney diseases and glomerulonephritis. In adults, diabetes mellitus and hypertension are the most common causes. These diseases can begin in childhood or adolescence but typically require at least ten years before irreversibly damaging the kidneys. Both diseases, if treated aggressively, can spare the kidneys.

Managing renal failure involves the ongoing monitoring of urine, blood, and nutritional status. If the teenager is not growing well, extra calories from carbohydrates and fats are generally recommended. Dairy and animal products are restricted because their protein is metabolized into wastes that the kidneys have difficulty processing. Salt intake is also restricted when the urine volume is low because it increases fluid retention.

Some teenagers with chronic renal failure are treated with "hemodialysis" two or three times weekly. This procedure requires filtering the blood through a special machine for four to five hours at a time. For other teenagers, "peritoneal dialysis" is used. A catheter, or small tube, is placed in the abdomen and fluid is allowed to flow into the abdominal cavity where it bathes the intestines and organs. The waste products in the blood move into the fluid, which is then drained out of the abdomen several hours later through the catheter. Peritoneal dialysis is done at home on a schedule designed to minimize the disruption of daily life.

In acute renal failure, dialysis may take over the kidneys' work until they can heal and begin functioning again. Once dialysis is required in chronic renal failure, the kidneys will not heal and either dialysis or a kidney transplant is essential to sustain life. The success of transplantation depends on the "match" between the donor kidney and the adolescent. A perfect match, as from an identical twin, means that the kidney is not recognized by the body as foreign so that no antibodies are produced to reject the kidney. A well-matched kidney from a brother or sister carries a 90 percent chance of good function ten years after the transplant. A kidney from a parent, who can never be as well matched as a sibling, carries a 70 percent chance of function after ten years. A kidney from a nonrelative carries a 50 percent chance of function at ten years. In all cases, medications are used after the transplant to suppress the immune system and protect the kidney. These medications have greatly improved the likelihood that a kidney transplant will be, and will remain, successful.

31

The Bones and Joints

Puberty is a time of rapid growth for the bones and joints. For most teenagers, this growth proceeds smoothly and, except for an occasional sports-related injury, the bones and joints are trouble-free.

This chapter addresses conditions of the bones and joints that are not caused by athletic injuries (Chapter 4). Most of this chapter is organized by the part of the body in which the symptoms appear—back, hip, knee, leg, ankle, foot. The last three sections discuss problems that may occur anywhere in the body: benign bone growths, bone infections, and arthritis.

First, a few basic terms and definitions:

Cartilage is gristle, or hard tissue, that covers some bones and joints. It has an elastic quality that diminishes friction and allows joints to bend smoothly.

Ligaments are tough connective bands that hold bones together and keep them in place.

Tendons are strong fibers that attach muscles to bones.

Vertebrae are the bones that form the spinal column.

The spinal column (spine or backbone) is the body's central trunk. Its upper end attaches to the skull and its lower to the pelvis at the "sacroiliac joints." The spinal column surrounds and protects the body's central nervous system.

Disks are flat pieces of cartilage between the vertebrae. They act as cushions to protect the vertebrae from rubbing against each other.

The Back

SCOLIOSIS

This condition is a curvature of the spine that affects 5 percent of adolescents. It progresses most rapidly during the growth spurt of puberty. It tends to run in families and is eight times more common in females than males.

Scoliosis generally is painless and unnoticeable when the teenager is dressed. A physician or nurse may first detect it on a routine physical examination. Less commonly, parents may notice that the teenager's skirt hems or pants are uneven or that one shoulder or hip is higher than the other. In a minority of cases, scoliosis is caused by an underlying condition such as cerebral palsy, rheumatoid arthritis, injury, spina bifida, or muscular dystrophy. In most cases, the cause is unknown.

The signs of scoliosis include a lateral (sideways) curve of the spine; uneven shoulders, breasts, or hips; a protruding shoulder blade; a sloping waistline; and a tilt to the back that makes one arm or leg seem longer than the other.

Many schools examine teenagers regularly for scoliosis as part of physical education classes or sports screenings. The teenager is asked to undress above the waist and to stand with the back facing the examiner. The symmetry of the spine is examined with the teenager standing straight and then bending over from the waist. If scoliosis is suspected, the adolescent should see a physician who is experienced in the evaluation and management of scoliosis.

The treatment of scoliosis depends on the degree of curvature. If the physical examination indicates significant scoliosis, the exact degree of curvature can be measured on an X-ray of the spine. A teenager whose curve is less than twenty-five degrees does not require treatment but should be examined every three months until growth is completed. An orthopedic surgeon should be consulted if the curve is greater than twenty-five degrees or increases rapidly.

Most adolescents with scoliosis have minor curves that remain stable without treatment throughout life. About 15 percent of adolescents with scoliosis require active intervention. Several types of braces are available to reduce the curvature or curtail its progress. Braces are worn twenty-three hours daily until the teenager's full growth is reached. With some braces, exercises supplement the treatment, but exercises alone will not correct or slow scoliosis.

Electrical stimulation of the muscles along the spine is an experimental method for slowing the progression of scoliosis in teenagers with minor curvatures. Long-term results are still unclear, and it is not the recommended form of treatment for most adolescents with scoliosis.

In severe cases, surgery is done to correct scoliosis. The vertebrae are fused together and held in a straight line by inserting a metal rod. This "Harrington rod" remains in place for life. The teenager must wear a body cast for several months after surgery.

Wearing a round-the-clock brace for years or a body cast for months presents tremendous psychological and social challenges to an adolescent. The alternatives, though, can be much worse. If significant scoliosis goes uncorrected, the consequences can include progressive deformity, chronic back pain, and impaired breathing. With treatment, the prognosis is excellent.

KYPHOSIS

Two forms of kyphosis, or rounded back, generally appear in teenagers: postural roundback and Scheuermann disease. Postural roundback is painless, and the vertebrae are normal. Scheuermann disease often causes back pain, particularly with physical activity, and the shape of the vertebrae is abnormal.

In addition to the rounded shape of the upper back, other signs of kyphosis are a forward slope of the shoulder, a slouching posture, a winglike appearance of the shoulder blades, a protruding abdomen, and a tendency to hold the head and neck forward. A doctor will diagnose kyphosis by the clinical signs and by X-ray.

Treatment involves exercises in milder cases and braces in more severe cases. If the spine is flexible, braces offer a good prognosis for correction. If the spine is rigid and the curve is pronounced, surgery similar to that for scoliosis may be necessary. The growth plates, or epiphyses, of the ribs in the upper back continue to grow until about age seventeen in females and nineteen in males, which makes correction of kyphosis possible even after the rest of the skeletal system has stopped growing.

Teenagers often bristle at parental reminders to "stand straight," "stop slouching," "sit up." Most adolescents are able to straighten up when reminded, and standing straight does help strengthen the muscles of the upper back and shoulders. Teenagers who cannot straighten the spine or maintain a straight posture should see a physician.

BACK PAIN

This problem is uncommon in adolescence. When it does occur, it is important to determine the cause. The pain can signal a serious problem, such as infection, herniated disk, arthritis, scoliosis, kyphosis, or tumor. More often, it is caused by muscle strain from heavy lifting, inadequate conditioning before exercise, or poorly fitting shoes. The most important causes of back pain in adolescents are the following:

Acute back strain begins suddenly, usually in the low back, and typically improves on its own within a few weeks. Some general guidelines can help prevent back strain:

• When lifting a heavy object from the ground, squat and use the legs to lift yourself and the object upright;
• When sitting, press your spine against the back of the chair and keep your knees higher than your hips;
• Sleep on a firm mattress on your side with hips and knees bent;
• Wear low-heel shoes;
• If you must stand for a long time, put one foot on a step to reduce the strain on the back, alternating feet every few minutes.

Exercises can help reduce the chance that acute back strain recurs. Once the pain has disappeared, begin the exercises slowly. Some simple exercises include the following:

• Stretch your back muscles by pulling your knees to your chest while lying on the floor or by arching your back to the ceiling while resting on your hands and knees;
• Strengthen your back muscles by lifting one leg at a time and then both shoulders while lying on your stomach;
• Strengthen the abdominal muscles that help support the back by pulling in your stomach muscles as you press your back flat against the floor;
• Check your posture by pressing your heels, buttocks, shoulders, and head against a wall. Try to hold that posture as you walk away from the wall.

Spondylolisthesis is the forwarding sliding of one vertebra upon another. The symptoms include pain in the lower back, buttocks, and thighs; tight hamstring muscles (those at the back of the thigh);

limping; and pronounced arching of the back with protrusion of the abdomen.

A diagnosis of spondylolisthesis is made by X-ray. Even when there is no pain, teenagers with spondylolisthesis should be examined every six months until growth is completed because the slippage may progress. If X-rays indicate that the spondylolisthesis is progressing, the treatment options include immobilization in a cast, wearing a brace, or surgery to fuse the slipped vertebra to an adjoining, stable one. After surgery, 95 percent of teenagers return to full activities with no symptoms.

Herniated disk is rare in adolescents, unlike adults. The disk slips, or "herniates," out of its normal place between two vertebrae and presses on nerves as they branch out from the spinal cord. This pressure causes irritation of the nerves with excruciating pain in the low back, buttock, or leg. In severe cases, there is numbness or weakness in a leg or foot. The diagnosis is best confirmed by an MRI of the back.

Treatment for a herniated disk begins with bed rest and analgesic medicines. If symptoms persist, surgery to remove the disk may be necessary.

Diskitis, or infection of the disk space between the vertebrae, is caused by bacteria that have spread through the bloodstream from the respiratory or urinary tract. Symptoms include back or leg pain, tenderness when the area is touched, and difficulty walking. Scans of bone and soft tissue can identify the infection earlier than X-rays, which generally do not reveal the problem until two to three weeks after symptoms first appear.

Treatment begins with bed rest and oral antibiotics. If symptoms persist, the adolescent may require hospitalization for intravenous antibiotics and removal of the infected material through a needle inserted into the disk space.

A much more serious problem than diskitis is vertebral osteomyelitis. This is an infection of a vertebra that causes pain, fever, and eventual destruction of the bone if untreated. Vertebral osteomyelitis always requires weeks of intravenous antibiotics, bed rest, and frequently a cast.

Ankylosing spondylitis is a chronic inflammatory disorder of unknown cause that tends to run in families. Symptoms include back stiffness in the morning and back pain at night that is partially relieved by walking around. Other diseases, such as inflammatory bowel disease (Chapter 29), may be associated with ankylosing spondylitis. Adolescents with the disorder typically have pain in joints as well as the back. Many have intermittent fever, fatigue, weight loss, and anemia. The treatment includes anti-inflammatory medication and physical therapy to promote back muscle strength.

The Hip

Unlike older adults, teenagers rarely have hip pain. The two most common hip disorders of adolescence are described below.

SLIPPED CAPITAL FEMORAL EPIPHYSIS

This disorder is the displacement of the growth plate (epiphysis) located between the thighbone (femur) and the hip. This problem is two to three times more common in males than females and tends to occur in early puberty. The exact cause is unknown, but it may be precipitated by the added stress on the epiphysis from excess body weight, rapid growth, or an injury.

Early signs of slipped capital femoral epiphysis include an ache in the groin, buttock, hip, or knee; limping with a foot turned outward; and limited mobility of the hip. Symptoms may appear gradually or suddenly. If a slipped hip is suspected, walking should be discouraged and immediate care sought. Once the diagnosis is confirmed by X-ray, surgery is done to pin the femur and hip permanently in the correct position. A delay in treatment can lead to progressive hip arthritis.

LEGG-CALVÉ-PERTHES DISEASE

In this hip disorder the blood supply to the upper end of the leg bone (the femoral head) is interrupted. It affects boys more often than girls and tends to run in families. Most cases are diagnosed in early childhood, but the disease seems to be increasing among young adolescents. The signs and symptoms include limp, thigh pain, hip stiffness, and muscle loss in the thigh or buttock. Once the diagnosis is confirmed by X-ray, treatment involves bed rest and exercises that do not put weight on the hip. In some cases, surgery is necessary.

The Knee

The knees could be called the body's heavy lifters. They are constantly called upon to bend, stretch, and bear weight. In a task such as climbing stairs, for example, a force greater than three times the body's weight is exerted on the knee by the quadriceps, the large muscles at the front of the thigh.

Knee pain is very common in teenagers. The pain usually originates in the knee itself, though it may signal a hip disorder. Knee problems tend to arise from misalignment or instability of the joint.

General symptoms of a knee disorder include pain (especially when climbing stairs or squatting), swelling, stiffness, creaking, clicking, and buckling (or giving way) of the knee. Locking of the knee, with inability to bend or straighten, usually indicates a sports-related tear of the cartilage in the knee.

The most common knee problem during adolescence include the following:

OSGOOD-SCHLATTER DISEASE

This disorder affects the large tendon that connects the front of the knee to the shinbone or tibia (the larger bone between the knee and ankle). It affects boys more than girls and is more common during early puberty. Osgood-Schlatter disease appears to be caused by repeated stress on the tendon during a period of rapid growth. Activities like basketball that require a great deal of knee turning and twisting can aggravate it. The signs and symptoms are pain and tenderness throughout the knee and a small, tender bump about an inch below the bend in the knee.

Osgood-Schlatter disease is uncomfortable, but it is not serious. The only treatment is to curtail physical activities or exercises that cause the pain. Other activities should be continued and encouraged. Only in rare instances does it require more aggressive treatment, such as a cast. Most teenagers with Osgood-Schlatter disease find that the knee pain disappears on its own as they progress through puberty.

CHONDROMALACIA

Chondromalacia is an instability or shifting of the kneecap (patella). It occurs most commonly in physically active teenage girls during early puberty. One or both knees may be involved, and the pain is worse after running, bicycling, jumping, climbing, or prolonged sitting. Less common symptoms include clicking of the knee, a sense that the knee "gives way" on exercise, and knee swelling.

Treatment begins with restricting activities that cause the pain. Specific exercises should be done to strengthen the thigh muscles that support the knee. For example, sit straight in a chair with your leg extended and hang a pocketbook over your foot. Raising your leg against the resistance of the weight will strengthen the quadriceps and help to keep the patella in place.

In some cases of chondromalacia, a cast or splint may become necessary to correct the misalignment. In the most serious cases, surgery may be required.

DISLOCATION OF THE KNEE

Like chondromalacia, dislocation of the knee is more common in girls than boys and peaks in mid-adolescence. The patella actually slips, or dislocates, to the side, causing pain and weakness. It usually responds well to the same types of stretching and strengthening exercises recommended for chondromalacia. Surgery is rarely necessary.

TEARS OF THE LIGAMENTS AND MENISCUS OF THE KNEE

These are common occurrences during adolescence, particularly from athletic injuries. The "meniscus" is a crescent-shaped piece of cartilage that surrounds the knee. A tear through a ligament or the meniscus causes pain, swelling, locking, clicking, and weakness of the knee. When cartilage is damaged, a small piece may detach and float freely within the knee joint. These "loose bodies" and significant tears often require surgical repair. Much of this surgery can be done through an "arthroscope," a scope with a magnifying lens that can be inserted into the joint. The procedure is done under general anesthesia.

FRACTURE OF THE KNEE

Knee fracture may be either a single, severe injury or repeated minor injuries to the partly bent knee (as in football). When there are no loose bodies in the knee joint and the bones are aligned, treatment may involve only limitation of activities. In many cases, though, surgery and immobilization in a cast are necessary.

The Leg

Leg problems during adolescence can originate from hip or knee disorders, injuries, bone infections, or bone tumors. When those possibilities are excluded, the diagnosis is often "growing pains."

Growing pains defy easy description. Their cause is unknown, though they may be associated with pubertal changes, rapid growth, weather, or psychological factors. Some doctors question their existence, but teenagers find the pain very real. It typically begins late in the day or evening and sometimes is bad enough to interfere with sleep.

Growing pains appear in late childhood or early adolescence, with a peak age of eleven for girls and thirteen for boys. The pains come and go in both legs, usually in the front of the thighs, the calves, and the backs of the knees. The back, shoulders, and arms also may ache. Physical examination, X-rays, and laboratory tests are normal. There is no loss or restriction of movement, no fever, no swelling, and no localized tender spot.

Growing pains are not a sign of any serious illness. They require no treatment, and will go away on their own within a year. The discomfort can be controlled with a heating pad and acetaminophen (Tylenol).

The Ankle

Sprains, strains, Achilles tendonitis, and fractures are common causes of ankle pain among adolescents. A sprain is an injury to a ligament. A strain is an injury to the muscle–tendon unit. Whether they occur on or off the athletic field, the treatment goal is the same: a return to full strength and range of motion of the ankle. The first step is to limit swelling and stabilize the joint. During the first thirty-six hours after an injury, the RICE plan (Rest, Ice, Compression, Elevation) should be followed (Chapter 4).

The Achilles tendon, which attaches the calf muscle to the heel, should be stretched as soon as possible after the swelling recedes and the ankle is able to move without pain. Swelling generally stabilizes within forty-eight hours of the sprain. Stretching exercises should begin with three or four twenty-second stretches at a time. The ankle's range of motion can be improved by placing the toes in warm water and tracing letters of the alphabet for several minutes; repeat the same in ice water for one minute; alternate the warm–cold pattern four times, but always stop if the swelling becomes worse.

As soon as the ankle can bear weight without pain, an exercise of heel and toe walking should be started. Walk on the heels for five minutes, then on the toes for five minutes, once or twice a day. Also, when free of pain, balance on the injured foot or stand on tiptoe while holding on to a table or chair. To prevent reinjury, wear high-top athletic shoes and tape the ankle during sports activities.

Teenagers with chronic ankle instability should see a doctor for evaluation. A physical therapist can be very helpful in designing an appropriate rehabilitation plan.

Achilles tendonitis results from repeated stress on the ankle, usually from athletics. Tendonitis of any joint refers to inflammation of the tendon. Small tears in the Achilles tendon cause pain and limping. The remedy is to avoid activities that require the tendon to be stretched. Aspirin or anti-inflammatory drugs can be used to decrease pain. In severe cases, a cast may be necessary.

The Foot

A protrusion or bump where a toe joins the sole of the foot can cause chronic pressure and pain. A pad inserted across the sole of the shoe by a podiatrist or physical therapist can help redistribute the body's weight on the foot and relieve the pain. In some cases, surgery is necessary.

Running and high-impact aerobic exercises can cause a small fracture of the foot that may be difficult to see on standard X-rays (occult fracture). The fracture usually heals on its own when activities are limited, but in some cases a cast may be necessary.

Hallux valgus is an abnormality in the shape of the foot. Instead of pointing straight forward, the big toe turns toward the second toe and a bunion, or bump, appears on the side of the foot. Pointed-toe shoes do not cause hallux valgus but do cause pain because of pressure on the bunion. In severe cases, surgery is required to straighten the toe and remove the bunion.

Benign Bone Tumors

Nonmalignant, or benign, bone tumors are not uncommon in older children and adolescents. (Malignant tumors are discussed in Chapter 36.) Benign tumors usually appear alone rather than in clusters. The most common site is the lower leg. A benign bone tumor often causes pain that becomes worse when the teenager is inactive—at night or while sitting still. Other signs may include swelling of the area or weakness of the surrounding muscles. A benign tumor in the spine can cause scoliosis and spasm of the muscles of the back.

Most benign tumors are visible on standard X-rays, but sometimes special scans are done to confirm the exact location and size. A benign tumor that causes no or mild symptoms requires no treatment in most cases. If symptoms are bothersome, the tumor is removed surgically.

Infection of the Bone (Osteomyelitis)

This very serious bacterial infection requires immediate medical care. In some cases, the only symptom is persistent fever, though usually there also is pain and swelling over the infected bone. Osteomyelitis can involve any bone, but the most common site is the upper arm or the lower leg.

Most cases of osteomyelitis in children and adolescents are caused by bacteria that have spread through the bloodstream to the bone. Less commonly, bacteria can spread directly from an infected skin wound into the bone. The diagnosis of osteomyelitis is made by history, physical examination, blood tests, X-rays, and bone scans. Blood cultures that grow bacteria are found in over half of patients with osteomyelitis. Correct identification of the bacteria causing the infection helps the physician decide which antibiotic to use. In many cases, it is necessary to obtain a sample of the infected bone through a special needle. This sample is cultured to determine the type of bacteria that is involved.

Osteomyelitis requires hospitalization for intravenous antibiotics, followed by oral antibiotics for four to six weeks. In chronic or prolonged cases, surgical drainage or removal of the infected bone may be required for a complete cure.

Arthritis

Arthritis is an inflammation of the tissues lining the joint and the "synovial fluid," which bathes and lubricates the joint. Normally, there is a very small amount of synovial fluid in the joint. As the inflammation progresses, the fluid increases and changes. The signs and symptoms of arthritis include pain, swelling, stiffness, warmth, and redness of one or more joints.

Arthritis during adolescence has a host of possible causes, including injury, infection, and autoimmune diseases. "Autoimmune" means that antibodies are produced against the body's own proteins. These antibodies may lodge anywhere in the body—joints, kidneys, heart, lungs, brain, or skin. Autoimmune diseases often are called rheumatologic or collagen vascular diseases. During adolescence, the most common autoimmune diseases involving the joints are juvenile rheumatoid arthritis (p. 417–18), systemic lupus erythematosus (p. 418–20), Reiter syndrome (Chapter 18), and inflammatory bowel disease (Chapter 29). The correct diagnosis and treatment of autoimmune diseases can be difficult. A physician should always be consulted for persistent arthritis, especially if there are other symptoms, such as fever, rash, or weight loss.

This section discusses the most common causes of arthritis in adolescents.

BACTERIAL (SEPTIC) ARTHRITIS

Bacterial, or septic, arthritis is a bacterial infection of the joint space and synovial fluid. The symptoms are fever, sudden joint pain without injury, stiffness, and swelling. It usually affects only one joint, such as the knee, hip, elbow, or wrist. Early treatment is important to prevent permanent damage to the joint.

In young children, septic arthritis usually is caused by either *Haemophilus influenza* or *Staphylococcus aureus*. In sexually active adolescents, gonorrhea is the most common cause of septic arthritis. The gonorrhea spreads through the bloodstream and causes arthritis of several joints, along with painful red skin bumps on the arms, legs, hands, and feet. Males may have some discharge from the penis. Most females have no genital symptoms.

Cultures of the blood and joint fluid should always be done when septic arthritis is suspected. When the cause is gonorrhea, these cultures are often negative. It is essential, therefore, to do urethral and cervical cultures in all sexually active teenagers with septic arthritis. When the cause is another bacteria, the joint fluid culture is nearly always positive. The treatment of septic arthritis involves intravenous antibiotics for several weeks.

VIRAL ARTHRITIS

Many types of viruses can cause this problem. Rubella (German measles) and hepatitis B are the most common. Less common causes are infectious mononucleosis, mumps, and chicken pox.

Viral arthritis typically affects only one or two joints and disappears without treatment within two to five days. In unusual cases, viral arthritis can be prolonged. Aspirin or anti-inflammatory drugs help to control the pain and swelling.

JUVENILE RHEUMATOID ARTHRITIS (JRA)

This noninfectious arthritis affects children and adolescents. JRA is divided into three major types, depending on the number of joints involved and the associated symptoms. "Pauciarticular JRA" is the mildest and most common form. "Polyarticular JRA" involves more joints, but usually does not cause problems elsewhere in the body. "Systemic JRA" is the most severe form, involving many systems throughout the body.

Pauciarticular JRA typically begins in early adolescence with painful swelling of the knee, ankle, or hip. Over the next few months, up to five other joints become inflamed. Most teenagers with pauciarticular JRA are otherwise well. For half of them, the disease ends by young adulthood. About 10 percent of boys with pauciarticular JRA develop a severe arthritis involving the low back. The tendency for this "ankylosing spondylitis" is inherited and can be detected by measuring an antibody in the blood called "HLA-B27." Girls who develop pauciarticular JRA in early childhood are at risk for an inflammation of the eye called "uveitis" (Chapter 25) during adolescence. Many of these girls have an antibody called antinuclear antibody, or ANA.

Polyarticular arthritis causes painful swelling of five or more joints and effects small joints, such as the hands and feet, more than large joints. As in pauciarticular JRA, there are usually no other symptoms and the flareups decrease in severity and frequency as the teenager approaches adulthood. About 10 percent of girls with polyarticular JRA have a more severe form of the disease that can cause progressive destruction of the involved joints. Many of these teenagers have an antibody called rheumatoid factor.

Systemic JRA, or "Still disease," is more common in younger children than in adolescents. It begins abruptly with afternoon or evening fevers, in the 102°–105°F range. A pink, raised rash, usually on the torso, may come and go with the fever. The arthritis begins days to months after the daily fever spikes and involves large joints, such as the knees or hips. Other complications may include enlarged lymph glands, liver, or spleen; anemia; and inflammation of the heart or lungs. Over time, these other systemic effects decrease and the arthritis waxes and wanes.

JRA is treated with medications, physical therapy, and psychological support. Anti-inflammatory drugs decrease the arthritis and the fever. In more severe cases, an oral medication containing gold or intramuscular injections of gold may be very helpful in controlling the joint pain and swelling. When gold therapy is inadequate, medications that suppress the immune system (such as methotrexate, cyclophosphamide, and azathioprine) may be added. Oral corticosteroids like prednisone are very effective but should be used only for short periods of time because of their many side effects.

The chronic nature of JRA makes it a trying disease for the maturing teenager. In addition to the pain and limitation of movement, adolescents are distressed by the changes in their appearance that accompany the joint swelling or result from taking certain medications. Physical therapy helps protect joint mobility and teaches teenagers how to adjust daily activities to their level of function. Psychological counseling, as with any chronic condition, helps the adolescent and family to deal with the emotions that accompany the illness.

SYSTEMIC LUPUS ERYTHEMATOSUS (SLE)

This disease can affect virtually any organ system of the body. The most common symptoms are arthritis and rash. SLE most often begins during the teens and twenties and is five times more common in females than in males. Its cause remains unknown, though genetic factors probably play a role. The underlying problem is the production of "autoantibodies," or antibodies that the body makes against its own tissues. These antibodies become entrapped and inflame small blood vessels throughout the body, causing organ damage.

SLE usually begins insidiously with fatigue and aching of the muscles or joints. The arthritis most commonly involves the hands and knees, comes and goes, and travels from one joint to another.

Unlike some forms of JRA, the arthritis of SLE does not permanently damage or deform the joints.

Hair thinning and skin rash often appear early in the course of SLE. The classic "butterfly" rash of SLE is a red rash over the cheeks and bridge of the nose that becomes worse with sun exposure and may last for several weeks.

The most serious complications of SLE are its potential effects on the kidneys and brain. Inflammation of the kidney, called glomerulonephritis (Chapter 30), occurs in half of teenagers with SLE. This may range from very mild abnormalities, such as small amounts of blood or protein in the urine, to kidney failure. The diagnosis of lupus glomerulonephritis is made on the basis of a kidney biopsy.

"Lupus cerebritis," or inflammation of the brain, also varies widely in severity. The manifestations include headache, mood or personality change, intellectual decline, visual problems, seizures, and stroke. Other complications of SLE include inflammation of the heart or lungs, abnormal liver function, abdominal pain, anemia, susceptibility to infection, and abnormal blood clotting.

When the history and physical examination suggest SLE, blood studies to measure autoantibodies can help confirm the diagnosis. Nearly all patients with SLE have high levels of antinuclear antibody, or ANA, and half have high levels of a specific component of ANA called the anti-DNA antibody.

Treatment of SLE depends on the severity of the disease. Mild skin and joint symptoms can be managed with anti-inflammatory drugs, sun avoidance, and topical steroid creams. More severe SLE usually requires oral corticosteroids. For lupus glomerulonephritis, drugs that suppress the immune system, such as cyclophosphamide, are added to the corticosteroids. Repeated kidney biopsies may be necessary to determine the response of the disease to treatment.

The course of SLE depends on the organs involved. The ten-year survival rate for all patients with SLE is over 90 percent, thanks to aggressive treatment with steroids and immunosuppressants, dialysis, and a kidney transplant for patients with kidney failure.

Teenagers with SLE need a great deal of psychological and social support. Despite the severity of the disease, it often is misunderstood by family and friends. SLE does not fit into the more clear-cut categories of heart disease or lung disease or cancer. At the very time when the teenager and family are trying to deal with the illness, they must explain its complicated course to friends and relatives. Local support groups for individuals with SLE can be very helpful both in dealing with the anxiety accompanying a chronic illness and in better understanding the illness and its ramifications.

In addition to JRA and SLE, other autoimmune diseases cause arthritis. Most, however, begin with problems outside the joints. Reiter syndrome, for example, causes inflammation of the urethra (Chapter 18), eyes, and joints. Psoriatic arthritis affects the skin (Chapter 24) and joints. Some diseases, such as Lyme arthritis and rheumatic fever, may have an autoimmune component that is triggered by an infection (Chapter 34).

The diagnosis and treatment of arthritis in adolescents are often difficult and complex. Always consult a physician when a joint becomes swollen and painful. Early treatment not only alleviates pain, it also may prevent permanent damage to the joint.

32

The Brain and Nervous System

The human nervous system is a highly complex communications network serving two vital purposes. It controls internal functions, such as breathing and heartbeat, and it reacts to external stimuli, such as a gust of cold wind.

The *central nervous system* (CNS) consists of the brain and the spinal cord. The *brain,* the body's most sophisticated organ, processes incoming information and sends out messages in the form of electrical–chemical impulses.

The brain has three distinct parts: the cerebrum, the cerebellum, and the brain stem (Figure 32.1). The *cerebrum* is the largest portion, accounting for 85 percent of the brain's weight. It is the upper part of the brain, extending from the forehead to the back of the skull. The cerebrum controls "higher" mental functions, such as thought and speech. It is divided into four lobes: frontal, temporal, parietal, and occipital. The frontal lobe controls thinking, behavior, speech, smell, and movement. The parietal lobe interprets touch and helps regulate body position. The temporal lobe coordinates hearing, the interpretation of sound, and speech. The occipital lobe interprets visual stimuli.

The *cerebellum,* at the lower back of the head, coordinates the body's reflexes, movement, and balance. The *brain stem* is the part of the brain that controls involuntary vital functions such as heart rate and breathing. It also coordinates the *cranial nerves,* which are critical for vision, eye movement, hearing, balance, taste, smell, facial movement, and swallowing. The brain stem connects the brain to the *spinal cord,* the main highway of the central nervous system. The spinal cord carries sensory information to the brain and transmits instructions from the brain to nerves throughout the body. The spinal cord is a cable of nerves from the neck to below the waist. It is protected by a bony cage called the *vertebral column,* or backbone.

The brain and spinal cord are covered by three thin, protective membranes, called the *meninges.* Between the layers of the meninges is a clear, shock-absorbing fluid called the *cerebrospinal fluid (CSF).*

The *peripheral nervous system* includes all of the nerves that transmit information between the CNS and the rest of the body. The peripheral nerves supply the internal organs, muscles, membranes, and skin. They are the messengers of sensations and the stimuli for muscle movement. The powerful coordinating capabilities of the brain and spinal cord work through the complex network of the peripheral nervous system.

Evaluating the Nervous System

The *neurologic examination,* which is part of the physical examination, is used to evaluate the function of the brain, CNS, and peripheral nerves. The neurologic examination is divided into seven main parts:

1. Mental status or thinking is tested by asking the adolescent a series of questions that involve some simple calculations, memory, judgment, and concentration.
2. The twelve cranial nerves are examined by testing vision, eye movement, sense of smell, facial sensation and movement, hearing, taste, tongue movement, and swallowing function.
3. Body sensation is checked by asking when the adolescent feels light touch or a gentle pinprick on different parts of the body.
4. Motor strength of the arms or legs is tested by having the teenager press hard against resistance.
5. Reflexes are checked by gently tapping the arms, knees, and ankles with a rubber hammer and watching for the normal, involuntary "jump."
6. Gait and stability are tested by asking the adolescent to walk normally, like a tightrope walker, on heels, and on toes.

THE BRAIN

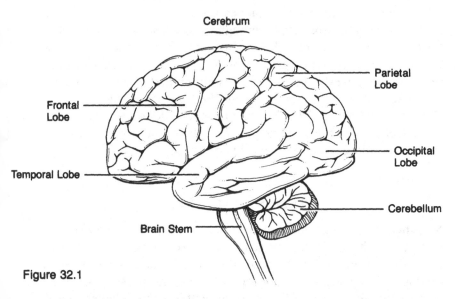

Figure 32.1

7. Coordination is tested by asking the teenager to do rapid hand movements, touch finger to nose, or run the heel down the opposite shin.

Sometimes the cause of a neurologic problem can be identified on the basis of the history and neurologic examination. Several neurologic tests, though, may be done to clarify or confirm the diagnosis. A *lumbar puncture* (or "spinal tap") is always done when an infection of the CSF is suspected. It is a simple, safe procedure that can be done in a doctor's office or emergency room. A needle is inserted through the skin of the low back, between the bones of the vertebral column, and through the meninges that surround the spinal cord. A small amount of CSF is pulled out through the needle and sent to the laboratory for testing. *Computed tomography (CT, or CAT scan)* is a diagnostic technique in which X-ray pictures of the brain and spinal cord are taken from many angles. *Magnetic resonance imaging (MRI)* also provides detailed pictures of the brain and spinal column, similar to CT, but does not use X-rays. An *electroencephalogram (EEG)* is a recording of the brain waves taken through electrodes that are pasted to the scalp. An EEG is done when a seizure or epilepsy is suspected.

Headache

Most adults and about half of all teenagers experience some headaches. For many people, headaches are infrequent and brief. For others, headaches are severe enough to interfere with daily functioning. Common causes of headaches range from the nasal congestion of a head cold to allergies, smoking, alcohol, physical exertion, jaw clenching, eyestrain, hunger, tension, premenstrual symptoms, and head injury. In rare cases, headaches are caused by tumors or bleeding in the brain. The pain of a headache does not begin in the brain itself, where there are no pain receptors, but from the sensory impulses coming from the meninges or scalp.

TENSION HEADACHES

Most headaches are related to stress or anxiety. Tension makes the muscles in the head and neck contract, resulting in a constant, dull pain that encircles the head like a tight elastic band. Tension headaches typically come on gradually and can persist for weeks without disrupting daily life. The treatment is a pain reliever (acetaminophen, ibuprofen, aspirin), rest, and relaxation techniques to alleviate the tension.

Tension headaches do *not* signal major illness. They do not endanger health. If tension headaches recur frequently, counseling can help identify the cause of the tension and biofeedback can help control the discomfort.

MIGRAINE

Migraine headaches are characterized by severe throbbing or pounding pain, often accompanied by nausea, vomiting, abdominal pain, light-headedness, and sensitivity to light or sound. An "aura," or warning sign, may precede the headache. The most common aura is a visual symptom, such as a sensation of flickering lights, spots, or lines before the eyes. Auras may also consist of unusual smells, ringing in the ears, numbness in an arm or leg, or mood changes. The aura typically starts ten to thirty minutes before the headache and stops when the pain begins. Most migraine headaches last four to six hours, but some can continue for days.

Migraine headaches tend to run in families. They are more common in females than males and often are associated with menstruation. One third of migraines begin in childhood, with the incidence increasing at puberty and peaking in late adolescence. Migraines that begin in childhood often decline with puberty, while those that begin in adolescence tend to continue into adulthood.

Migraines are sometimes called vascular headaches because they are caused by constriction and dilation of the blood vessels within the head. Certain factors may trigger migraines. For example, some people find that caffeine, alcohol, foods containing nitrites (such as hot dogs), or aged cheeses may precipitate their migraines. Others find that fatigue, stress, strenuous exercise, or changes in eating and sleeping patterns may contribute to their headaches.

Migraine headaches are diagnosed on the basis of these symptoms and a normal neurologic examination. Laboratory tests are all normal and, in most adolescents, need not be done. It is important to see a doctor when migraine headaches are suspected. Once a correct diagnosis is made, treatment can help prevent the headaches entirely or decrease their frequency and severity.

The first step in treatment is identification of the triggers. Adolescents may find it is useful to keep a diary of the headaches, noting when they occur in relation to eating and activities. When the triggers can be avoided, the headaches may improve dramatically. There are times, though, when the trigger—such as menstruation—cannot be avoided. In these situations, the physician may suggest a trial of medication.

The types of medication used to treat migraines fall into three groups: analgesics, or pain relievers; medications that block the crescendo pattern of the migraine; and medications that decrease the frequency of migraines.

Adolescents with mild migraines often find that acetaminophen, aspirin, ibuprofen, or naproxen are effective. Sometimes a physician may prescribe a mild sedative because sleep usually ends the migraine. Many teenagers find that resting in a quiet, dark room helps relieve migraines.

If the headaches are more severe but not too frequent, the physician may suggest a prescription medication that blocks the progression of the pain. The most commonly used are ergotamine (Cafergot, Ergostat), Midrin, and sumatriptan. All work best when taken with the aura or soon after the pain begins. These medications can cause significant side effects, such as nausea, vomiting, jitteriness, and anxiety. They must not be used during pregnancy or by adolescents with high blood pressure or heart disease.

When migraines occur several times a week, the doctor may suggest "prophylactic medication," which is taken on a daily basis to decrease the frequency of migraines. The most commonly prescribed medication for migraine prophylaxis is a "beta-blocker" such as propranolol (Inderal) or atenolol (Tenormin). Other types include "calcium channel blockers" such as verapamil (Calan), diltiazem (Cardizem), and nifedipine (Procardia); and tricyclic antidepressants (Chapter 13). All of these medications have side effects that teenagers and parents should discuss with the physician when deciding whether and which to use.

HEAD INJURY

Trauma to the head can cause headache because of bleeding within the skull, a bruise to the brain (concussion), or injury to the muscles of the neck (whiplash) or skull.

The most serious cause of post-traumatic headache is bleeding or hemorrhage. The bleeding can occur between the meninges or within the brain itself. If the bleeding stops quickly and the amount of blood is small, no treatment is necessary other than close observation by parents and physician. If the bleeding is severe, emergency surgery may be lifesaving.

Head trauma always should be taken seriously. If the adolescent loses consciousness—even momentarily—emergency care should be sought. Even if there is no loss of consciousness and the adolescent seems fine immediately after the injury, close observation over the next twelve to twenty-four hours is important. Call your doctor or go to an emergency room if the teenager develops excessive sleepiness, confusion, severe headache, change in vision, or vomiting.

BRAIN TUMORS AND ANEURYSMS

Although many people worry that a headache signals one of these major problems, they are rarely the cause of a headache during adolescence. A tumor can produce a dull headache that comes and goes, but there usually are other symptoms such as change in vision, vomiting, muscle weakness on one side of the body, poor coordination, or changes in personality. Unlike tension headaches or migraines, tumors usually cause pain that is worse on lying down or first awakening in the morning. Malignant brain tumors are discussed in detail in Chapter 36.

An aneurysm is a weakness in the wall of an artery that can expand and cause pressure in the brain, leak blood slowly, or rupture suddenly. If there is an expanding mass or a small, slow leak, the headache increases over a few days. If there is a sudden rupture, the headache peaks within minutes. The pain may then decrease, but other serious signs will appear, such as stiff neck, drowsiness, confusion, seizures, trouble speaking, visual changes, partial paralysis, or coma. *Always* call a physician or go to an emergency room immediately if an adolescent develops a sudden, severe headache with any of these signs. The diagnosis of bleeding within the head is usually made by CT or lumbar puncture.

PSEUDOTUMOR

Another cause of increased pressure within the skull that causes headache is "pseudotumor cerebri." This condition is most common in adolescent and young adult females who are obese. It is *not* a brain tumor but is called a pseudotumor because the symptoms may mimic a tumor. The teenager typically complains of a constant, dull headache, worse on lying down, and visual problems, such as blind spots, blurring, or dimming of vision. These symptoms result from an increase in the cerebrospinal fluid that bathes the brain. The diagnosis is made by neurologic examination, CT or MRI, and lumbar puncture. The pain usually improves after the lumbar puncture because withdrawal of the cerebrospinal fluid reduces the pressure. Oral medications are used to control the pressure and the symptoms.

Infections of the Brain

MENINGITIS

The meninges and spinal fluid can become infected by bacteria, viruses, or fungi. The symptoms of meningitis include headache, fever, stiff neck, sensitivity to light, confusion, mood changes, and lethargy.

Viral meningitis clears on its own and does not require antibiotics. Bacterial meningitis is a medical emergency and requires hospitalization and intravenous antibiotics. The diagnosis is made by lumbar puncture. The spinal fluid withdrawn is tested for white blood cells, protein, and glucose (sugar), and is cultured to identify the type of bacteria. If there are seizures, vomiting, or a change in the level of consciousness, a CT or MRI may be done before the lumbar puncture to look for a mass within the brain.

When bacterial meningitis is suspected, intravenous antibiotics will be started in the emergency room or doctor's office, even before the results of the laboratory tests are known. Without prompt treatment, bacterial meningitis can lead to lifelong neurologic problems and even death. Antibiotics are continued in the hospital for at least ten days.

When meningitis is caused by bacteria called meningococci, oral antibiotics are recommended for household members and classmates. This is because meningococcal infection is highly contagious and the resulting meningitis is very severe. Prompt antibiotic treatment will prevent the development of illness in others.

ENCEPHALITIS

Encephalitis is an inflammation or infection of the brain itself. It typically is preceded by fever and symptoms of an upper respiratory infection (cough, runny nose, sore throat). Like meningitis, encephalitis usually is caused by a virus. However, encephalitis causes less stiff neck and sensitivity to light and more changes in mental status than meningitis. The diagnosis is made on neurologic examination and lumbar puncture. A CT or MRI often is done to confirm the diagnosis. Most types of viral encephalitis clear on their own without treatment. Bacterial encephalitis is treated with intravenous antibiotics.

BRAIN ABSCESS

An abscess (a small collection of pus) in the brain can cause headaches, fever, vomiting, and seizures. It is more likely than either meningitis or encephalitis to cause specific abnormalities on the neurologic examination, such as weakness in an arm or leg. A brain abscess is nearly always caused by bacteria, usually spreading from a sinus, ear, or lung infection. The diagnosis is confirmed by CT or MRI. A brain abscess usually is cured with several weeks of treatment with intravenous antibiotics. If it is very large, surgical drainage may be necessary.

Light-headedness, Dizziness, and Fainting

Light-headedness is a feeling of being off balance without a sense of motion. It is a common complaint of teenagers, usually caused by a rapid change in position (such as jumping out of bed), rapid breathing, anxiety, hunger, or dehydration. A single episode of light-headedness that lasts seconds and does not cause fainting does not require medical evaluation. Repeated episodes, even if brief, should be discussed with a physician. More serious causes of recurrent light-headedness include irregular heart rhythms and neurologic problems.

An unusual symptom during adolescence is *vertigo,* a sensation of spinning motion. There may be a feeling of twirling round and round in circles or a feeling that the room is spinning rapidly around. Vertigo should always be discussed with a physician, even if it occurs only once, because its causes generally are more serious than those of light-headedness. The doctor will pay particular attention to examination of the ear, nervous system, and heart.

The most common cause of vertigo in a teenager is a problem in the ear. The "labyrinthine" system in the inner ear is responsible for maintaining the body's sense of balance. Infection of this system, or "labyrinthitis," causes the sudden onset of vertigo that peaks over the next day. The infection usually is caused by a virus and clears on its own without treatment over several days to weeks. Another cause of vertigo is a tear in the labyrinthine system following head trauma. The tear usually heals on its own within several days but may require surgery if the vertigo persists. Ménière disease is a common cause of chronic vertigo in the elderly but is quite rare in teenagers. It involves both the balance and hearing functions of the inner ear, resulting in hearing loss and tinnitus (ringing in the ears) as well as vertigo. "Benign positional vertigo" also is uncommon in teenagers. This type typically occurs with rapid changes in head position. Its cause is unknown, and it may begin and end suddenly. It is not a serious condition but is very bothersome because the vertigo recurs every few weeks. It usually clears on its own within six to twelve months.

Other causes of vertigo outside the ear are rare. They include seizures, migraines, brain tumors or bleeding, certain medications, illegal drugs, and meningitis or encephalitis. The evaluation and treatment of vertigo are complex and depend on the adolescent's history and physical examination. In some cases, the diagnosis requires no additional tests. In other cases, MRI or CT scan, hearing tests, or evaluation of inner ear function may be recommended.

The symptoms of vertigo can be controlled with Antivert, Bonine, or Dramamine. All cause drowsiness and should not be used without a doctor's knowledge.

Fainting, or *syncope,* occurs when blood flow to the brain is insufficient. Light-headedness usually precedes syncope. People who faint should immediately be placed on their backs with their legs slightly elevated to help the blood flow to the brain. Breathing and heartbeat continue during syncope. If the breathing has stopped or a pulse cannot be felt in the neck, CPR (cardiopulmonary resuscitation) should be started immediately and a rescue squad should be called. The vast majority of teenagers with fainting have normal heart and lung function and will wake up within a few seconds or minutes.

Syncope has many possible causes: intense emotion, stress, or pain; rapid breathing (hyperventilation) from exercise or anxiety; drugs and alcohol; long periods of standing that cause blood to pool in the legs; dehydration; heat stroke; low blood sugar; migraines; a seizure disorder; and heart problems (such as an irregular heartbeat or narrowing of a heart valve). Among these many causes, four are typically seen in teenagers:

• "Vasovagal syncope" is a simple faint that may follow excitement, stress, injury, pain or fear of pain, the sight of blood, or fasting. Just before a simple faint, the teenager develops light-headedness, nausea, blurred vision, rapid heartbeat, and weakness.

During the faint, the adolescent is unresponsive and limp. After regaining consciousness, the teenager is fully alert but may continue to feel weak, dizzy, or nauseated for ten or twenty minutes. If the feeling of faintness recurs, the teenager should lie down or sit bent forward with the head between the knees.

• "Orthostatic hypotension" is an episode of light-headedness or syncope that occurs when the teenager sits up or stands quickly. It is caused by a sudden drop in blood pressure. Orthostatic hypotension in adolescents usually is associated with dehydration from inadequate fluid intake during exercise, hot weather, or illness. A doctor should always be seen if it persists.

• Hyperventilation, or rapid breathing, can be caused by stress, anxiety, panic attacks (Chapter 13), pain, or strenuous exercise. Breathing in and out of a paper (*never* plastic) bag held tightly around the nose or mouth will help restore a normal breathing pattern and prevent a faint. If the adolescent does faint, it will resemble a vasovagal (simple) fainting episode.

• Heat stroke occurs when someone exercises in hot weather without drinking enough water to replace the body's losses through perspiration. Fainting is just one sign of heat stroke; it can also involve neurological disorders (such as twitching, seizures, and coma) and heart problems. *Heat stroke is a medical emergency.* The adolescent should be taken immediately to an emergency facility.

Seizures

Seizures are convulsions, or sudden episodes of involuntary movement, with or without a loss of consciousness. *Epilepsy* is a recurrent pattern of seizures caused by an abnormality in the brain. Epilepsy affects less than 1 percent of the entire population but has its highest prevalence in children and teenagers. The peak years for the appearance of epilepsy are the first year or two of life and adolescence.

Epilepsy is particularly troubling to teenagers because it represents a loss of control at a time when increasing autonomy is the developmental norm. The unpredictable nature of the seizures and dependence on others for help when they do occur can produce feelings of helplessness, frustration, anger, and embarrassment. Seizures can necessitate constraints—on driving or certain sports, for example—that may add to the adolescent's frustration and translate into rebellious behavior or noncompliance with medical therapy. Families and health professionals can work together to develop a regimen that controls the seizures and maximizes the teenager's independence and coping.

Seizures are a sign of an underlying problem. In most cases, especially in youth under sixteen, the cause is idiopathic, or unknown. Possible causes include infection, such as meningitis, encephalitis, or brain abscess; malformed or inflamed blood vessels in the brain; an aneurysm or tumor in the brain; injury to the head; low blood sugar; alcohol or drug overdose; liver disease; and kidney failure. The probability that a seizure is caused by a tumor, abscess, or hemorrhage is rare during adolescence, but the physician will always do a thorough evaluation before making a diagnosis of idiopathic seizure disorder.

Even when an exact cause is not apparent, certain factors may be associated with seizures. For example, puberty, menstruation, fever, particular foods or medications, stress, sleep deprivation, and flashing lights may increase the likelihood that a seizure will occur in someone with epilepsy. These factors are *not* the cause of epilepsy; there is an underlying disorder within the brain that predisposes the individual to seizures. This lowered threshold for seizures makes the individual especially susceptible to outside stimuli that have no effect on individuals without epilepsy.

TYPES OF SEIZURES

The basic categories of seizures are simple partial, complex partial, and generalized. "Partial" means that the seizure begins in a particular part of the brain. "Generalized" means that the seizure involves the whole brain from the start. Partial seizures may progress to generalized seizures. "Simple" means that there is no loss of consciousness. "Complex" means there is a loss of consciousness.

Simple partial seizures begin locally, cause specific symptoms, and do not cause loss of consciousness. They often are heralded by an aura of sensory disturbances, such as blinking lights, buzzing sounds, tingling sensations, or changes in smell and taste. There may be a feeling of anger, fear, a dreamy state, hallucinations, or a sense of déjà vu (flashback). Motor symptoms include jerking movements of one part of the body (such as the arm), difficulty speaking, or abnormal posturing (positioning) of the body.

Complex partial seizures begin as simple partial seizures and progress to unconsciousness. Complex partial seizures may begin with unresponsiveness, an empty stare, or repetitive involuntary actions, such as lip smacking, picking at clothing, wandering, humming, etc. The seizure lasts up to several minutes. When it ends, the teenager has no memory of it and may appear confused, sleepy, or combative.

There are two major types of generalized seizures: "grand mal" and "petit mal." Grand mal seizures start with an aura of flashing lights, odd tastes, ringing or buzzing in the ears, or nervous anticipation. The aura is followed quickly by convulsions, rhythmic muscle jerking, irregular breathing, tongue-biting, incontinence, and partial or complete unconsciousness. It usually ends within five minutes, leaving the teenager feeling sleepy and with no memory of the event. Grand mal seizures can occur as often as several times a day or as infrequently as once every few years.

Petit mal, or "absence" seizures are recurrent, brief (less than a minute) lapses in consciousness without an aura or convulsions. They may be accompanied by repetitive movements, such as eye blinking, or the adolescent may remain still with a fixed, blank stare. Petit mal seizures typically begin between ages four and eight and disappear by the mid-teens.

EVALUATING SEIZURES

An observer's report of what happens during a seizure is very important information. Did the adolescent complain of strange sensations before the seizure? Were there jerking movements? Where did they begin? Was there loss of consciousness? How long did it last? Was there urinary or bowel incontinence during the seizure? Any injury during the seizure? How did the teenager seem on awakening? All of this information can help the physician determine if a seizure occurred and, if so, what type of seizure it was. The adolescent will not recall these details; only a witness can provide the information.

The physician will ask the teenager and parents for a thorough medical history. This will begin with any known injury during the teenager's birth, and include questions about childhood development, past seizures, head injury or CNS problems, alcohol and drug use, emotional and physical stress, sleeping patterns, and family members with seizures. Teenagers with epilepsy will be asked to keep a written diary of their seizures to help identify potential triggers.

A thorough physical examination, with particular attention to the neurologic examination, will be done whenever a seizure occurs. The doctor will look for possible causes outside the brain, such as decreased blood flow to the brain because of a heart or lung problem. Blood studies may be done looking for imbalances in glucose or electrolytes that could precipitate a seizure. A urine or blood drug screen will be done if there is any question of drug use—either legal or illegal.

An EEG can be a very helpful test when seizures are suspected or to determine if medication is effectively suppressing the abnormal brain waves that cause seizures. The patterns of the brain waves differ between the various types of seizures, and the location of the abnormal pattern within the brain helps identify the beginning site of the seizure. Triggers, such as light stimuli, may be used during the EEG to elicit the abnormal pattern. In some cases, the adolescent may be kept awake for a "sleep-deprived EEG" in an attempt to bring on the abnormal wave patterns. These triggers are used within the very controlled environment of the neurology office or clinic; should a seizure develop, a physician is always there to control it quickly.

The decision about whether to do a CT or MRI of the brain will depend on what has been found on the preceding evaluation. These studies are done to look for *structural* problems within the brain, such as tumors, abnormal blood vessels, or bleeding. Adolescents with idiopathic epilepsy have normal CT and MRI scans.

TREATMENT

The most successful treatment approach to seizures involves two key elements: education and prevention. First, families must know what to do when a seizure occurs. A petit mal seizure requires no first aid. For generalized convulsions, take the following steps:

Do not apply physical restraint. Help the teenager lie down. Turn the head to the side to permit saliva to drain from the mouth. Do not put anything in the mouth. Loosen any tight clothing. Remove glasses if worn. Move any sharp or dangerous objects from the immediate area. If the seizure lasts more than ten minutes, call an ambulance or take the adolescent immediately to an emergency room. Persistent seizure activity, called status epilepticus, is a medical emergency and requires intravenous medication.

Education begins with several basic facts. Seizures are not contagious. They do not cause tongue swallowing. They do not mean that someone is dangerous. They do not affect intelligence. They do not exclude participation in most sports. They can be prevented and controlled with medication.

Until seizures are under good control with medication, certain precautions are essential and should be discussed with the doctor. An adolescent at risk for seizures should not drive a car, ride a motorcycle, swim unattended, deep-sea dive, engage in activities at heights (such as rope climbing or gymnastics), or operate hazardous equipment.

One of the most important parts of education about seizures is understanding the importance of compliance with medication. The vast majority of seizures can be prevented by medication, but it must be taken regularly to be effective. If there are side effects that are bothersome or the dosing schedule is inconvenient, talk it over with your doctor.

Many types of medication are available to prevent seizures. The preferred approach is to use a single drug, but sometimes more than one is required. The treatment regimen is highly individualized. The choice of medication depends on the type of seizure and the drug's side effects. Some debate exists about when to begin anticonvulsant medication, with some doctors initiating it after the first seizure and others waiting until the second or third episode.

Commonly prescribed antiseizure medications (with their trade names) include: carbamazepine (Tegretol), phenobarbital, phenytoin (Dilantin), ethosuximide (Zarontin), primidone (Mysoline), and valproic acid (Depakene).

For an estimated 80 percent of children and teenagers with epilepsy, medications prevent seizures completely or control their frequency. For some adolescents whose seizures are not controlled by medication, surgery may be an option. It usually involves the removal of tissue from either the part of the brain that is the focus of the seizure activity or a part of the brain that is responsible for spread of the seizure. The success of the surgery depends on very careful screening to select individuals who are most likely to benefit from it. The evaluation and the surgery are done at specialized medical centers with extensive experience in seizure management.

Weakness, Paralysis, and Numbness

These symptoms may indicate a problem in the brain, spinal cord, nerves branching off from the spinal cord, or smaller nerves supplying a certain part of the body. Numbness or tingling that comes and goes often is caused by hyperventilation. Symptoms that localize in one extremity (arm or leg) or on one side of the body may be caused by a migraine, injury to a nerve, or a seizure. The list of all possible causes of weakness, paralysis, and numbness is extensive. Those that may appear during adolescence include the following:

GUILLAIN-BARRÉ SYNDROME

This syndrome involves inflammation of peripheral nerves, and usually appears one to three weeks after a respiratory or gastrointestinal infection. Its earliest symptoms are tenderness and weakness in the legs, which may then spread to the arms, torso, head, and face. It may progress to complete paralysis and, less commonly, to sensory loss. The most serious complications of Guillain-Barré syndrome are difficulty breathing because of paralysis of the respiratory muscles, blood pressure problems, and irregular heart rate.

The treatment of Guillain-Barré syndrome focuses mostly on close observation of the adolescent's respiratory function. Temporary use of a ventilator (breathing machine) in an intensive care unit may be necessary until the disease begins to improve. Use of medications, such as steroids or gamma globulin, remains controversial. Plasmapheresis, a process of filtering the blood, also is controversial.

The prognosis for Guillain-Barré syndrome is good. The symptoms begin to abate within several days or weeks in 90 percent of individuals. Over 75 percent of individuals have no long-term neurologic symptoms, but complete recovery may sometimes take over a year.

MULTIPLE SCLEROSIS (MS)

This disease is caused by the destruction of myelin, a protein that insulates nerve fibers in the CNS. Hard, or "sclerotic," plaques form where the myelin disintegrates. The resulting symptoms depend on the location of the affected myelin and can include vision problems, numbness, impaired sensation, muscle weakness or paralysis, changes in gait, and urinary problems. The symptoms typically appear in young adulthood, though it is not uncommon for MS to be diagnosed during adolescence. MS affects more females than males and more whites than other racial groups. The precise cause of MS is unknown, but it is a genetically based autoimmune disorder in which the body's immune cells attack the myelin.

A diagnosis of MS is made on the basis of the history of symptoms, neurologic examination, MRI, and laboratory tests of the spinal fluid. There is no cure for MS, but medications such as corticosteroids are used to manage the symptoms. The course of the disease and the prognosis are highly variable between individuals. In some people, symptoms come and go. In others, the symptoms may progress over months or years. Teenagers with MS tend to have milder disease than adults who are diagnosed later in life.

BELL PALSY

This condition is a weakness or paralysis of one side of the face. It develops quickly over a few hours and leaves the teenager unable to smile or close the eyes tightly. It also affects the sense of taste and may cause ear pain. Bell palsy involves inflammation of the nerve that controls the muscles of the face, but the cause of the inflammation usually is unclear. The most common cause in teenagers probably is Lyme disease (Chapter 34).

Most people with Bell palsy recover completely and spontaneously within a few weeks or months. Between 10 and 20 percent have permanent effects, such as weakness of one side of the face. Treatment involves protecting the eye by keeping it moist with eyedrops and using an eye patch to prevent injury. If Lyme disease is suspected, antibiotics will be prescribed.

MYASTHENIA GRAVIS

This autoimmune disorder affects the junction of nerve and muscle. The result is muscle weakness, particularly around the eyes, mouth, and throat. Early signs are subtle. The face becomes less expressive, the eyelids droop, the voice becomes weak, and chewing and swallowing become tiresome. The symptoms are worse late in the day and when the teenager is tired or stressed. The early signs of facial weakness may progress to generalized fatigue, muscle weakness, or difficulty breathing.

Treatment involves daily use of medication that enhances stimulation of muscles by the nerve endings. If the disease flares up while the adolescent is on the medication, a brief course of corticosteroids (prednisone) may be recommended. Some adolescents with myasthenia gravis improve after surgical removal of the thymus gland, located beneath the breastbone.

MUSCULAR DYSTROPHY

Muscular dystrophy refers to a variety of disorders in which muscles weaken and degenerate. These conditions are genetically inherited. Most cases are identified in childhood, but one type, Becker muscular dystrophy, begins in adolescence. It is characterized by muscle weakness, heart disorders, and impaired mental functioning. There is no cure for muscular dystrophy. Treatment focuses on helping the teenager maintain muscle function through physical rehabilitation. The prognosis is variable, depending on the specific disorder.

CEREBRAL PALSY

This condition results from brain injury before birth and is usually diagnosed in early childhood. The signs and symptoms include abnormal movements of the face, arms, or legs; poor muscle development; muscle spasms; and impaired speech. Cerebral palsy does *not* mean mental retardation. Intelligence often is completely normal.

NEUROFIBROMATOSIS

This genetic disorder, also called von Recklinghausen disease, may produce benign tumors of the skin, nerves, and other organs. The disorder may first be recognized because of flat, light brown spots on the skin. Neurofibromatosis is a very unpredictable disease. Some people experience no symptoms, while others develop severe complications, including vision and hearing problems, seizures, and malignancies.

Chronic neurologic and muscular diseases are difficult during the adolescent years when peer interaction is increasing and individual self-image is developing. Families and health professionals can work together to support the adolescent and ease the transition to adulthood (Chapter 9).

33 | The Hormonal System

Hormones are chemical messengers that control virtually all body functions. Some hormones affect sexual maturation. Some regulate physical growth. Others govern metabolism, the process of transforming nutrients and fluids into energy. Hormones are manufactured by the glands of the endocrine system. They are released into the bloodstream and travel to individual cells throughout the body.

The endocrine system includes the following major glands: The *thyroid* gland, located in the neck, produces thyroid hormone, which controls the body's rate of metabolism. The *parathyroid* glands are behind the thyroid gland and make parathyroid hormone, which controls calcium balance. The *adrenal* glands are located above the kidneys and produce many hormones, including cortisol (p. 450–51). The *ovaries and testes* make predominantly the sex hormones: estrogen, progesterone, and testosterone. The *pancreas* is located in the abdomen and produces insulin and digestive hormones. The *pituitary* gland is in the brain and is sometimes called the master gland because it makes hormones that regulate the thyroid, adrenal glands, ovaries, and testes. It also produces growth hormone, prolactin (which controls breast milk production), and antidiuretic hormone (ADH), which determines the body's water balance.

Hormonal conditions may appear as disorders of a single gland or several glands. This chapter discusses problems that may have a hormonal basis, such as delayed growth and development, and specific disorders of the thyroid, adrenal glands, and pancreas. Ovarian and testicular function are discussed in Chapters 15, 17, and 18.

Delayed Growth and Development

During childhood, growth hormone and thyroid hormone are the primary regulators of growth. During puberty, the production of estrogens and androgens increases, contributing to both growth and sexual development. Ninety-five percent of adolescents grow and develop normally and within an expected time frame. The other 5 percent experience either delayed or early maturation. Growth and development follow five sequential stages of puberty (Tanner stages, Chapter 2), but each teenager goes through these stages at an individual pace. Although many teenagers worry about that pace, the vast majority fall well within a range of normal variation.

Puberty is considered delayed if it starts too late or proceeds too slowly. In females, delayed puberty is the absence of any breast development by age thirteen or the absence of menstruation by age fifteen. In males, the definition of delayed puberty depends on testicular size. In both females and males, puberty is also considered delayed if more than five years elapse between the beginning and end of puberty or if there is more than a two-year plateau at any single Tanner stage.

Some causes of delayed puberty include the following:

• *"Constitutional" delay* (Chapter 2). Teenagers with constitutional delay of puberty enter puberty later and often are shorter than average. Once puberty starts, they move through its stages at a normal rate and ultimately reach a normal adult height. Constitutional delay accounts for 90 to 95 percent of delayed puberty and is diagnosed by excluding other causes.

• *Deficiencies in pituitary hormone production.* Low body weight or inadequate body fat (as in anorexia nervosa, Chapter 7) can cause the pituitary gland to produce low amounts of follicle-stimulating hormone (FSH) and luteinizing hormone (LH). These hormones instruct the ovaries and testes to make estrogen, progesterone, and androgens, which are essential to sexual development. Other causes of FSH and LH deficiency include chronic illness, excessive exercise, heavy substance abuse, head injury, and infections of the brain (Chapter 32). *Kallmann syndrome* is a rare inherited cause of FSH and LH deficiency manifested by pubertal delay and a decreased sense of smell.

• *Congenital abnormalities of the ovaries or testes.* The most common inherited cause of delayed puberty with normal height is *Klinefelter syndrome,* which occurs only in males at a rate of 1 in 600. Boys with Klinefelter syndrome develop normally during childhood but do not progress normally through puberty during adolescence. Height is normal, or even tall, but the testes remain small, and the penis and pubic hair are underdeveloped for age. Half of males with Klinefelter syndrome develop gynecomastia (Chapter 26), and nearly all are sterile. The treatment involves testosterone administration throughout life, testicular prostheses, and surgery if necessary for gynecomastia.

The most common genetic cause of pubertal delay and short stature in females is *Turner syndrome,* in which the ovaries fail to develop during fetal life. It affects 1 in 2,000 females and usually is diagnosed during childhood because of short stature and characteristic physical findings such as malformed ears, short neck, or abnormal hearing and vision. Puberty does not occur unless hormonal medications are administered.

• *Damage to the ovaries or testes.* Puberty does not occur if the ovaries or testes are unable to produce adequate amounts of estrogen or testosterone. Complete absence of these hormones, especially in boys, may be associated with short stature as well as pubertal delay. Partial function may result in pubertal delay with normal stature. The ovaries or testes may be damaged by injury, infection (as with mumps, Chapter 18), and some forms of chemotherapy or radiation therapy (Chapter 36). Puberty will progress normally once the appropriate hormonal medications are begun.

• *Pituitary failure.* An infection, head injury, or brain tumor can cause abnormal production of one, several, or all pituitary hormones. When growth hormone, FSH, and LH levels are low, pubertal delay and short stature result. Both problems are treated with hormonal medications.

• *Long-term corticosteroid use.* When certain chronic illnesses, such as lupus (Chapter 31) or inflammatory bowel disease (Chapter 29), are treated with corticosteroids for long periods, the functions of the endocrine glands can be suppressed, resulting in short stature and delayed puberty.

• *Chronic illness.* Even without corticosteroid use, chronic illnesses can inhibit physical growth and postpone or delay the progression of puberty. The most common examples are inflammatory bowel disease, chronic kidney disease (Chapter 30), sickle cell disease (Chapter 35), cystic fibrosis (Chapter 27), and anorexia nervosa (Chapter 7).

Evaluating delayed puberty depends on several factors: the teenager's growth record, family history, nutritional history, eating patterns, and a review of body systems. It is very important to keep a record of a child's growth into adolescence—even if it is dated height marks on the wall. The doctor will use the record to determine when the growth delay began. The physical examination will include assessment of the adolescent's height, weight, overall nutrition, arm span, ratio of upper to lower body length, and sexual maturity rating (Tanner stages, Chapter 2). The external genitalia will be examined in all adolescents with pubertal delay, and a pelvic examination may be done for females (Chapter 3).

Laboratory studies used to evaluate delayed puberty include blood and urine tests and an X-ray to determine bone age (Chapter 2). In some instances, blood tests may be done for chromosomal, or genetic, analysis. If a pituitary problem is suspected, computed tomography (CT) or magnetic resonance imaging (MRI) of the brain often will be performed.

The psychological consequences of delayed growth and development must be addressed while the medical evaluation is underway. Some adolescents with delayed puberty withdraw from friends and social activities because of feelings of inferiority. Some become anxious, depressed, or overly dependent on parents. Others become angry or aggressive in an attempt to compensate for their feelings. The decision about if and when to begin hormonal medication depends on both the medical cause of the delay and its psychological consequences.

Some of the emotional problems will respond to counseling and parental support. When they persist, hormonal therapy for the pubertal delay may be indicated regardless of cause. In cases of constitutional delay—the most common cause—full pubertal development eventually will occur. But if the psychological cost of waiting becomes too great, hormonal therapy should be started. With other causes, such as congenital absence of the ovaries or testes, full puberty will result only if hormonal therapy is used. Treatment for these adolescents should begin early, so that puberty progresses on schedule.

The goal of hormone therapy in boys and girls with delayed puberty is to stimulate maturation. The choice of which hormonal medication to use depends on the cause of the delay and the adolescent's sex. Three types of sex hormones can be used: androgens (such as testosterone), estrogens (such as Premarin), and progesterone (such as Provera).

Androgens have the greatest effect on height growth. Although they are considered the "male hormones," significant amounts are normally made by the female ovaries and adrenal glands. Androgens are used for three to six months in both boys and girls with constitutional delay and short stature to stimulate growth in height. Oral androgens, which have fewer masculinizing effects, are used in females. Testosterone, which is injected every two to four weeks, is often used in males.

Estrogen and progesterone have little effect on growth and are used only in females. Their major role is to promote breast development and menstruation. They may be given together in one pill, as in the oral contraceptive, or separately. Estrogen is available as either a pill or a skin patch. Progesterone is available as either a pill or an injection.

Replacement sex hormones should be given in the smallest doses and for as short a period as possible. Adolescents with constitutional delay of puberty require only a few months of treatment. Adolescents with anorexia nervosa may require several years of treatment. Adolescents with absent ovaries or testes require lifelong treatment.

In addition to promoting puberty, hormones have other protective effects, especially for females. Estrogen is important to help protect a female against osteoporosis (thinning of the bone) and adult heart disease. In both males and females, sex hormones may improve self-image and mood.

The side effects of hormonal therapy depend on the dosage and length of treatment. The most common side effect for males who are treated with testosterone is gynecomastia. This happens because some of the testosterone is changed by the body into estrogen, which stimulates breast development. Short-term androgen therapy in girls with constitutional delay usually is well tolerated, but side effects can include acne, weight gain, and growth of body hair. All of these side effects go away when the hormones are stopped.

Females with delayed puberty who require long-term hormone treatment usually begin therapy when puberty is expected, about age eleven to twelve. The lowest possible daily dose of estrogen is given for one year to stimulate development of the breasts and uterus. The dose is then increased for another six to twelve months, followed by the addition of progesterone to produce menstruation. The major side effects of estrogen and progesterone therapy include irregular vaginal bleeding, breast tenderness, weight gain, and mood change. If the estrogen and progesterone are taken as two separate pills (Premarin and Provera), adolescents with ovaries who are sexually active may not be adequately protected against pregnancy. Adolescents who are sexually active may prefer to take the estrogen and progesterone in one pill, the oral contraceptive (Chapter 19).

Precocious Puberty

Precocious puberty is the early arrival of puberty—before the age of eight in girls and nine in boys. The physical growth and secondary sex characteristics develop in the same sequence as they do when puberty normally begins. Girls start with breast budding, pubic hair development, and menstruation. Boys begin with growth of the testes and penis, deepening voice, erections, and ejaculation. For both girls and boys, precocious puberty is marked by changes in hair and skin: increased perspiration, oiliness of skin, acne, growth of underarm hair, and emotional changes.

There are two types of precocious puberty, "central" and "peripheral." Central precocious puberty results from an abnormality in the hypothalamus and/or pituitary gland, located in the brain (Chapter 15). The problem may be caused by head injury, a tumor in the brain, or hydrocephalus (an accumulation of fluid around the brain). When central precocious puberty is suspected, a head CT or MRI will be done. Peripheral precocious puberty is caused by a problem in the adrenal glands, ovaries, or testes. It is confirmed by blood tests to measure the levels of the hormones produced by these organs. Abdominal CT, MRI, or ultrasound is often done to look for abnormalities of the adrenal glands or ovaries.

The treatment of precocious puberty depends on its cause. The most common cause of central precocious puberty is a benign tumor of the hypothalamus. It can be treated with medication and does not require surgery. Tumors of the adrenal glands, ovaries, or testes usually are removed surgically, both to stop early puberty and to determine if the tumor is benign or malignant. Many other causes of peripheral precocious puberty are treated with medication.

Children with precocious puberty have important psychosocial needs that must be considered. Although their bodies are maturing early, their intellectual and social development is not advanced. They appear bigger and older but are no more ready to handle teenage responsibilities than their same-age peers. They may be teased by classmates and may cause confusion for adults who do not understand what to expect of them intellectually. Parents should talk with teachers and other involved adults to explain the problem. Parents and physicians must work together with the child to explain the body changes that are happening.

Excessive Height

For many teenagers, tall stature is desirable. Boys rarely complain about it. While some girls welcome tallness, others worry about excessive height. The definition of "excessive" is highly individualized. One girl believes that five-feet-ten-inches is "too tall," while another is perfectly happy at six feet. A great deal depends on family height and the adolescent's own self-image.

Most tall adolescents come by their height genetically—they have a family history of tall relatives. Possible causes of nonfamilial tallness include excessive growth hormone (acromegaly), abnormal hormone production by the adrenal glands, tumors of the ovaries or testes, Klinefelter syndrome (see above), and Marfan syndrome. It is not unusual for children with Marfan syndrome to reach puberty before the diagnosis is made. This is a genetic disorder that primarily affects the bones and joints, cardiovascular system, and eyes. The characteristic findings are a tall, thin appearance; long, narrow fingers and hands; scoliosis (Chapter 31); and a sunken breastbone. The major complication of Marfan syndrome is a defect in the aorta, the major vessel that carries blood from the heart.

The evaluation of nonfamilial tallness includes a thorough history, physical examination, sexual maturity rating (Chapter 2), blood and urine tests, and an X-ray for bone age (Chapter 2). The sexual maturity rating and bone age are especially important. If both are advanced for the teenager's chronological age, growth will probably slow down and stop before it does in same-age peers. The adolescent may be taller than peers now, but probably will be a normal-height adult. If the bone age is not advanced and the adolescent has not reached a sexual maturity rating of (Tanner stage) five, growth will continue.

The treatment of excessive height depends on the cause. Females who are concerned about excessive height may consider estrogen therapy. Estrogen can diminish growth potential but it carries side effects that should be discussed thoroughly with a physician. If estrogen treatment is to have an effect, it must start early in puberty, before bone growth starts to slow.

Thyroid Conditions

The thyroid gland regulates body metabolism. Too much thyroid hormone generally causes a felling of being wound up. Too little causes a feeling of sluggishness. Females are eight to ten times more likely to have thyroid problems than males. An early finding may be an enlarged thyroid gland (goiter) or a lump in the thyroid. Frequently, though, the signs and symptoms of a thyroid problem appear slowly and are misinterpreted as the typical mood swings or bodily changes of adolescence.

The pituitary gland in the brain stimulates the thyroid gland in the neck to make thyroid hormone. Blood tests can be done to measure the levels of thyroid-stimulating hormone (TSH) made by the pituitary and the level of thyroid hormone made by the thyroid gland. These blood tests are called *thyroid function tests*. The size, shape, and function of the thyroid gland can be assessed by a *thyroid scan*, in which a tiny, safe amount of radioactive iodine is given by mouth. The thyroid concentrates the iodine, and a scanner passed over the neck gives a picture of the radioactive iodine within the gland. An ultrasound examination of the thyroid can be done to determine if a lump felt in the neck is a cyst filled with fluid or is solid. Some diseases of the thyroid gland are "autoimmune," meaning that the body makes antibodies that attack the thyroid gland. The levels of these antibodies can be measured by blood tests.

THYROID ENLARGEMENT

Enlargement of the thyroid, or goiter, is usually discovered by a physician during a routine health screening examination. A "simple goiter" is "euthyroid," meaning that normal amounts of thyroid hormone are produced. Most adolescents with euthyroid goiter have no symptoms. If the gland is very large, there may be a sense of fullness in the neck or difficulty swallowing. The causes of euthyroid goiter include viral infections of the thyroid, autoimmune diseases of the thyroid, multiple benign lumps in the thyroid, and—rarely in the United States—dietary iodine deficiency. If the thyroid gland is very large or increasing in size, thyroid hormone is given orally as a pill (Synthroid) to "turn off" the gland and allow its size to shrink. If the enlargement is mild and stable, no treatment is necessary.

HASHIMOTO THYROIDITIS

In this autoimmune disorder the body produces antibodies that attack the thyroid gland. It is a common disorder of adolescent females and is responsible for 80 percent of euthyroid goiters of adolescence. The gland in Hashimoto thyroiditis is enlarged, firm, and usually nontender. There also may be some enlargement of the lymph nodes in the neck.

The course of Hashimoto thyroiditis is difficult to predict. The enlarged size may diminish after a few months, or the gland may remain enlarged throughout life. Some adolescents with Hashimoto thyroiditis produce normal amounts of thyroid hormone, while others produce too much (hyperthyroid) or too little (hypothyroid). Treatment with Synthroid for up to a year generally is recommended for all euthyroid and hypothyroid adolescents to shrink the goiter. The medication then can be tapered by a physician who is examining the gland and measuring thyroid function periodically. Teenagers with Hashimoto thyroiditis who are hyperthyroid will require antithyroid medications for several months. Most will eventually become euthyroid or hypothyroid and the antithyroid medication can be stopped. Those teenagers who become hypothyroid will require Synthroid.

HYPERTHYROIDISM

Hyperthyroidism is overactivity of the thyroid gland with production of excess thyroid hormone. Its symptoms include nervousness, insomnia, mood swings, tremor, moist skin, a staring appearance of the eyes, heat intolerance, pounding or fast heartbeat, weight loss, increased appetite, diarrhea, hair loss or thinning, and irregular menstrual periods. Most people with hyperthyroidism have an enlarged thyroid gland.

The most common cause of hyperthyroidism is *Graves disease*. It affects females more than males and tends to run in families.

Graves disease is an autoimmune condition that may involve the eyes and skin as well as the thyroid gland. In addition to the stare of hyperthyroidism, the eyes in Graves disease frequently are bulging or prominent. This can be a very serious problem that affects vision; management by an experienced ophthalmologist is essential. The skin involvement, in addition to the changes of hyperthyroidism, usually is on the legs. The affected areas appear thickened, discolored, and wrinkled. Teenagers are far less likely than adults to have the eye and skin complications of Graves disease.

Other, less common causes of hyperthyroidism include Hashimoto thyroiditis, viral infection of the thyroid gland, and benign or malignant tumors of the gland. Treatment, regardless of cause, usually begins with antithyroid medication, such as propylthiouracil (PTU) or methimazole, to block the gland's production of thyroid hormone. If the cause is a tumor or Graves disease, the hyperthyroidism usually persists when the medication dose is diminished.

A nodule or tumor causing hyperthyroidism often is removed surgically. Graves disease can be treated with long-term antithyroid medications, radioactive ablation (below) of the thyroid gland, or surgery. Some teenagers respond to antithyroid drugs within a few weeks, while others do not respond for several months. Once the medication reduces the size of the gland and its hormone production, some teenagers may require no treatment for years.

The unpredictable course of Graves disease has led many physicians to recommend radioactive ablation. This is an outpatient procedure in which a large dose of radioactive iodine is given by mouth. The iodine concentrates in the thyroid gland, and the radioactivity destroys the gland. The goal is to destroy all the thyroid tissue so that hyperthyroidism does not recur. The adolescent then takes Synthroid daily throughout life. There is no evidence that the radioactive iodine places the adolescent at risk for future cancer, infertility, or genetic damage.

People taking antithyroid medications require close supervision by a physician. The dosage necessary to control the hyperthyroidism can change over time, and the drugs have serious side effects, such as a fall in white blood cells, which fight infection. The adolescent should notify a physician immediately if fever, mouth sores, or rash develop.

HYPOTHYROIDISM

Underactivity of the thyroid gland, or hypothyroidism, is not common during adolescence. When it does occur, the usual cause is Hashimoto thyroiditis. The symptoms of hypothyroidism include weakness, lethargy, intolerance to cold, weight gain, swelling of the face and eyes, constipation, hoarseness, skin dryness, thinning of the hair and eyebrows, and brittle nails. Females may notice heavy, irregular menstrual periods and cramping. Hypothyroidism can delay puberty, physical growth, and bone maturation.

Hypothyroidism is diagnosed by thyroid function tests and is treated by Synthroid taken once daily.

THYROID NODULES

These growths or lumps within the thyroid can be benign or malignant. The chance of malignancy is higher in males than females and higher when there is a single nodule rather than many nodules. Blood tests, ultrasound, and thyroid scans are commonly used to evaluate thyroid nodules, but none distinguish benign from malignant. In most cases, an office procedure called fine-needle aspiration biopsy is done. A thin needle is inserted through the skin into the nodule and a sample of fluid and cells is withdrawn for microscopic examination. If the cells are benign, the adolescent may be followed closely without treatment. If the cells are malignant, surgery is indicated to remove the tumor and most of the thyroid gland. After surgery for thyroid cancer, the adolescent may be treated with radioactive iodine to destroy any remaining thyroid tissue. Synthroid then is taken daily for life. The prognosis for adolescents with thyroid cancer treated in this way is excellent.

Adrenal Conditions

The two adrenal glands, located above each kidney in the back of the abdomen, produce two major hormones: cortisol (hydrocortisone) and aldosterone. Through a complex series of steps, the adrenal glands take the body's own cholesterol and convert it into these two hormones. The major effect of cortisol is to increase the body's production and storage of carbohydrates. The major effect of aldosterone is to maintain salt and water balance.

In the process of producing cortisol and aldosterone, the adrenals make different types of androgens, estrogens, and progestins (such as progesterone). A block in any one of the many steps can tip the balance, leading to excessive production of these intermediary hormones and inadequate amounts of cortisol and aldosterone. The adrenal glands receive instructions from the pituitary gland, which produces adrenocorticotropic hormone (ACTH). When the body needs more cortisol, ACTH production increases. When there is enough cortisol, it diminishes.

CORTISOL EXCESS

Cushing syndrome, or cortisol excess, has the following signs and symptoms: weight gain in the torso more than the legs and arms; full, rounded face; delayed growth; high blood pressure; high blood sugar; muscle weakness and wasting; thin skin; easy skin bruising; red-purple stretch marks; changes in personality; osteoporosis (thinning of bone); acne; and excessive body hair (hirsutism).

Cushing syndrome has several causes. The most common is extended use of corticosteroids (such as prednisone) to treat chronic illnesses. It also may result from overproduction of ACTH by the pituitary or from adrenal tumors, which are rarely malignant.

The diagnosis is made by measuring cortisol and ACTH levels in the blood or urine. If the levels are high, additional tests may be done in which medication is given to suppress the body's production of cortisol. If the cortisol levels remain elevated, Cushing syndrome or an adrenal tumor may be suspected. CT or MRI scans of the brain and abdomen then will be done to examine the pituitary and adrenal glands.

Treatment methods depend on the cause of the excess cortisol. If the cause is corticosteroid medication, the doctor will try to taper the medication. If the cause is a pituitary tumor, the treatment is "microsurgery" in which a small part of the pituitary gland is removed. If the cause is an adrenal tumor—especially if there is concern about malignancy—abdominal surgery and removal of the tumor is done.

CORTISOL DEFICIENCY

If the adrenal glands do not produce sufficient cortisol, the signs and symptoms include weakness, lethargy, loss of weight and appetite, abdominal pain, low blood pressure, low blood sugar, and patchy changes in skin color. A pronounced deficiency in cortisol can lead to severe electrolyte imbalance, seizures, shock, coma, and death.

The diagnosis of cortisol deficiency is suggested by the teenager's history of symptoms, physical examination, and blood tests. It is confirmed by giving the adolescent a dose of ACTH intravenously and measuring the blood cortisol level thirty to sixty minutes later. Normally, the ACTH should stimulate the adrenal glands to make cortisol and the level should increase. If it does not, a diagnosis of "adrenal insufficiency" is made.

The most common cause of adrenal insufficiency is rapid withdrawal of corticosteroid medication that the adolescent has been taking for a long time. When taken for longer than a week, corticosteroid medication suppresses the normal production of cortisol by the adrenal glands. When the medication is stopped, it takes weeks or even months for the adrenal glands to "wake up" and make normal amounts of cortisol. The symptoms of steroid withdrawal include headache, low fever, muscle aches, nausea, vomiting, and loss of weight and appetite. If corticosteroid medication is going to be stopped, the doctor usually will taper the dose slowly rather than stop it abruptly.

If the adolescent has not been taking corticosteroid medication, the most common cause of adrenal insufficiency is *Addison disease,* a chronic autoimmune condition in which antibodies destroy adrenal tissue. Less commonly, adrenal insufficiency is caused by congenital abnormalities of adrenal function, infections of the adrenal glands, or bleeding into the adrenal glands.

Adolescents with adrenal insufficiency must take corticosteroid medication every day. The usual regimen is oral hydrocortisone taken once in the morning and once in the evening. If the adolescent is injured or ill, the dose is increased. Teenagers with adrenal insufficiency should wear a Medic Alert bracelet or necklace in case they ever need emergency medical care. This lets the treating doctor know that the adolescent must be given higher doses of corticosteroid until the crisis is over. *Acute adrenal insufficiency is an emergency.* Intravenous fluids containing glucose and salt must be given immediately, along with a high dose of intravenous hydrocortisone.

CONGENITAL ADRENAL HYPERPLASIA (CAH)

A series of enzymes convert cholesterol to cortisol in the adrenal glands. When a genetic disorder causes the enzymes to be diminished or absent, the adrenal glands produce too little cortisol. The pituitary gland then produces too much ACTH in an effort to stimulate the adrenals. The result is hyperplasia, or overgrowth, of the adrenal glands. "Classic CAH" becomes apparent shortly after birth because the enzymes are nearly absent. If the enzymes are only partly diminished, the diagnosis may not become clear until adolescence when mild hormonal disturbances appear. This is called late-onset, or nonclassic, CAH.

The most common type of CAH is a deficiency of the 21-hydroxylase enzyme with resulting excess production of androgens. In the classic form, male and female children will show early virilization, or masculine characteristics, and rapid growth. Early treatment with hydrocortisone results in normal growth and development. The steroid must be taken for the rest of life. Partial 21-hydroxylase deficiency often is not recognized until adolescence. In both females and males, it causes acne, early growth of body and pubic hair, and rapid growth in height. In females, it also causes menstrual irregularities. In males, it causes enlarged penis and small testes. Like the classic form, partial 21-hydroxylase deficiency is treated with daily oral corticosteroids.

Diabetes Mellitus

Diabetes mellitus is a chronic disorder in which the pancreas produces too little insulin, the hormone responsible for controlling the body's blood sugar (glucose) level. Diabetes mellitus is one of the most common hormonal problems of children and adolescents. There are three forms of the disease:

• *Insulin-dependent diabetes mellitus (IDDM)*, also known as juvenile diabetes, tends to appear in normal-weight children between ages ten and fourteen. Its cause is unknown, but there probably is a strong autoimmune component. It is possible that there is an infectious trigger because more cases begin in the cooler months of the year. Siblings and children of someone with IDDM have a 5 percent chance of developing IDDM in their youth and a slightly higher chance later in life. IDDM must be treated with insulin injections.

• *Noninsulin-dependent diabetes mellitus (NIDDM)* is most common in older adults. When it develops during adolescence, it usually is associated with obesity and a strong family history. NIDDM may be treated with diet, oral medication, or insulin.

• *Maturity-onset diabetes of the young (MODY)* is similar to NIDDM but obesity generally is not present. It begins in childhood or adolescence but is less severe than IDDM. Treatment to control the glucose level is important, though, because the long-term complications of diabetes can develop later in adulthood.

NIDDM and MODY are rare during adolescence. The following discussion pertains mainly to IDDM.

SYMPTOMS

The symptoms of diabetes mellitus include increased thirst and appetite, frequent urination, bedwetting, weight loss, and fatigue. Later signs and symptoms include marked wasting, dehydration, nausea, vomiting, abdominal pain, excessive sleepiness, and coma.

The diagnosis of diabetes mellitus is confirmed by measuring the level of blood glucose. As the level increases above normal, glucose will appear in a urine test as well. In adults, the diagnosis may be "borderline," and blood tests may need to be repeated frequently before and after eating. In children and adolescents, the diagnosis usually is clear-cut after a single blood glucose measurement.

The most serious complication of IDDM is *diabetic ketoacidosis (DKA)*. Without treatment, the risk of death is high. With prompt treatment, the prognosis is excellent. DKA happens when the insulin level is so low that glucose does not move from the blood into the cells, where it is needed for fuel. The body responds by accumulating ketones and acids, which are by-products of the fat that is burned when glucose is unavailable to the cells. These ketones and acids can be measured in the blood and urine. The symptoms of DKA include rapid breathing, dehydration, pronounced lethargy, weakness, fruity-smelling breath, shock, and coma. Immediate treatment and hospitalization are required to replace insulin, fluids, and nutrients.

DKA may be precipitated by missed doses of insulin, illness, infection, dehydration, or stress. About 15 percent of teenagers with IDDM are first diagnosed following an episode of DKA. Once diagnosed, the best treatment for DKA is prevention, through insulin, diet, and frequent blood sugar checks.

The long-term complications of diabetes mellitus tend to develop a decade after the illness starts. Some people have no long-term effects, while others develop progressive disease of the eyes, kidneys, blood vessels, and nerves. The most serious complications include blindness, kidney failure, severe nerve damage, heart disease, stroke, and loss of blood flow to the legs. Many of these complications can be prevented by good control of the blood glucose, as discussed below.

HYPOGLYCEMIA

There is often confusion about diabetes mellitus, which causes hyperglycemia, or high blood sugar, and hypoglycemia, or low blood sugar. Hypoglycemia can happen in diabetes when too much insulin is used. The symptoms of hypoglycemia include light-headedness, shakiness, headache, hunger, anxiety, confusion, rapid heartbeat, sweatiness, and pallor. These symptoms clear quickly with sugar intake—such as drinking juice or eating candy. If the symptoms are allowed to continue, seizures and coma can result.

Hypoglycemia in a nondiabetic teenager is rare. Occasionally, it occurs three or four hours after a meal and lasts less than thirty minutes. This is called an exaggerated normal response and is due to an outpouring of insulin following a large carbohydrate (sugars and starches) load. If these episodes recur frequently, the teenager should try a lower-carbohydrate, higher-protein diet that is divided into five or six smaller meals daily.

MANAGEMENT OF DIABETES MELLITUS

The goals of treatment are threefold: to eliminate symptoms, to achieve normal growth and development, and to prevent long-term complications. The hormonal changes of puberty can make management of diabetes difficult. It is important that the adolescent and family work with health professionals who understand both the disease and the normal processes of adolescence. Doctors and nurses can provide information and medical direction, but the ultimate responsibility for the control of diabetes lies with the teenager and family. Diabetes depends on daily self-care: administering insulin, checking glucose levels, and monitoring diet and exercise.

IDDM presents a real challenge to adolescents. It is hard to give yourself injections, prick your finger (to check your blood sugar level), watch your diet. Teenagers should be encouraged to assume responsibility for their own care. Initially, parents should monitor the day-to-day care. As the adolescent demonstrates competence and responsibility, parents must relinquish daily control of the disease to the adolescent.

The treatment of IDDM centers around daily insulin injections. Most adolescents with IDDM give themselves injections twice daily, before breakfast and dinner. The insulin dose is adjusted by checking the blood glucose levels several times a day. The teenager uses a small, sterilized lance or special needle to prick the finger. A drop of blood is collected on a strip and placed in a hand-held machine that measures the glucose level in minutes. The best practice is to take a measurement before each meal and before the bedtime snack. Keeping a record at home is important as a basis for deciding when and how to adjust the insulin dosage.

Insulin therapy is affected by two important factors during adolescence: (1) Many teenagers have erratic eating and sleeping patterns. If mealtimes and bedtime vary from day to day, smaller doses of insulin can be injected three or four times a day rather than larger doses once or twice a day. (2) Insulin requirements typically increase during puberty. Once growth is completed, insulin requirements may decrease.

Glucose levels and the amount of insulin needed may change dramatically when the adolescent is ill. For example, a gastrointestinal illness with vomiting will decrease the needed dose of insulin because less food is being digested. Other illnesses, though, may increase the needed dose because of physical stress. The bottom line is to measure glucose levels every four to six hours during any illness and to stay in touch with your doctor about how to adjust your insulin dose.

Diet is a key factor in controlling diabetes mellitus. The optimal diet is one that keeps glucose levels as normal as possible, while providing enough nutrients for healthy growth and development. Teenagers have varying caloric requirements, depending on their sex, activity levels, and stage of growth. Adolescents with IDDM generally do well when calories are distributed over three meals and three snacks daily. The American Diabetes Association recommends that the daily diet consist of 50 percent carbohydrate, 20 percent protein, and 30 percent fat.

Body weight also enters the picture. IDDM generally is easier to control in normal-weight than overweight individuals. The frequent small meals are important to control the glucose, but they may make it difficult to maintain a desirable body weight. Many teenagers with IDDM find it helpful to talk with a nutritionist who is familiar with both the caloric needs of puberty and diabetes.

Athletic participation should be encouraged for teenagers with IDDM. Regular exercise eventually can lower insulin requirements and helps the adolescent maintain a normal body weight and cardiovascular fitness. Exercise may require adjustments in insulin dosage and diet. By burning calories, exercise lowers the glucose level and, consequently, requires a lower insulin dosage, greater food intake, or both. As a general rule, an hour of moderate to rigorous exercise demands an extra 100 to 150 calories from carbohydrates. In real terms, that amounts to an apple and an orange.

All adolescents should exercise, watch their diets and weight, and avoid smoking. These factors are especially important in adolescents with IDDM, however, because of their increased risk of heart disease. The benefits of a healthy life-style become immediately apparent in good glucose control. Just as important, though, is the reduced risk for the long-term complications of diabetes mellitus.

34

Infections

Infection is the presence and growth of a pathogen anywhere in the body. A pathogen is a virus, bacteria, fungus, or parasite that invades a host, resists the host's defense mechanisms, grows, and causes harm. The infection caused by a pathogen can involve an area as small as a skin pore or can spread through the bloodstream to all parts of the body.

This chapter addresses infections, such as mononucleosis, that involve more than one system of the body. Infections that primarily affect a single body system are discussed elsewhere. For example, pneumonia is described in Chapter 27, The Lungs. Sexually transmitted infections are discussed in Chapter 21.

Some definitions and background information are useful before addressing individual diseases:

Bacteria are microscopic, one-cell organisms. Some do not cause infection and live normally on the skin, in the mouth, in the vagina, and in the intestines. Some bacteria help the body function (by aiding digestion, for example), while others cause illness.

A *virus* is an organism smaller than a bacterium that reproduces in the cells of the body. A virus is parasitic; that is, it requires a host cell to survive.

A *fungus* is a one-cell or many-cell organism that may survive in or outside the human body. In other words, not all fungi are parasitic and not all cause disease.

An *antibody* is a protein molecule produced by white blood

cells that creates immunity to, or protection against, specific organisms and foreign substances.

The *immune system* is the body's defense system against harmful microrganisms and foreign substances. It produces antibodies directed against these threatening intruders and sends white blood cells to the site of infection.

Immunodeficiency is the inability of the immune system to protect against infection.

An *antibiotic* is a medication such as penicillin that is prescribed by a physician to counteract a bacterial infection. Antibiotics either destroy bacteria or inhibit their growth and spread.

Viral Infections

Everyone has had viral infections such as the common cold or the flu. Once a virus invades the body's cells, it may quickly cause illness—such as measles—or may remain quiet for years—such as HIV (Chapter 22). Some viruses disappear from the body shortly after the illness develops. Other viruses, such as herpes (Chapters 21 and 25), cause an acute illness, seem to disappear, but then periodically "wake up" and cause recurrent illness.

Several important viral diseases—measles, mumps, rubella (German measles), and hepatitis B—can be prevented by immunization. Many adolescents, though, have not been fully immunized and are at risk of infection. Hepatitis B (Chapter 29) can cause severe illness at any age. Measles, mumps, and rubella tend to cause more severe illness in adolescents and adults than in children. All teenagers should have been immunized during childhood against measles, mumps, and rubella with two "MMR" injections (Chapter 3).

Measles (rubeola) begins ten to sixteen days after exposure to the virus. It starts with fever, headache, runny nose, cough, sensitivity of the eyes to light, and conjunctivitis, or redness of the eyes. Within three to four days, a rash of reddish spots appears on the face and then spreads to the torso, arms, and legs. Within a week, the rash turns a brown color and begins to peel.

Most cases of measles are uncomplicated, but serious problems can arise. The fever can be very high, ear involvement can cause hearing loss, and pneumonia can impair breathing function. There is no special treatment for measles, but a doctor should *always* be seen if measles is suspected. All cases must be reported to the local health department. Measles is a highly contagious disease that will spread quickly among unprotected individuals. All people who neither have been immunized nor have had the disease are at high risk of infection. If exposed to someone with measles, they must be immunized immediately.

Rubella (German measles) is a milder disease than measles. It begins sixteen to twenty-two days after exposure to the virus with mild fever, muscle or joint aches, fatigue, and a rash of small spots that begins on the face and spreads to the torso, arms, and legs. There is no specific treatment for rubella and it generally is not a serious disease—with one exception. If a woman contracts rubella during the first trimester of pregnancy, there is considerable risk of injury to the fetus, including mental retardation, deafness, cataracts, and heart defects. *All* children and adolescents—male and female—should be immunized against rubella long before pregnancy is a possibility.

Mumps begins fifteen to twenty-five days after exposure to the virus with "swollen glands" at the sides of the face, beneath the jaw, and under the ears. The symptoms include fever, difficulty swallowing, headache, and fatigue. The swelling increases over two or three days and subsides within a week.

There is no specific treatment for mumps, but acetaminophen can help relieve the pain. Foods that are hard to chew or that stimulate the glands to produce saliva (such as citrus fruits) may increase the pain of mumps.

One of the most serious complications of mumps is orchitis, or inflammation of the testes (Chapter 18), which can cause scarring and infertility. Approximately 40 percent of adolescent males with mumps develop orchitis. Other complications include infection of the spinal fluid, brain, and pancreas. A doctor should always be consulted if mumps is suspected.

Varicella, or chicken pox, is caused by a type of herpes virus. It is one of the most common viral infections of childhood, but up to 10 percent of people have not been infected by adolescence. When the disease occurs during the teenage or adult years, there is an increased risk of complications such as pneumonia or infection of the brain. A blood test for immunity generally is done prior to immunization because up to 15 percent of adolescents who have been infected never had symptoms of the illness.

The first symptoms of varicella appear eleven to twenty days after exposure and include a low fever, fatigue, and headache. A day or two later, small red spots appear on the torso and quickly fill with a clear fluid. The rash, described as "dewdrops on a rose petal," spreads to the face, arms, legs, scalp, mouth, and genitalia. As older lesions crust over, crops of new fluid-filled lesions appear daily. The adolescent remains contagious until all lesions have crusted over (usually about five days). It takes about two weeks for the lesions to disappear completely.

The itching of chicken pox can be relieved with cool washcloths or baths, calamine lotion, and antihistamines. Scratching can cause bacterial infection of the sores that leaves permanent scars.

Most adolescents with chicken pox do not require specific treatment. If complications such as pneumonia develop, an antiviral medication called acyclovir may be prescribed. If someone who has never had chicken pox is exposed to it, an injection of varicella-zoster immune globulin given within ninety-six hours decreases the risk of illness.

The varicella-zoster virus that causes chicken pox can lie dormant in nerve cells for many years. It may then suddenly reactivate, causing a painful skin rash called shingles in the skin area supplied by the nerve (Chapter 24).

Infectious mononucleosis is a very common viral illness of high school and college students. "Mono" is caused by the Epstein-Barr virus (EBV), which is carried in secretions of the nose, mouth, and throat and is easily transmitted through kissing and shared eating utensils. The symptoms of infectious mononucleosis include extreme fatigue, fever, swollen glands, sore throat, and headache. Less common signs and symptoms are rash, abdominal pain, nausea, vomiting, loss of appetite, and muscle and joint aches. About a third of adolescents with EBV infection have very mild or even no symptoms. A few are ill enough to require hospitalization, usually because severe throat pain or vomiting interferes with eating and drinking.

The diagnosis of infectious mononucleosis is suggested by the history and physical examination and confirmed by blood tests. The physical examination typically shows an inflamed throat; swollen glands in the neck, under the arms, and in the groin; and—in some cases—enlargement of the liver and spleen. A blood test called the Monospot is positive in 90 percent of adolescents within three to four weeks after the illness begins and becomes negative within two to three months. The Monospot can give false results, especially early or late in the illness. Another blood study that measures antibodies against EBV is more reliable but also is more expensive and more difficult to interpret.

The symptoms of infectious mononucleosis usually last four to six weeks and improve slowly without specific treatment. The most persistent symptom is fatigue. It is difficult for busy teenagers to slow their pace. If they feel well and the liver and spleen are back to normal, they can return to full activity.

Enlargement of the spleen and inflammation of the liver are common complications of mono and must not be ignored. A swollen spleen can bleed or even rupture, so sports should be avoided as long as it persists. The hepatitis (liver inflammation) of mono usually clears within seven to ten days, but it should be managed with limited physical activity and close physician follow-up. Hepatitis is probably the most common cause of nausea, vomiting, and weight loss in adolescents with mono. Unlike other types of hepatitis, liver inflammation caused by mono does not result in permanent liver damage.

One of the most common complications of mono is severe pain and swelling of the throat. In about a third of cases, there may be a streptococcal infection of the throat as well as the EBV infection. All adolescents with strep throat—whether or not they have mono—should receive antibiotics. Ampicillin or amoxicillin should be avoided because they commonly cause rashes in individuals with mono. If the sore throat of mono is so severe that drinking and breathing are impaired, a one-week course of oral corticosteroids (prednisone) may be prescribed. This usually results in prompt improvement of the symptoms. There is much controversy about whether infectious mononucleosis and EBV infection are the cause of chronic fatigue syndrome. (CFS). Little direct evidence supports this hypothesis. CFS is discussed in Chapter 8.

Influenza is an acute respiratory illness caused by three major types of viruses, influenza A, B, and C. The protein coating of these viruses can change, which means that someone immune to one type of influenza may be susceptible to another type. Peak flu season in the United States is October through March. In any given flu season, several virus types predominate. The immunization against influenza changes each year, depending on which virus types are involved. Yearly flu shots are recommended for adolescents with asthma, heart or lung disease, and other chronic diseases.

Influenza is very contagious; it is spread easily through the air by sneezing and coughing or by hand contact (such as on doorknobs). Symptoms typically appear eighteen to seventy-two hours after exposure and include fever, headache, sore throat, cough, runny nose, muscle and joint aches, and fatigue. Most symptoms disappear within five days, though the cough can persist for weeks.

There is no specific treatment for influenza. Rest, fluids, and acetaminophen for the fever and achiness help. Aspirin should never be used to treat influenza during childhood or adolescence because it has been associated with a severe disease of the liver and brain called Reye syndrome (Chapter 29).

The complications of influenza include high fever, dehydration, and pneumonia. The pneumonia usually is caused by the influenza virus itself, but occasionally a bacterial pneumonia can accompany the influenza. Antibiotics are prescribed when a bacterial pneumonia is suspected.

Bacterial Infections

Bacterial infections vary widely in severity. Minor infections often clear on their own without treatment. More severe bacterial infections require aggressive treatment with appropriate antibiotics. Different types of bacteria are sensitive or resistant to particular antibiotics. "Sensitive" means that the antibiotic kills the bacteria or inhibits its growth. "Resistant" means that the antibiotic has no effect on the bacteria. These characteristics are determined by taking a sample from the infected site and sending it to the laboratory for a culture in which the bacteria are grown. The bacterial species can be identified from the culture, and its response to various antibiotics can be tested.

The decision to begin antibiotic therapy is a serious one that requires medical expertise. Antibiotics are prescription medications that should never be used without a doctor's knowledge. An incorrect antibiotic or inappropriate dosage may delay healing or cause serious side effects. It may mask the symptoms of another problem that requires different treatment. Even when you are sure there is an infection and you have an antibiotic at home, talk with a physician before beginning treatment.

Antibiotics can cause allergic reactions. The antibiotics most likely to do this are the penicillins (such as Pen-Vee K, amoxicillin, ampicillin, Augmentin) and the sulfas (such as Bactrim, Septra, Gantrisin). The signs and symptoms of an antibiotic allergy include an itching rash, usually on the torso; swelling of the face, tongue, or mouth; and difficulty breathing. Some allergies are very mild, with only a faint rash, while others are life-threatening, with shock and airway obstruction. Once an allergy to a specific antibiotic is confirmed, that antibiotic should be avoided for life. Allergies to penicillin can be documented by skin testing. Allergies to sulfas and other antibiotics cannot be documented by skin testing, and their confirmation depends on a good description of the symptoms. Always discuss the symptoms with a physician before deciding that they represent an allergic reaction. If the physician cannot be reached before the next dose is due, it is always safest to withhold the antibiotic.

Normally, the human body is inhabited by hundreds of different types of bacteria that do not cause disease. For example, there are over three hundred species of bacteria in the mouth and throat and nearly five hundred species in the large intestine. On the skin, bacteria cling to the surface cells, living in small crevices and niches. As long as the cells or the mucus linings of the mouth, throat, and intestine remain intact, the bacteria do not cause illness. When these surfaces are injured, though, the bacteria invade and multiply. The damage done depends on the bacteria, the site, and the overall health of the individual.

The body fights bacterial infections by making antibodies against the bacteria and by sending white blood cells to the site of infection. These antibodies help to inactivate the bacteria or the toxins produced by them and attract the white blood cells that destroy the bacteria. The pus at an infected site is caused by the influx of white blood cells. When the bacterial infection becomes severe, the body responds by making more white blood cells. This increase in the white blood cell count can be measured on a routine blood test and is one sign of a bacterial infection.

Staphylococcal infections are caused predominantly by two species, *Staphylococcus aureus* and *Staphylococcus epidermidis*. About 20 percent of normal people carry *S. aureus* in their nasal passages, and everyone carries *S. epidermidis* on their skin. Most staphylococcal infections are caused by bacteria that an individual normally carries. The specific type of bacteria is important because each type is sensitive to different antibiotics.

The major illnesses caused by *S. aureus* in adolescents are skin infections (Chapter 24), bone and joint infections (Chapter 31), food poisoning (Chapter 29), and toxic shock syndrome (Chapter 17). With the exception of food poisoning, which disappears on its own, all should be treated with antibiotics. If the infection is mild, the usual antibiotic is dicloxacillin taken by mouth. If the illness is severe, the adolescent may be hospitalized for more aggressive treatment, including intravenous antibiotics.

S. epidermidis is an uncommon cause of infection in healthy adolescents. It can cause severe blood infections in intravenous drug users and in individuals who have artificial heart valves. These infections are very serious and require weeks of intravenous antibiotic therapy.

Streptococcal infections can be caused by many different species of streptococci. The most common causes of illness in children and adolescents are *Streptococcus pyogenes* and *Streptococcus pneumoniae*. Nearly all types of streptococci are sensitive to penicillin.

S. pyogenes is the cause of several skin infections (Chapter 24), strep throat (Chapter 25), rheumatic fever (Chapter 28), a kidney disease called acute glomerulonephritis (Chapter 30), and scarlet fever (see below). *S. pyogenes* spreads easily among schoolchildren and families through skin contact, coughing, and sneezing. About 25 percent of family members exposed to strep throat develop symptoms within forty-eight to seventy-two hours. Strep throat can cause serious complications and should be treated with antibiotics. Family members or classmates should not be treated unless they develop symptoms or their throat cultures are positive for the bacteria.

Scarlet fever, or scarlatina, can follow strep throat or strep skin infections. A rash appears within one to two days, usually on the neck, and then spreads to the torso, arms, and legs. The rash often has a rough "sandpaper" quality and is reddest in the skin folds. The face is flushed, but there often is a ring of pale skin around the mouth. The tongue is redder than usual and may have a white coating. Scarlet fever can cause joint aching, swollen glands, nausea, and vomiting. Even if untreated, the infection usually clears in seven to ten days. Antibiotics should be started as soon as the diagnosis is made, though, because scarlet fever can go on to cause rheumatic fever or glomerulonephritis.

S. pneumoniae, or pneumococcus, is a common cause of pneumonia (Chapter 27) and ear infections (Chapter 25) in teenagers. Ten to 30 percent of healthy people carry *S. pneumoniae* in their mouths and throats and do not require treatment unless they develop signs of an infection. Nearly all infections with *S. pneumoniae* are thought to begin in the mouth and throat.

Mycoplasma infections are caused by a group of organisms that are smaller than bacteria but larger than viruses. *Mycoplasma pneumoniae* is the most common cause of pneumonia among adolescents and is especially prevalent in camps, boarding schools, and colleges. The organism spreads quickly from person to person through nose and mouth secretions that are propelled into the air by coughing or sneezing. It persists in the secretions for weeks after the symptoms are gone, even when antibiotics have been taken.

Mycoplasma can cause bronchitis or pneumonia (Chapter 27). The symptoms of mycoplasma pneumonia develop more slowly than those of pneumococcal pneumonia or influenza. The hallmark of the disease is a disabling, hacking cough that begins two or three days after the appearance of fever. Other symptoms include headache, achiness, and sore throat. If the infection is not treated with antibiotics, most of the symptoms disappear within one to three weeks, though the cough may persist longer. Early treatment with erythromycin or tetracycline shortens the duration of symptoms by about half.

Two other species of mycoplasma, *M. hominis* and the ureaplasmas, can cause genital infections that are transmitted through sexual intercourse. Both organisms can cause urethritis or prostatitis in males (Chapter 18) and vaginitis or pelvic inflammatory disease in females (Chapter 21). Treatment is with doxycycline or tetracycline.

Tick-Borne Diseases

The primary diseases caused by tick bites in the United States are Lyme disease and Rocky Mountain spotted fever (RMSF). As yet, no vaccine is available for either disease, so it is important to learn preventive measures, recognize the signs of infection, and seek prompt medical attention if disease is suspected. These precautions apply to all teenagers—not just those who camp or hike in the woods. RMSF, for example, has been reported in the Bronx, New

York. The ticks that carry Lyme disease can spread from animals that live in wooded or grassland areas to domestic animals, such as dogs and cats, to humans.

Some preventive measures can help protect against tick-borne illnesses:

• When walking in the woods or tall grass, wear long pants with cuffs tucked into socks and long-sleeve shirts. Light-colored clothing reveals ticks more readily than dark colors.
• Use insect repellents on pant legs, socks, and exposed parts of the body. Read the labels for instructions on correct application.
• Use tick- and flea-repellent collars on pets.
• Brush off clothing and pets before coming inside.
• Learn to recognize ticks and look for them when undressing.
• Know how to remove ticks.

There are several kinds of ticks. The deer tick that causes Lyme disease is much smaller than the common wood or dog tick. It is about the size of the period at the end of this sentence.

A tick bite is not painful and may go unnoticed. Most tick bites do *not* cause disease, but prompt and correct removal of the tick is always wise:

• Use fine-point tweezers to grasp the tick where it entered the skin. Pull it gently but firmly until it releases its hold. Try not to squeeze the tick's body. Take your time; the tick will not give up easily.
• Do not use lighted cigarettes, matches, Vaseline, alcohol, or other methods. They can cause the tick to regurgitate infected material before removal.
• Wash your hands after the tick is removed. Wipe the bite area with an antiseptic or rubbing alcohol.
• Save the tick in a covered jar of alcohol. Note the date, where the tick was acquired, and the location of the bite. This information, along with the tick, can be helpful if a rash or other symptoms develop.
• If a tick is found but there is no bite, destroy the tick in a sealed jar of alcohol.

Rocky Mountain spotted fever (RMSF) is caused by tiny bacteria called rickettsiae that are carried on dog ticks. Only one in twenty dog ticks is infected with rickettsiae, and it takes up to twelve hours after a bite for the tick to release the organisms. The only treatment that is recommended after a dog tick bite is removal of the tick and cleansing of the area. Preventive antibiotics for RMSF should not be used because the risk of infection is low.

RMSF has been reported primarily in children and adolescents during warm months (April to September). The highest rates occur in the south-central and southeastern parts of the United States. The classic indicators of RMSF are history of a tick bite, fever, and rash, but not all of these features are always present and—even when they are present—the infection can mimic other illnesses.

The symptoms of RMSF begin two to fourteen days after the tick bite with fever, headache, achiness, and a flat pink rash on the wrists and ankles. Over the next few days, the rash spreads to the palms, soles, and torso and changes to red splinterlike dots under the skin. Other symptoms may include nausea, vomiting, abdominal pain, diarrhea, eye inflammation, and cough. The diagnosis is confirmed by a blood test in which antibodies to rickettsiae are measured.

RMSF progresses slowly, over a period of one to two weeks. Treatment with tetracycline or doxycycline should be started as soon as the disease is suspected, even before the blood test results return. Without treatment, serious complications can result, including insufficient platelets in the blood and involvement of the heart, lungs, and brain. With treatment, the likelihood of full recovery is excellent.

Lyme disease is caused by small, coiled bacteria called spirochetes that are carried on three types of ticks in the United States. All of these ticks, which have been called deer, sheep, and bear ticks, are much smaller than the common dog tick. Ticks that carry the spirochetes usually are found on animals that live in the woods or grasslands, but the ticks can spread to domestic animals such as dogs, cats, and horses. Lyme disease was first identified in Old Lyme, Connecticut, in 1976, but cases have since been reported throughout the United States. The months of greatest risk, especially in the northeast and midwest, are the warm summer months.

The tick that transmits Lyme disease is so small that its bite may go unnoticed. Not all deer ticks carry Lyme disease, and even those that are infected may not transmit the spirochete during a bite. The longer the tick remains on the skin, the more likely it is that a bite will result in human infection. Prompt removal is the most important prevention. Because most ticks do not carry Lyme disease, preventive antibiotics after a bite are not recommended. Prompt antibiotic therapy is recommended, though, if the signs and symptoms of Lyme disease develop.

The earliest symptom of Lyme disease is a red rash that begins as a flat or slightly raised single spot that slowly expands. Less commonly, there may be several spots. After a few days, the middle of the rash may clear or a blister or scab may appear in the center. The rash usually fades away without treatment within one to two weeks. Twenty to 40 percent of people with Lyme disease never develop—or do not recall—a rash. Other symptoms of early Lyme disease include fatigue, headache, stiff neck, muscle and joint achiness, low fever, and swollen glands. Antibiotic treatment at this early stage is highly effective in preventing the development of later symptoms and complications.

The late manifestations of Lyme disease involve the joints, nervous system, and heart. Lyme arthritis (painful joint swelling) may occur as early as a few weeks after the tick bite, but the average delay is six months. The arthritis usually begins in the knee, may come and go, and may spread to other large joints such as the hip. Sixty to 90 percent of people with Lyme arthritis improve after treatment with antibiotics.

The neurologic complications of Lyme disease vary from mild symptoms, such as headache and irritability, to nerve paralysis or severe brain inflammation. One of the most common complications is Bell palsy, or paralysis of the nerve that controls the face muscles (Chapter 32). Over 90 percent of individuals with Bell palsy due to Lyme disease have full recovery of the nerve function within one month, even without treatment. Other complications include meningitis, encephalitis, and inflammation of the peripheral nerves supplying different parts of the body (Chapter 32). The symptoms may be persistent headache, stiff neck, paralysis, numbness of a part of the body, or changes in mood, personality, or thinking. The treatment for these neurologic manifestations of Lyme disease usually is intravenous antibiotics.

Lyme carditis, or heart involvement, occurs in less than 10 percent of people with Lyme disease. The symptoms appear about three weeks after the tick bite and include irregular heartbeat, lightheadedness, fainting, and shortness of breath. Even without treatment, Lyme carditis usually clears within a few days or weeks. It is treated with intravenous antibiotics.

The possibility of Lyme disease should be considered when there is a history of a tick bite in someone who develops any of the symptoms described above. The diagnosis can be confirmed by a blood test. The decisions about when to begin an antibiotic, which antibiotic to use, and whether to give it by mouth or injection are complex ones. Adolescents, parents, and physicians need to work together to reconstruct the story of the illness. Appropriate, prompt treatment generally leads to an excellent outcome.

35

The Blood

Blood is essential for life. No cell in the human body can survive without the nourishment and oxygen carried in the bloodstream. Blood bathes and lubricates, fights infection, promotes metabolism, and transports wastes. It has four main components:

Red blood cells (RBCs) are the most plentiful cells in the bloodstream. A special protein within the RBC, called *hemoglobin,* binds oxygen in the lungs and delivers it to tissues throughout the body. RBCs are made in the *bone marrow,* or soft inner core of bone.

White blood cells (WBCs) fight disease and infection. There are two major types of WBCs: neutrophils and lymphocytes. Neutrophils, the most numerous type, attack invading bacteria. When a bacterial infection develops, the bone marrow makes extra neutrophils that travel through the bloodstream to the site of the infection and destroy the bacteria. Lymphocytes are produced in both bone marrow and the lymph nodes, or glands, of the lymphoid system. They are the soldiers of the immune system, making antibodies that counteract foreign organisms and particles.

Platelets are small, disk-shaped cells produced in the bone marrow that travel through the bloodstream, accumulate at the site of a cut or damaged blood vessel, stick to each other, and seal off the injury. They are critically important in normal blood clotting.

Plasma is the fluid in which the RBCs, WBCs, and platelets float. Plasma is mostly water and makes up almost two thirds of the total blood volume. It also carries carbohydrates, lipids, proteins, minerals, waste products, dissolved gases, hormones, and special proteins that work with the platelets to help the blood clot.

EVALUATING THE BLOOD

The first laboratory test used to evaluate the blood is the *complete blood count* (CBC). This simple test is part of the routine health screening examination and can be done on a very small quantity of blood collected either from a finger prick or a vein in the arm. The CBC includes the RBC, WBC, and platelet counts. It also measures the amount of *hemoglobin* in the blood and the *hematocrit*, which is the proportion of the blood made up of RBCs.

The RBC count and hemoglobin and hematocrit values change during adolescence—especially in males. Androgen hormones, which increase during puberty, stimulate the bone marrow to make more RBCs. Boys have higher androgen levels than girls, resulting in higher RBC counts. Most girls either have no change in the RBC count or may even have a decrease because of the blood loss associated with menstruation. In both girls and boys, the WBC count stabilizes by age eight and the platelet count by age one.

Other tests, in addition to the CBC, are done if a blood clotting problem is suspected. The evaluation begins with a *prothrombin time (PT), partial thromboplastin time (PTT),* and *bleeding time.* The PT and PTT are measured on a small sample of blood collected from an arm vein. The bleeding time is done by making a very short, shallow, painless scratch on the arm and measuring how long it takes for the bleeding to stop. The PT and PTT reflect the special proteins (clotting factors) in the plasma. The bleeding time reflects both the platelets and the clotting factors.

If an abnormality in the production of RBCs, WBCs, or platelets is suspected, a *bone marrow aspirate and biopsy* may be performed. A needle with a hollow core is inserted through the skin into the hip bone. Once the tip of the needle reaches the bone marrow, fluid (the aspirate) and tissue (the biopsy) are drawn into the core of the needle. The fluid and the tissue are then examined under a microscope to determine if the blood cells are normal in appearance and number. A bone marrow aspirate and biopsy can be done in the doctor's office with local anesthesia. It usually is done by a hematologist, a doctor who specializes in disorders of the blood.

Anemias

The term "anemia" refers to insufficient or impaired RBCs. When anemia is mild, there usually are no symptoms. As the RBC count drops further, fatigue and pallor develop. When anemia is severe or sudden, symptoms such as light-headedness, rapid heartbeat, headache, and fainting may develop.

Understanding the causes of anemia begins with some knowledge about normal RBCs. The bone marrow releases young RBCs, called *reticulocytes*, into the bloodstream. The reticulocytes develop quickly into mature RBCs that survive in the bloodstream for about 120 days. The bone marrow continually releases new reticulocytes to replace the old RBCs. If the body loses excess RBCs, the marrow responds by releasing extra reticulocytes.

There are four main causes of anemia:

• Insufficient RBC production by the bone marrow. This is the most common cause of anemia in adolescents. It usually is due to dietary deficiency of iron, a key component of hemoglobin.

• Bone marrow failure. This is rare but very serious. In addition to anemia, there may be low WBC and platelet counts, resulting in infection and bleeding.

• Hemolysis, or destruction of RBCs. The hemoglobin that is released from the destroyed RBCs may cause jaundice (a yellow tint to the skin) and dark urine.

• Blood loss. This is common in adolescent girls who have irregular or heavy menstrual periods. In an attempt to replace the lost blood, the bone marrow uses up its iron stores. Unless the teenager takes supplemental iron tablets, iron deficiency anemia follows the blood loss.

IRON DEFICIENCY ANEMIA

The diet of the average American youth contains inadequate iron to keep pace with the demands of growth during puberty. This is especially true in girls who lose iron each month with menstruation. Nearly one quarter of children and teenagers in the United States have iron deficiency anemia, though in most it is mild with few, if any, symptoms. Because of its insidious progression, all teenagers should have their hemoglobin or hematocrit level checked as part of a routine examination.

The earliest symptom of iron deficiency anemia is fatigue, especially with exercise. As the anemia becomes more severe, the adolescent may complain of headache or may appear pale. There may be cracking at the corner of the mouth, irritation of the tongue, or a concave shape to the nails. These signs warrant prompt medical attention.

Iron deficiency anemia is diagnosed by measuring the hemoglobin, hematocrit, and iron level in the blood. Within five days of beginning prescribed iron medication, healthy reticulocytes appear in the bloodstream and the hemoglobin and hematocrit levels begin to increase. It typically requires one to two months of iron medication to restore the body's iron supply and increase the hemoglobin level to normal. Adolescents then should try to maintain a normal iron level by eating foods that are rich in iron: fish, meat, fortified cereals and breads, eggs, spinach, and other green, leafy vegetables.

Iron medication can cause side effects, such as nausea, abdominal pain, constipation, and black stool. It also can interfere with the absorption of tetracycline, doxycycline, and minocycline—antibiotics that are commonly used to treat acne and sexually transmitted diseases. The iron and antibiotic, therefore, should be taken at least two hours apart.

FOLIC ACID AND B$_{12}$ DEFICIENCY

These dietary vitamins are essential for normal RBC production. They are contained in many foods, and deficiencies are rare causes of anemia in teenagers. Folic acid deficiency can be caused by inadequate dietary intake, intestinal malabsorption, or increased utilization—as in pregnancy. Folic acid comes from leafy green vegetables, liver, whole grains, and eggs. If folic acid is eliminated from the diet, the body depletes its stores within four months and anemia results. Within days of adding folic acid back to the diet, the anemia begins to improve. The absorption of folic acid can be impaired by chronic diseases of the small intestine (such as inflammatory bowel disease, Chapter 29) and by medications (such as Dilantin for control of seizures, Chapter 32). Folic acid deficiency is corrected with folic acid tablets taken once daily for at least three months. Most over-the-counter multivitamin tablets contain folic acid and will prevent its depletion.

Vitamin B$_{12}$ deficiency is harder to develop and harder to treat than folic acid deficiency. The cause of B$_{12}$ deficiency is less likely to be dietary insufficiency because the body's stores of B_{12} last three years, even if B_{12} intake ceases. B_{12} deficiency eventually will develop if there is no intake of meat, eggs, or dairy products. In this case, changing the diet will correct the problem. A more common cause is malabsorption of the vitamin, resulting from inflammatory bowel disease (Chapter 29) or intestinal surgery. Treatment then involves monthly injections of the vitamin throughout life.

ANEMIA OF CHRONIC DISEASE

Anemia can accompany many chronic conditions, including kidney failure, chronic infectious or inflammatory disorders, autoimmune diseases, cancer, and anorexia nervosa. Anemia of chronic disease does not respond to vitamins. As the underlying illness improves, the anemia improves.

SICKLE CELL ANEMIA

Normal RBCs are shaped like round, flat disks and contain hemoglobin A, hemoglobin A_2, and small amounts of hemoglobin F. In the hereditary blood disease sickle cell anemia, the RBCs are shaped like curved sickles because of an abnormal hemoglobin called hemoglobin S (Hb S). When the level of Hb S increases or when there is a physical stress—such as an infection—the abnormal RBCs stick to the walls of the blood vessels, blocking the flow of blood and the delivery of oxygen to the tissues. The result is episodes of pain called sickle cell crises.

Sickle cell anemia occurs throughout the world but predominates in Africa, the Mediterranean, the Near East, and India. In the United States, 1 of 400 African-American babies is born with sickle cell anemia, and 8 of 100 have sickle cell trait. People with sickle cell anemia carry two genes for Hb S, while people with sickle cell trait carry only one gene for Hb S.

People with sickle cell trait do not have painful crises and live normal lives, without anemia or other problems. In rare cases, they may experience pain when deprived of normal amounts of oxygen. This can occur when exercising at high altitudes (as in mountain climbing), scuba diving, or flying in unpressurized planes. Teenagers with sickle cell trait can participate in all athletic activities but should understand that they can pass the gene for Hb S on to their children. If both parents have sickle cell trait, they face a one in four chance of having a child with sickle cell anemia.

The complications of sickle cell anemia vary with age. Young children experience frequent bacterial infections, painful crises, and enlargement of the spleen (located in the upper left side of the abdomen) because of "sequestration," or trapping, of the sickled RBCs. Repeated episodes of sequestration damage the spleen and cause it to scar so that little blood flows into it. By adolescence, the spleen shrinks to a very small size and no longer traps RBCs. The bacterial infections of childhood also become less frequent during adolescence, but the painful crises continue.

The symptoms of sickle cell anemia vary in severity and frequency between individuals, but they tend to have a consistent pattern in any one person from late childhood on. Between crises, a teenager with sickle cell anemia usually feels well. The unpredictable nature of the crises, though, and the severity of the pain means that the disease is always at the forefront of the adolescent's life.

A painful crisis typically lasts several days and tends to localize to the abdomen, low back, arms, or legs. The pain may be accompanied by fever, though frequently there are no other symptoms. Milder crises can be managed at home with analgesics (acetaminophen, codeine). More severe crises require hospitalization for both pain control and close monitoring for complications.

Sickle cell crises can be life-threatening. For example, *acute chest syndrome* is a crisis that causes pain, fever, and breathing difficulty due to pneumonia or trapping of the sickled RBCs within the lung tissue. It requires hospitalization for intravenous fluids, antibiotics, pain control, and RBC transfusions to decrease the proportion of Hb S in the bloodstream. Another life-threatening complication, called *aplastic crisis*, occurs when the bone marrow is unable to keep pace with the demand for new RBCs and shuts down completely. *Priapism,* or trapping of the sickled RBCs within the penis, causes prolonged, painful erections that can lead to impotence. Sickle cell anemia can involve the central nervous system and can cause strokes during childhood and adolescence. Once a stroke has occurred, the adolescent is given RBC transfusions monthly in an attempt to prevent recurrences.

Sickle cell anemia causes many chronic problems as well as acute, painful crises. Growth and pubertal development often are delayed. The repeated destruction of sickled RBCs causes the hemoglobin to form stones in the gallbladder (Chapter 29). Sickled RBCs within the kidneys can cause blood in the urine or difficulty concentrating the urine, resulting in frequent urination or bedwetting. Pregnancy can be complicated by an increased frequency of painful crises, miscarriage, low birth weight, and premature delivery.

Early diagnosis is important in the management of sickle cell anemia. All African-American babies should be screened for Hb S using a simple blood test called a sickle prep. If this test is positive, another blood test is done to measure the proportion of Hb S in the bloodstream. Once the diagnosis is made, a major goal of management is the prevention and aggressive treatment of infections, which can trigger painful crises. A well-balanced diet, supplemented with iron and folic acid, helps provide the minerals and vitamins necessary for RBC production.

The adolescent with sickle cell anemia needs the support of family, friends, and health professionals. A clear plan should be made to manage painful crises, including when to begin pain medications and how much to take. This plan works best when it carries over from home to hospital and is reviewed periodically with a physician whom the adolescent trusts and likes.

Thalassemia

Thalassemia is a group of RBC disorders of markedly different severity. All are inherited abnormalities in hemoglobin production. Normal hemoglobin is made up of two "beta" chains and two "alpha" chains. Beta-thalassemia results from decreased beta chains. Alpha-thalassemia results from decreased alpha chains.

BETA-THALASSEMIA MAJOR

Beta-thalassemia major, or Cooley anemia, is the most severe type. It primarily affects people of Mediterranean ethnicity, but it also appears in Africans and Asians. The disorder is inherited when each parent passes one abnormal beta-thalassemia gene on to a child. Within the first year of life, there is marked anemia requiring frequent RBC transfusions for survival. Children who receive adequate, regular transfusions grow normally. If the transfusions are inadequate, many problems develop, including severe anemia, poor growth, enlargement of the liver and spleen, and bone abnormalities. The bone marrow, which works overtime in an attempt to counteract the anemia, grows rapidly and causes thinning of the outer layer of hard bone. As result, some bones become brittle and fracture easily, while others (such as the forehead) appear overgrown and prominent.

A life-threatening consequence of the frequent RBC transfusions required in thalassemia major is a buildup of iron that the body cannot excrete. This accumulation can be prevented by desferoxamine, a medication that binds and removes the excess iron. Without it, iron accumulates in organs throughout the body, including the heart, liver, pancreas, ovaries, and testes. The most serious complication of iron overload—and the most common cause of death among adults with beta-thalassemia—is heart failure and irregularities in the heartbeat.

A new approach to the treatment of beta-thalassemia is bone marrow transplantation, which has been done successfully in children before the complications of the disease develop. Because of the complexity of the disease and evolving new treatment options, people with beta-thalassemia should be treated by hematologists (blood specialists) at major medical centers whenever possible.

BETA-THALASSEMIA TRAIT

This trait does not cause illness and is associated with a normal life span. It is caused by the inheritance of one gene for beta-thalassemia. There typically is a mild anemia that initially may be attributed incorrectly to iron deficiency. People with beta-thalassemia trait should receive genetic counseling about the likelihood of passing the gene on to their children.

THALASSEMIA INTERMEDIA

This condition is less severe than beta-thalassemia major and much more serious than beta-thalassemia trait. It causes moderate anemia, enlargement of the liver and spleen, and some expansion of the bone marrow. Most individuals with thalassemia intermedia are managed with RBC transfusions and desferoxamine.

Bleeding

Every teenager has experienced bleeding after a cut or injury. The bleeding normally lasts only a few minutes and responds to some simple measures:

• Clean the cut gently with soap and water or rinse it thoroughly with clean water alone if soap is unavailable.

• Cover the cut with a clean cloth or bandage and press firmly with the fingers or palm. If the blood soaks through the cloth, place another over the first and continue pressing. It is better to add new bandages because removing the soaked one can pull away coagulated blood cells from the cut and reopen the wound.

• If the cut is on an arm or leg, raise it above the level of the heart while applying the pressure.

• When the bleeding stops or slows, wrap the cut to maintain pressure but not so tightly that blood flow is cut off. The circulation can be checked by squeezing the fingernail or toenail nearest the cut. The nail should turn white when squeezed, then pink when released. If it does not turn pink, loosen the bandage.

• Seek medical attention if the bleeding persists. At the same time, find a pressure point near the cut, between it and the heart. Good pressure points are those where pulses are felt: the inside of the wrist, the inside of the elbow, the groin. Apply continuous pressure to the appropriate point until the bleeding has stopped for one minute. If bleeding resumes, reapply pressure.

• Keep tetanus immunizations up to date. The guidelines for prevention of tetanus are described in Chapter 3.

Prolonged bleeding, or bleeding from no apparent cause, can represent a problem in the body's normal clotting mechanism. The possibilities include the following:

• The blood vessels at the injury site do not constrict properly;
• The platelets are either deficient or abnormal;
• The proteins, or "clotting factors," in the blood are deficient or abnormal; or
• A medication, such as aspirin, is interfering with the normal blood clotting mechanism.

The signs and symptoms of a bleeding disorder include:

• recurrent, heavy nosebleeds;
• gum bleeding;
• prolonged bleeding after minor injury, surgery, or dental work;
• painful bleeding into the joints;
• heavy vaginal bleeding;

- rectal bleeding;
- urinary bleeding;
- bleeding into the skin.

"Purpura" is a brownish-red or purple discoloration caused by bleeding into the skin. "Petechiae" are tiny capillary bleeds, resembling red dots or pinpricks. "Ecchymoses," or purple bruises, are caused by collections of blood in the skin. All can be caused by platelet dysfunction, insufficient platelets, or inflamed blood vessels. A physical examination, medical history, family history, and blood tests help diagnose the cause and determine treatment.

HEMOPHILIA

The term "hemophilia" refers to a group of inherited disorders in which the blood fails to clot correctly. The most prevalent type, "classic hemophilia," is a deficiency of a clotting substance called Factor VIII. The severity of hemophilia varies between individuals, depending on the level of Factor VIII in the plasma.

Severe hemophilia becomes apparent during infancy. Moderate hemophilia causes several bleeding episodes during childhood and is usually diagnosed by adolescence. Mild hemophilia causes excessive bleeding only with major injury or surgery and may not be diagnosed until adulthood.

The leading sign of moderate to severe hemophilia is painful bleeding into a joint. This may follow a minor injury or may occur spontaneously. This leads to swelling and limited movement in an elbow, shoulder, hip, knee, or ankle. The knee is the primary site in younger teenagers, while the elbow is often affected in older adolescents. Repeated episodes of bleeding cause destruction of the joints, decreased mobility, and chronic pain. Other complications of hemophilia include hematuria (blood in the urine) and bleeding into muscles. Head injury, with bleeding into the brain, is the most frequent cause of death among people with hemophilia.

Management of hemophilia relies heavily on injury prevention. When bleeding occurs, Factor VIII concentrates are given intravenously at home. People with severe disease may give themselves periodic infusions to prevent bleeding. All blood products—including Factor VIII concentrates—used in the United States are now pretreated with heat or detergents to eliminate HIV and are screened for HIV prior to use. (Before 1985, many hemophilia patients were exposed to HIV through transfusions and blood products.) All blood products, including Factor VIII concentrates, also are screened for hepatitis B. Nevertheless, all people with hemophilia should be immunized against hepatitis B (Chapter 3).

Hemophilia is inherited through a defective gene on the X chromosome. Males have one X and one Y chromosome; females have two X chromosomes. A male who inherits the hemophilia gene on his X chromosome has the disease. A female who inherits it on one of her X chromosomes is a carrier without symptoms, but she can pass the gene on to her children. She will not have hemophilia because her other X chromosome ensures the production of clotting factors. In very rare instances, a female inherits the hemophilia gene on both of her X chromosomes and develops the disease. All teenagers with a family history of hemophilia should receive genetic counseling, whether or not they have the disease.

VON WILLEBRAND DISEASE

Both males and females can have von Willebrand disease, but it predominates in females. It is caused by insufficient or abnormal production of a blood protein that makes platelets sticky and that transports Factor VIII.

Teenagers with von Willebrand disease have symptoms such as nosebleeds, gum bleeding, prolonged bleeding from superficial cuts or surgery, and excessive menstrual bleeding. Unlike hemophilia, bleeding into joints or the brain is rare. Persistent bleeding is treated with infusion of normal plasma that contains clotting factors. Aspirin and products containing it (such as Alka-Seltzer) must be avoided. Teenagers with excessive menstrual bleeding should discuss with their physicians hormonal therapy to regulate their periods.

IDIOPATHIC THROMBOCYTOPENIC PURPURA (ITP)

This is the most common bleeding disorder of adolescents and is caused by increased destruction of platelets. *Acute ITP* appears suddenly and clears on its own within three to twelve months. *Chronic ITP* begins more gradually and lasts longer. In both types, the first signs are petechiae or ecchymoses (see above), gum bleeding, nosebleeds, heavy menstrual bleeding, and blood in the stool or urine. ITP can cause prolonged bleeding from superficial cuts, but the bleeding usually can be controlled with pressure or ice.

Though the cause of acute ITP is unknown, a respiratory infection often precedes it by two to four weeks. Acute ITP requires no specific treatment if bleeding is minor and the platelet count is not too low. Heavier bleeding may require corticosteroids, transfusions of RBCs and platelets, or surgical removal of the spleen (which traps platelets). In most cases, corticosteroids increase the platelet count and control the bleeding within a few days.

Chronic ITP is associated with an immunologic problem in which antibodies are made against the platelets. Up to 80 percent of teenagers with chronic ITP are cured with surgical removal of the spleen. Other forms of therapy, including corticosteroids, also may be effective.

White Blood Cell Disorders

The most common disorder of white blood cells is *neutropenia,* which means an abnormally low number of neutrophils, one of the major types of WBCs. Severe neutropenia increases the risk of life-threatening bacterial infections. Neutropenia may be caused by decreased production of WBCs by the bone marrow or by increased destruction of WBCs in the bloodstream. It can accompany autoimmune diseases (such as lupus), infections, nutritional deficiencies, malignancies, chemotherapy, and radiation therapy. Chronic neutropenia may be a congenital problem, present from birth, or may appear for the first time later in life.

Adolescents with chronic neutropenia typically have recurrent infections, fevers, and ulcers of the mouth and lips. Neutropenia is cyclic in some cases, meaning that the WBC count rises and falls in a regular, periodic pattern.

With diminished WBCs to fight infection, teenagers must pay close attention to good hygiene of the skin, mouth, and genitalia. Fever demands immediate evaluation and usually prompt treatment with antibiotics. The newest treatment for neutropenia is the use of intravenous medications that increase the production of WBCs by the bone marrow.

Another set of WBC disorders involves the function rather than the number of WBCs. Unlike neutropenia, these disorders are rare in adolescents. Disorders of WBC function cause recurrent fungal as well as bacterial infections. The treatment of children and teenagers with disorders of WBC function is difficult and should be handled by a hematologist at a major medical center.

36

Cancer

The subject of cancer is somber, yet promising. About 11,000 Americans under age twenty are diagnosed with cancer each year. The diagnosis frightens teenagers and families, but new treatments have led to steadily increasing survival rates. Two thirds of young people with cancer survive at least five years, and many are considered cured. Over the last three decades, the death rates for children under age fifteen have declined 80 percent for Hodgkin disease, 50 percent for leukemia and bone cancer, and 31 percent for all other types combined.

Cancer is a disease of the cells that make up body tissues. Cells normally divide just enough to replace themselves and, during childhood and puberty, to allow growth. Cancerous cells multiply too rapidly, replacing healthy cells and forming tumors. Although the primary cause of cancer is still unclear, scientists know that genetics is an important part of the puzzle. When normal genes mutate, or change in a harmful way, they may cause cells to multiply too fast and increase in number. This is called malignancy.

Cancer demands a great deal of teenagers and their families. Adolescents must limit some activities, comply with strict medical regimens, undergo therapies that have undesirable side effects, and face an uncertain future. Families experience denial, discouragement, anger, grief, and guilt. They must balance the medical and emotional needs of the teenager with the ongoing demands of work and home life. Both adolescents and parents can feel lost in a medical maze of complex tests, treatments, and procedures.

It is helpful if the adolescent and family can work with a team of knowledgeable, supportive health professionals. Ideally, the team should include physicians, nurses, social workers, and psychologists. If professional support is not forthcoming, the family needs to seek it. Many medical centers have cancer treatment programs designed specifically for adolescents. Some special considerations include:

• Teenagers deserve full, accurate information about their diagnoses and treatments. They should be actively involved in managing the disease and consenting to procedures and therapy.
• They should be told about the side effects of therapy (such as hair loss, nausea, vomiting), how long the symptoms will last, and what can be done to alleviate them.
• Adolescents with cancer need ways to cope with their emotional turmoil. They should be encouraged to talk with family, friends, and health professionals. Teenagers also can learn relaxation techniques, hypnosis, and other methods that help with stress reduction during chemotherapy.
• Returning to school may be difficult for some adolescents who have had changes in appearance from therapy. Others may want to participate fully in all activities but, because of temporary suppression of the immune system, cannot risk exposure to infections. Flexibility is necessary in both situations—by adolescents, parents, and physicians. The goal should always be to regain a normal lifestyle as soon as possible.

There are more than 100 types of cancer that affect humans. The prevention and detection of several types have been discussed elsewhere in this book: testicular self-examination (Chapter 18); breast self-examination (Chapter 26); tobacco and lung cancer (Chapter 12); Pap smear screening and sexually transmitted diseases (Chapter 21). This chapter addresses the four most common cancers diagnosed during adolescence: leukemia, lymphoma, brain tumors, and bone tumors.

Leukemia

Leukemia, or cancer of the white blood cells (WBCs), is the most common malignancy of adolescents. It develops when abnormal precursor (very young) WBCs multiply and fill the bone marrow where blood cells are manufactured (Chapter 35). The abnormal cells overwhelm the normal precursor cells, depleting the bone marrow's store of normal WBCs, red blood cells (RBCs), and platelets. The leukemic cells, or "blasts," eventually spill over into the bloodstream and can infiltrate the lymph nodes, liver, spleen, central nervous system (CNS), skin, bone, and testes.

Normal blood contains several types of WBCs (Chapter 35). Neutrophils are the most numerous and protect the body against bacterial infections. Myelocytes are the precursor cells that mature into neutrophils. Myeloid or myelocytic leukemia refers to cancer of the myelocytes and neutrophils. Lymphocytes, another group of normal WBCs, make antibodies and help regulate immunity. There are two kinds of lymphocytes: T cells and B cells. Lymphoid or lymphocytic leukemia refers to cancer of either T-cell or B-cell origin.

In addition to the classification as myeloid or lymphoid, leukemias also are characterized as acute (sudden appearance) or chronic (slower development). Acute lymphoblastic leukemia (ALL) is the most common type during adolescence. Acute myeloid leukemia (AML), also called acute nonlymphocytic leukemia (ANLL), is somewhat less common. Chronic myelocytic leukemia (CML) accounts for only 3 percent of leukemia in adolescents. A fourth type, chronic lymphocytic leukemia (CLL) is primarily a disease of the elderly.

The cause of leukemia remains unclear, but certain factors have been linked to specific types of leukemia. For example, ALL is associated with some genetic disorders (such as Down syndrome), exposure to high-dose radiation (the atomic bomb), and exposure to certain chemicals (such as benzene). AML is associated with other genetic disorders, chemotherapy for previous malignancy, and radiation exposure. People with CML usually have an abnormal chromosome called the *Philadelphia chromosome* in the malignant cells.

ACUTE LEUKEMIA

Early signs and symptoms of acute leukemia include anemia, fever, bruises and pinprick bleeding into the skin, infection, bone pain, fatigue, pallor, and loss of appetite or weight. The lymph glands in the neck, under the arms, and in the groin may be enlarged, and there may be upper abdominal pain from swelling of the spleen and liver.

A blood test (CBC, Chapter 35) may reveal inadequate RBCs and platelets, excessive WBCs, and leukemic blasts. The diagnosis of acute leukemia is confirmed when blasts are found on the bone marrow aspiration and biopsy (Chapter 35). ALL is differentiated from AML by microscopic examination of the blast cells. The correct treatment and prognosis of acute leukemia depends on an accurate diagnosis.

When leukemia is diagnosed, the doctor will look beyond the blood and bone marrow. For example, both ALL and AML can invade the central nervous system (brain, spinal cord, and spinal fluid). A standard procedure for all people with acute leukemia is a "lumbar puncture," in which a sample of spinal fluid is withdrawn through a needle inserted into the lower back. The sample is then examined microscopically for abnormal cells. Blood tests to examine liver and kidney function, chest X-rays, and special scans of the bones or abdomen may also be done.

Both ALL and AML can spread to the testes in males, especially during adolescence. ALL is more likely than AML to involve the liver and spleen, and AML is more likely to involve the bones. AML also can cause solid tumors of blasts, called chloromas, that appear as lumps most commonly on the head or back. An unusual complication of acute leukemia is infiltration of leukemic cells into the gums or skin.

The treatment of acute leukemia is divided into three phases called induction, consolidation, and maintenance. The goal of induction therapy is to achieve *remission,* or control of the proliferating leukemic cells. Complete remission is reached when the bone marrow has less than 5 percent blasts, the blood count is normal, and there are no leukemic cells outside the bone marrow. The goal of consolidation therapy is to decrease the likelihood of *relapse,* or flare, of the leukemia. Different chemotherapy is used during consolidation than induction to avoid resistance of the leukemic cells to the medications. Maintenance therapy, which consists of monthly chemotherapy for two to three years, has been shown to decrease the risk of relapse and to increase long-term survival.

Chemotherapy can involve an array of medications given orally, intravenously, or directly into the spinal fluid through a needle in the low back (intrathecal chemotherapy). Radiation of the head (cranial radiation) is usually a part of the standard treatment of acute leukemia. The goal of intrathecal chemotherapy and cranial radiation is to decrease the chance of central nervous system relapse. The brain and spinal cord are sometimes called a "sanctuary" site because the leukemic cells may be protected there from standard chemotherapy given orally or intravenously.

Induction chemotherapy brings 90 percent of individuals with ALL and 75 percent with AML into remission. Until recently, though, over half had relapses of the leukemia. Treatment today has become more aggressive, with a broader combination of medications used for longer periods of time. The result is improving survival, but there also is an increased chance of complications from the treatment. An early problem is called tumor lysis syndrome. As the leukemic cells are destroyed by the chemotherapy, they release their contents, causing imbalances in electrolytes and minerals. Treatment to prevent tumor lysis syndrome often begins even before induction therapy.

Chemotherapy and radiation therapy typically cause neutropenia, or a fall in the number of WBCs (Chapter 35). The goal of therapy is to destroy the leukemic cells, particularly in the bone marrow. Unfortunately, this means that normal bone marrow cells are destroyed as well. After successful therapy, the normal blood cells—but not the leukemic cells—proliferate. Until this happens and the neutropenia improves, the teenager is at risk for serious infections. Antibiotics will be started immediately if an adolescent with neutropenia develops a fever. In most cases, antibiotics to prevent pneumonia will also be given.

Suppression of the bone marrow during chemotherapy causes low RBC and platelet counts as well as neutropenia. Transfusions may be needed to support the adolescent during the period of bone marrow suppression. The risk of any blood loss, including menstruation, is high during aggressive chemotherapy. Hormonal medication often is given to females to prevent menstrual periods until the blood counts improve.

When remission is achieved in acute leukemia and after therapy is completed, adolescents may face some late complications of the disease and its treatment. Cranial radiation can cause problems with learning. It can permanently damage hormone production by the hypothalamus and pituitary gland in the brain, resulting in delayed growth and puberty. Chemotherapy may cause infertility by damaging the ovaries or testes. There also is a risk of second malignancies following chemotherapy and radiation. All of these problems are serious and real, but they should not outweigh the decision to treat acute leukemia promptly and aggressively. Without treatment, the risk of rapid death is high.

The prognosis for adolescents with acute leukemia depends on several factors. ALL has a higher likelihood than AML of both remission (90 versus 75 percent) and cure (60 versus 35 percent). Cure means no evidence of any malignant cells for at least five years. In ALL, teenagers and infants do not do as well as children, and males do not do as well as females. Other factors associated with poor outcome include a very high WBC count and the presence of disease in the central nervous system, chest, or abdomen.

There is much less agreement among doctors about the favorable, or unfavorable, features of AML. Because the prognosis for AML is less promising than that for ALL, the treatment regimens for AML tend to cause more side effects. Once remission is achieved in AML, an alternative to continued chemotherapy may be bone marrow transplant (see below). As more is learned about the predictors of AML outcome, doctors will be better able to help families decide which type of treatment is likely to be most successful.

CHRONIC LEUKEMIA

During childhood and adolescence, chronic leukemia is far less common than acute leukemia. When it does occur, the most likely form is CML (chronic myelocytic leukemia). CML develops far less abruptly than ALL or AML, but the average survival is only three to four years.

CML is a disease of two stages: the initial, or chronic, stage, which lasts an average of three years, and a later, accelerated stage called blast crisis, which has an average survival time of three to six months. The first signs and symptoms of CML are those of the chronic phase: fatigue, weakness, anemia, fever, bone pain, and abdominal pain. The physical examination nearly always shows marked swelling of the spleen on the left side of the abdomen.

A routine blood count demonstrates the hallmark of CML: a very high WBC count, usually more than ten times normal. A low RBC count (anemia) and a high platelet count typically are seen. The diagnosis of CML is confirmed by bone marrow aspiration and biopsy (Chapter 35). Most individuals with CML also have the abnormal Philadelphia chromosome, which is discovered on genetic testing of the leukemic cells.

The second, accelerated phase of CML looks like acute leukemia. The blood counts become worse, leukemic blast cells fill the marrow, and the spleen enlarges even further. Unlike ALL and AML, the accelerated phase of CML responds very poorly to treatment. Until recently, the chronic phase of CML was controlled, but not cured, by the use of single chemotherapy medications to limit the number of WBCs.

Bone marrow transplant during the chronic phase has provided new hope for people with CML. This is a procedure in which the diseased bone marrow cells of the "host" (the person with the malignancy) are replaced with healthy bone marrow cells from a "donor." Before the transplant is done, the host is treated very aggressively with chemotherapy and radiation to the entire body. This is done both to destroy malignant cells and to decrease the chance that the body will reject the donor cells. This treatment essentially destroys the host's own bone marrow, which is then "rescued" (or replenished) by the infusion of donor cells.

There are severe, and sometimes fatal, complications for the host of a bone marrow transplant. The new cells can be rejected and destroyed (graft versus host disease). The malignancy may recur. Infections are common and difficult to treat. The pretreatment chemotherapy and radiation therapy cause many uncomfortable side effects. But, when the adolescent with CML has a well-matched sibling donor, bone marrow transplant may offer the best chance of survival. Cure rates have been as high as 40 to 50 percent in CML when there is a sibling donor whose cell type matches that of the person with CML.

Lymphoma

Lymph nodes are located throughout the body. They cluster together in the neck, under the arms, in the groin, and near organs and blood vessels. The lymph nodes produce lymphocytes, white blood cells that make antibodies and help fight infection.

"Lymphoma" refers to a group of cancers that begin in the lymph nodes or other lymphatic tissues. As the malignant cells proliferate, they form tumors that may be felt in the neck, underarm, or groin, or that may interfere with organs deep in the chest or abdomen. Lymphoma is diagnosed in thirteen of every million children and teenagers annually in the United States and is the third most common childhood malignancy. The incidence rates for the two major types of lymphoma, Hodgkin disease and non-Hodgkin lymphoma, are about equal.

HODGKIN DISEASE

About 7,000 cases of Hodgkin disease are diagnosed in America each year. There are two peak ages of onset, the mid-twenties and the sixties. Among children and adolescents, 60 percent of cases are diagnosed between the ages of ten and fifteen. Hodgkin disease is one of the most curable types of cancer. With treatment, teenagers have a 90 percent chance of cure.

The earliest sign of Hodgkin disease typically is an enlarged, firm, painless lump in the neck, armpit, or groin. In some people, a tumor in the chest can cause symptoms of cough, shortness of breath, chest pain, or difficulty swallowing. Other symptoms may include fever, night sweats, weight loss, fatigue, and itching all over the body, especially after a hot bath or shower. On physical examination, the doctor may find enlargement of the lymph nodes, liver, or spleen.

Hodgkin disease is usually diagnosed by a biopsy (tissue sample) of a lymph node. The prognosis and treatment of Hodgkin disease depend on both the appearance of the cells under the microscope and the "stage," or spread, of the cancer through the body. Microscopic cell types, from best to poorest prognosis, are *lymphocyte predominance, nodular sclerosing, mixed cellularity,* and *lymphocyte depleted.* Nodular sclerosing is the most common cell type in young people with Hodgkin disease. It is seen in females more than males and usually begins in the neck or chest. The mixed cellularity type is seen in about 30 percent of adolescents with Hodgkin disease, and the lymphocyte predominance type in about 15 percent. Lymphocyte depletion is the least common type, affecting about 5 percent of young patients.

The four stages of Hodgkin disease are defined according to the parts of the body that are affected by malignant cells:

- *Stage I:* only one lymph node region (such as on one side of the neck);
- *Stage II:* two or more regions on the same side of the diaphragm (the division between the chest and abdomen);
- *Stage III:* regions on both sides of the diaphragm;
- *Stage IV:* scattered sites throughout the body involving organs as well as lymph nodes.

After the biopsy that confirms the diagnosis of Hodgkin disease, several tests are done to determine the stage: blood tests, chest X-ray, scans of the chest and abdomen, and bone marrow aspiration and biopsy (Chapter 35). Sometimes, bone scans or other special imaging tests are necessary. Until recently, the stage of Hodgkin disease was determined surgically. This involved general anesthesia and surgery to remove the spleen and explore the abdomen for tumors. The advent of better radiographic techniques (CT and MRI scans) allows determination of the stage without the direct look of surgery. In addition, the treatment used today makes removal of the spleen unnecessary.

Hodgkin disease can be successfully treated with radiation therapy, chemotherapy, or a combination of both. The best choice depends on many factors, including the cell type, the stage, the adolescent's age, and the symptoms.

Hodgkin disease is very sensitive to radiation, meaning that it usually causes the tumor to shrink. Radiation alone may be the choice for some adolescents with stage I disease. If the disease is more severe or widespread, the high dose of radiation required to destroy the tumor could not be tolerated by the rest of the body. Treatment then will be either radiation combined with chemotherapy or chemotherapy alone.

Chemotherapy for Hodgkin disease involves a combination of medications. The most commonly used combinations are abbreviated as MOPP (Mustargen, Oncovin, procarbazine, and prednisone) and ABVD (Adriamycin, bleomycin, vinblastine, and dacarbazine). MOPP has resulted in remission in 70 to 80 percent of individuals with advanced disease, and cure (no evidence of malignancy for at least five years) in over 50 percent. ABVD probably is as effective but has not been used as long as MOPP. Still other regimens combine several of these drugs, alternate ABVD and MOPP, or introduce other drugs altogether.

There is still some question about how long chemotherapy should continue in Hodgkin disease. Most oncologists (cancer specialists) recommend at least six cycles, or months, but in some cases this may be decreased when combined with radiotherapy. The goal is to rid the body of the tumor (remission) and prevent recurrence of the tumor (relapse). It is common to achieve remission yet experience relapse months or years later. Unlike some other cancers, relapsing Hodgkin disease is still sensitive to treatment and even curable. The prognosis is best when the relapse occurs more than a year after complete remission.

Bone marrow transplant is another treatment option for people with disease that has relapsed or proven resistant to therapy. Remission can be achieved in nearly all bone marrow recipients, but there are substantial relapse rates. Bone marrow transplant therefore is not the first treatment used for Hodgkin disease.

There are both acute and long-term complications of the treatment of Hodgkin disease. Side effects during radiation therapy include nausea, vomiting, skin redness, anemia, infection, and bleeding. The side effects during chemotherapy tend to be more severe and include nausea, vomiting, burning pain when the drugs are given intravenously, hair loss, and bone marrow suppression (inadequate production of blood cells). Fever should receive prompt medical attention because of the risk of infection.

The long-range impact of radiation and chemotherapy on a young, growing body is complex. Treatment approaches that are routine for an adult patient with Hodgkin disease require special consideration when used for an adolescent. Potential problems include impaired skeletal growth; delayed puberty; and damage to the lungs, heart, thyroid, ovaries, or testes. Some specific long-range complications include the following:

• Lung inflammation and possible scarring when bleomycin (as in ABVD) is given along with radiation to the chest area;
• Heart damage caused by either high-dose Adriamycin (as in ABVD) or radiation to the chest area;
• Thyroid problems, such as hypothyroidism (Chapter 33), following radiation to the neck;
• Reproductive problems due to both chemotherapy and radiation, including decreased fertility, decreased hormone production, and menstrual irregularity. Sterility occurs in nearly all males who receive MOPP six times, in 50 percent who receive it three times, and in 50 percent who receive ABVD. The risk of sterility in females is less, and pregnancies do occur.
• Second malignancies later in life occur in 1 percent of people treated with radiation, 5 percent with MOPP, and 10 percent with both MOPP and radiation. The types of cancers are solid tumors following radiation (especially of soft tissues, thyroid, and bone) and leukemia or non-Hodgkin lymphoma following MOPP.

These complications are serious, but usually are accepted given the likelihood of cure with treatment. Scientists continue to explore treatment options that retain high cure rates for Hodgkin disease but avoid both the short- and long-term problems.

NON-HODGKIN LYMPHOMA (NHL)

Like Hodgkin disease, NHL is a group of malignancies of varying severity. The incidence of NHL increases from late childhood through adulthood, and the types of NHL differ between adolescents and adults. NHL in adolescence usually begins in lymphatic tissues outside lymph nodes rather than within lymph nodes as it does in adults.

With appropriate therapy, NHL is curable in two thirds of children and teenagers. There are some types of NHL, however, that are particularly aggressive and carry a poor prognosis. Teenagers with immune system deficiencies, including HIV infection and AIDS, are at high risk for severe forms of NHL that respond poorly to treatment.

NHL in adolescents usually begins as a mass in the abdomen or chest that causes cough, shortness of breath, chest pain, weight loss, fever, or abdominal pain. These symptoms can appear very suddenly or may develop gradually as the tumor grows. Less commonly, the first symptoms of NHL appear after the cancer has spread to other parts of the body, such as the central nervous system or the bone marrow.

NHL in teenagers may progress very quickly and therefore requires rapid diagnosis. The earlier treatment begins, the better the prognosis. NHL in children and adolescents is divided into three main types. *Lymphoblastic lymphoma* usually begins with a mass in the chest. It causes enlargement of the lymph nodes, liver, and spleen and may involve the lung and central nervous system. Lymphoblasts, similar to those of ALL, are found in the bone marrow and lymph nodes. Lymphoblastic lymphoma eventually may evolve into ALL.

The second type of NHL in children and teenagers is *Burkitt lymphoma*, which usually begins as a mass in the abdomen. Involvement of the tonsils, central nervous system, and bone marrow is common in Burkitt lymphoma. The third type is *large cell lymphoma*, which typically begins as a mass in the chest or a swelling of the lymphatic tissue in the throat or neck. Unlike lymphoblastic or Burkitt lymphoma, early involvement of the central nervous system and bone marrow is uncommon in large cell lymphoma.

The diagnosis of NHL depends on a tissue biopsy (of a lymph node, for example) or a fluid sample (such as cerebrospinal fluid, Chapter 32) that shows the characteristic malignant cells. The following tests then are done to determine the stage of the lymphoma:

blood and urine tests, bone marrow aspiration and biopsy (Chapter 35), a sample of spinal fluid from a lumbar puncture (p. 485), chest and abdominal x-rays and scans (CT or MRI), and bone scan. Surgery rarely cures the disease and generally is not done because it delays treatment.

Combined chemotherapy drugs are the prime weapons in treating NHL. Radiation therapy may be used when the cancer is localized to one or two areas, but even then chemotherapy is given for at least six months to prevent relapse. More advanced, or widespread, disease may be treated with chemotherapy alone, often involving up to twelve different medications given over a two-to-three-year period. Lymphoblastic and Burkitt lymphomas are also treated with intrathecal (injected directly into the spinal fluid) medication and/ or radiation of the central nervous system because of the high risk of brain and spinal cord involvement.

Teenagers with lymphoblastic and Burkitt lymphomas are at particularly high risk of rapid breakdown of the tumor (tumor lysis syndrome, p. 486) during treatment. As described for ALL and AML, tumor breakdown is a desirable, but potentially dangerous, goal of treatment. When the malignant cells are destroyed, they release their contents and cause shifts in the body's fluid, electrolyte, and mineral balance. Doctors watch very closely for these shifts early in the course of treatment.

The other short- and long-term complications of treatment depend on the specific chemotherapy and whether radiation is used. Most regimens carry risk of heart damage, ovarian or testicular damage, and second malignancies. The risk of not treating, though, far outweighs the complications of treating, and the decision to proceed quickly should not be delayed.

The overall prognosis for teenagers with NHL is good, but specific outcome depends on the type and extent of the tumor. Over 90 percent of teenagers with localized tumor who are treated survive at least two years with no recurrence. Longer-term data is not yet available because the aggressive regimens described above are relatively recent. It is likely that many of these young people are cured of the malignancy. For more advanced disease, such as lymphoblastic lymphoma, the disease-free survival rates are 75 percent with aggressive treatment.

The prognosis is poor for adolescents with NHL who relapse after chemotherapy. If treatment can bring the disease back into remission, bone marrow transplant offers the best chance of cure.

Brain Tumors

Brain tumors are the second most common malignancy of adolescents, after leukemia. They constitute a highly varied group of different severity, location, and prognosis. Some brain tumors are benign. Others, though malignant, are very slow growing. Still others grow quickly and cause disabling symptoms. Malignant brain tumors of childhood and adolescence are best managed at medical centers with experienced teams of oncologists (cancer specialists) and neurosurgeons.

Tumors of the brain and spinal cord usually are classified according to their location: the cerebrum, or upper hemisphere of the brain: the cerebellum, or lower back portion; the brain stem, or lowest part of the brain that emerges from the skull; and the spinal cord. The major types of brain tumors during adolescence are as follows:

• *Cerebral astrocytomas* tend to increase in severity through adolescence into adulthood. "High-grade," or extremely malignant, astrocytomas have a poor prognosis with only a 25 percent five-year survival rate despite surgery, radiation, and chemotherapy. "Low-grade" cerebral astrocytomas have a 60 to 80 percent five-year survival rate.

• *Cerebellar astrocytomas* decrease in frequency from childhood through adolescence. Some forms can be removed entirely at surgery, resulting in a 90 to 100 percent cure rate. Nearly all forms respond well to radiation therapy.

• *Medulloblastomas* are usually located in the cerebellum and are more common in children and young adolescents than in older adolescents and adults. When treated with surgery, radiation, and chemotherapy, there is a 50 percent five-year survival rate.

• *Brain stem gliomas* are extremely aggressive tumors that are more common in young children than in teenagers. Despite surgery, radiation, and chemotherapy, the five-year survival rate is less than 20 percent.

• *Ependymomas* often involve the spinal cord during adolescence. They vary in their aggressiveness. Ependymomas usually are treated either with surgery alone or surgery and radiation.

The location of a brain tumor determines the symptoms, which can include headache, abnormal gait, numbness or weakness in an arm or leg, seizures, vision problems, vomiting, disturbed eating and sleeping patterns, stiff neck, tilting of the head, personality changes, depression, lethargy, and a decline in school performance. The headaches may be dull throughout the head or may localize to a particular area. They often occur on awakening and are worse when lying down than sitting up.

The major tools for the diagnosis of brain tumors are MRI and CT scans. MRI is superior to CT for the detection of tumors in the base of the brain, the brain stem, and the spinal cord. A lumbar puncture (p. 485) to examine the spinal fluid for malignant cells is done only when spinal cord involvement is suspected. Unlike other forms of cancer, additional tests usually are not needed before proceeding to surgery. The best approach to treatment and rehabilitation can be offered by a team of neurosurgeons, oncologists, nurses, social workers, and psychologists who are experienced in the special needs of teenagers with brain tumors.

Treatment takes three paths: surgery, radiation, and chemotherapy. The first goal is to remove surgically as much of the tumor as possible without harming healthy brain tissue. If the tumor is in an area of the brain that would be seriously damaged by surgery, only a small sample of the tumor will be removed (a biopsy) to make a diagnosis. Some brain stem tumors may be in such critical areas that even biopsy is unsafe, and treatment will begin without a tissue sample. Most malignant brain tumors are treated with both surgery and radiation therapy.

The role of chemotherapy has changed dramatically since the early 1980s when it was thought—incorrectly—that the medications would not reach the brain tissue. Doctors today increasingly add chemotherapy to surgery and radiation therapy in the management of brain tumors. Chemotherapy now is considered especially important for high-grade astrocytomas, medulloblastomas, and brain stem gliomas. Some doctors are using it before radiation in an attempt to shrink the tumor quickly. Many different combinations of drugs are being tested to determine the best treatments for specific tumor types.

Until recently, the prognosis was poor for teenagers with brain tumors that recurred after treatment. Aggressive chemotherapy followed by bone marrow transplant has yielded promising results, especially for high-grade astrocytomas. Before the chemotherapy, samples of the teenager's own healthy bone marrow are removed and saved. Very high dose chemotherapy then is given, which destroys both the brain tumor and the bone marrow. The saved samples of bone marrow are returned to the adolescent, providing new cells that replenish the bone marrow. Many serious complications accompany bone marrow transplant, but it provides a potentially lifesaving option for teenagers with an otherwise fatal disease.

Improved diagnostic and treatment methods have reduced many of the consequences of therapy. For instance, CT and MRI help doctors pinpoint the tumor's location, which allows more precise surgical removal with less damage to normal brain tissue. Even before treatment, though, the brain tumor may permanently damage intellect, vision, hearing, or motor function. These problems can be compounded by the side effects of both radiation and chemotherapy.

Radiation to the head carries some specific risks. Within hours of treatment, there may be swelling of the brain tissue around the tumor. Much of this swelling can be prevented by corticosteroids given before treatment. Radiation can also cause lethargy, weight loss, fever, and vomiting for one to two months following treatment. Unlike radiation to other parts of the body, radiation to the head tends to cause permanent hair loss. It can damage the hormone-producing glands in the brain (hypothalamus and pituitary), resulting in poor growth and delay in puberty. An insidious complication is progressive intellectual decline that begins months or years after treatment. An uncommon complication is the development of a secondary malignancy in the area treated with radiation years later. This may be a second brain tumor or cancer of the thyroid gland (Chapter 33).

The complications of treatment for brain tumors are very real and frightening. The risks of treatment must be weighed against the prognosis without treatment. The hope for life and even cure usually results in a decision to proceed with the most effective treatment available.

Malignant Bone Tumors

Benign bone tumors, which are common in children and adolescents, are discussed in Chapter 31. This section describes the two most common malignant bone tumors of adolescents: osteogenic sarcoma and Ewing sarcoma.

Nearly 25 percent of adolescent cancers are bone tumors that begin in the hard, outer portion of bone. Unlike bone tumors in adults, which often begin elsewhere (such as the breast) and spread to the bone, most bone tumors in teenagers are "primary," meaning that they begin in the bone. Until the 1970s, primary bone tumors were fatal in over 50 percent of cases. The only hope was aggressive surgery (usually amputation) in an attempt to remove the tumor. This approach often failed because of spread beyond the primary tumor. Today, early diagnosis and a combination of surgery, radiation, and chemotherapy result in cure without amputation for most adolescents with primary bone tumors.

OSTEOGENIC SARCOMA

This is the most common bone cancer of teenagers. It tends to appear during the growth spurt, around age twelve to thirteen in girls and fourteen to fifteen in boys. In order of declining frequency, these tumors occur in the lower part of the thighbone (femur), the upper part of the shinbone (tibia), and the upper arm bone (humerus).

The earliest symptom of osteogenic sarcoma is pain, which often is attributed to an injury. Swelling begins later, when the tumor erodes through the bone and forms a mass of soft tissue. In some cases, the tumor is first recognized when the weakened bone breaks after a minor injury.

A doctor often can determine from an X-ray whether a bone tumor is benign or malignant. Nevertheless, a biopsy of the tumor should always be done to confirm the diagnosis. A CT scan of the chest and bone scans should also be done to assess whether the malignancy has spread to the lungs or to other bones. Spread beyond the primary tumor does not exclude the chance of cure.

Treatment of osteogenic sarcoma begins with chemotherapy. The regimens may involve single medications, such as ifosfamide or methotrexate, or several drugs used in combination. Chemotherapy before surgery is very effective at shrinking the size of the tumor and sparing many adolescents amputation of a limb. Even when surgery is needed, the limb often can be saved when the procedure is performed by an experienced orthopedic oncologist (bone cancer specialist).

About 20 percent of teenagers with osteogenic sarcoma have evidence of malignant nodules in the lungs before any treatment is given. These nodules often disappear following chemotherapy. If they persist, chest surgery is performed to remove them. After limb and/or chest surgery, an additional one to two months of chemotherapy is given.

Over 50 percent of teenagers with osteogenic sarcoma are cured when treated with chemotherapy and surgery. When the malignancy has spread to the lungs, the cure rate is 25 to 50 percent. All teenagers with osteogenic sarcoma should be followed closely after treatment with bone X-rays and CT scans of the chest for several years.

The cause of osteogenic sarcoma usually is unknown, though it can follow childhood radiation for other malignancies by an average of ten years. This risk may decline for future generations as lower doses of radiation are used in combination with more effective chemotherapy. Tumors caused by previous radiation can be treated successfully with chemotherapy before and after surgery.

EWING SARCOMA

This is the second most common bone tumor in teenagers. It reaches a peak incidence in adolescence and is very rare in adults. Ewing sarcoma usually develops in the thighbone or in flat bones such as the pelvis, ribs, and shoulder blades.

Pain is the first symptom. Within a few weeks, a lump appears in the soft tissue surrounding the bone. In many teenagers, persistent fever also develops. Ewing sarcoma often can be diagnosed by an experienced radiologist by examining an X-ray of the bone, but a biopsy is always required to confirm the diagnosis.

Once the diagnosis is established, tests are done to determine the spread of the tumor. The most likely areas of spread are the lungs and other bones. Tests therefore include chest X-ray and CT scan, bone X-rays, CT scan of the primary tumor, bone scan of the other bones, and bone marrow aspiration and biopsy (Chapter 35).

Radiation therapy is no longer used alone for Ewing sarcoma because of the high rate of recurrence. Like osteogenic sarcoma, Ewing sarcoma is treated first with chemotherapy, though the medications used are different. One the tumor size shrinks from the chemotherapy, the involved bone is treated with radiation. After this, the area of the tumor is surgically removed. Chemotherapy is used again after the surgery.

The aggressive combination of preoperative chemotherapy, radiation, surgery, and postoperative chemotherapy has yielded over an 80 percent cure rate for Ewing sarcoma. After completing treatment, teenagers with Ewing sarcoma must be followed with chest X-rays, CT, and bone scans.

A long-term risk of the radiation used to treat Ewing sarcoma is second malignancies in the treated area. The risk may decrease in the future as teenagers are treated with aggressive chemotherapy and lower doses of radiation.

Survivors of Childhood Cancer

Childhood cancer refers to malignancy diagnosed before age twenty. Many children and teenagers today have been cured of cancer and look forward to normal life spans. But cure carries with it some long-term complications and risks. The specific risks depend on the type of treatment and are described in each of the preceding sections.

The family is told of the potential risks when the treatment is administered. The child, though, may be too young or ill at the time of treatment to understand the possible implications of cure. The goal, quite appropriately, is to save the child's life. Years later, once cure has been achieved, the teenager and parents may need to review the risks with their doctor. Understanding these risks may promote early detection if a problem develops.

Adolescents who have survived childhood cancer may face special difficulties or concerns during puberty. For example, growth and sexual maturation may be delayed. Fertility may be impaired. Appearance may be altered by the effects of treatment. Most importantly, all teenagers must begin to think ahead and plan for the future. This task may be difficult for adolescents who, as children, faced the possibility of early death and who now, as young adults, must cope with the consequences of their past illness and treatment.

Many medical centers have programs that follow young people with cancer into adulthood. Survivors need both ongoing medical care and help in making the transition to adulthood with grace and ease.

NOTES

1. Katchadourian, Herant, *The Biology of Adolescence* (San Francisco: W. H. Freeman and Co., 1977), p. 6.
2. Ibid., p. 8.
3. Kett, Joseph F., *Rites of Passage: Adolescence in America, 1790 to the Present* (New York: Basic Books, 1977).
4. Ibid.
5. Mead, Margaret, *Coming of Age in Samoa* (New York: William Morrow and Company, 1928, 1973), pp. 8–9.
6. Ibid, pp. 175–6.
7. Neinstein, Lawrence S., M.D., and Lonnie Zeltzer, M.D., "Chronic Illness in the Adolescent," *Adolescent Health Care: A Practical Guide*, 2nd ed. (Baltimore: Urban & Schwarzenberg, 1991), p. 988.
8. Holder, A.R., "Minors' Rights to Consent to Medical Care," *Journal of the American Medical Association*, 1987; 257 (No. 24): 3400–3402.

RESOURCES

The following organizations, hotlines, support groups, books, and materials are not intended to be a comprehensive list but a starting point for obtaining further information. General resources are listed first, followed by chapter-specific subjects. We have attempted to provide the most current information about organizations, but addresses and phone numbers may have changed since publication. Many national organizations have state and local offices; it is helpful to check your telephone book for local information. Some phone directories also provide a special section for health services.

GENERAL RESOURCES

American Academy of Family Physicians
8880 Ward Parkway
Kansas City, MO 64114
1-800-274-2237

The American Academy of Pediatrics
Department of Publications
141 Northwest Point Blvd.
P.O. Box 927
Elk Grove Village, IL 60009-0927

American College of Obstetricians and Gynecologists
409 12th St. SW
Washington, DC 20024

American College of Physicians
Sixth and Race Sts.
Philadelphia, PA 19106-1572
1-800-523-1546

American Medical Association
515 N. State St.
Chicago, IL 60610
1-800-262-3211

American Psychiatric Association
1400 K St. NW
Washington, DC 20005
1-202-682-6000

Society for Adolescent Medicine
Suite 120
19401 E. 40 Highway
Independence, MO 64055
1-816-795-8336

Congress of the United States, Office of Technology Assessment. *Adolescent Health—Vol. 1: Summary and Policy Options.* Washington, D.C.: Superintendent of Documents, U.S. Government Printing Office, 1991.

Dryfoos, Joy G. *Adolescents at Risk: Prevalence and Prevention.* New York: Oxford University Press, 1990.

Elkind, David. *All Grown Up and No Place to Go: Teenagers in Crisis.* Reading, MA: Addison-Wesley, 1984.

Erikson, Erik. *Identity: Youth and Crisis.* New York: W.W. Norton, 1968.

Ginott, Haim G. *Between Parent and Teenager.* New York: Avon, 1971.

Greydanus, Donald E., M.D., editor, for The American Academy of Pediatrics. *Caring for Your Adolescent.* New York: Bantam Books, 1991.

Katchadourian, Herant. *The Biology of Adolescence.* San Francisco: W.H. Freeman and Co., 1977.

Kett, Joseph. *Rites of Passage: Adolescence in America, 1790 to the Present.* New York: Basic Books, 1977.

Offer, Daniel. *The Psychological World of the Teenager.* New York: Basic Books, 1969.

Steinberg, Laurence. *Adolescence.* New York: Alfred A. Knopf, 1989.

Steinberg, Laurence, and Ann Levine. *You and Your Adolescent.* New York: Harper & Row, 1990.

EXERCISE AND SPORTS—CHAPTER 4

American College of Sports Medicine
P.O. Box 1440
Indianapolis, IN 46206-1440
1-317-637-9200

Griffith, H. Winter, M.D. *Complete Guide to Sports Injuries.* Price, Stern, 1986.

President's Council on Physical Fitness and Sports
701 Pennsylvania Ave. NW, Suite 250
Washington, DC 20004

NUTRITION—CHAPTER 5

Brody, Jane. *Jane Brody's Good Food Book.* New York: Bantam Books, 1987.

American Dietetic Association Nutrition Hotline
1-800-366-1655
(Toll-free hotline staffed by registered dietitians who answer questions about nutrition weekdays between 10 A.M. and 5 P.M.; also recorded nutrition messages are accessible 24 hours a day, changing each month to incorporate seasonal issues and scientific breakthroughs.)

ANOREXIA NERVOSA AND BULIMIA—CHAPTER 7

American Anorexia/Bulimia Association
418 E. 76th St.
New York, NY 10021
1-212-734-1114

Byrne, Katherine. *A Parent's Guide to Anorexia and Bulimia.* New York: Henry Holt, 1987.

Jablow, Martha M., for The Children's Hospital of Philadelphia. *A Parent's Guide to Eating Disorders and Obesity.* New York: Delta Publishing, 1992.

The National Anorexic Aid Society
445 E. Granville Road
Worthington OH 43085
Hotline: 1-614-436-1112 from 8 A.M. to 5 P.M., Mon.–Fri.

National Association of Anorexia Nervosa and Associated Disorders
    (ANAD)
P.O. Box 7
Highland Park, IL 60035
Hotline: 1-708-831-3438 from 9 A.M. to 5 P.M., Mon.–Fri.

Valette, Brett. *A Parent's Guide to Eating Disorders*. New York: Avon
    Books, 1988.

DEALING WITH CHRONIC CONDITIONS—CHAPTER 9

The Arc, National Organization on Mental Retardation
500 E. Border St., Suite 300
Arlington, TX 76010
1-817-261-6003; 1-817-277-0553 (TDD)
(Provides information, including *HIV and AIDS Prevention Guide for
    Parents*, a 16-page brochure designed to be used with disabled
    youth and adults.)

The Association for Persons with Severe Handicaps (TASH)
11201 Greenwood Ave. N.
Seattle, WA 98133
1-206-361-8870

Administration on Developmental Disabilities
U.S. Dept. of Health and Human Services
200 Independence Ave. SW
Room 329D
Washington, DC 20201
1-202-690-5504

Down Syndrome Center
630 W. Fayette St.
Baltimore, MD 21201
(Publishes quarterly newsletter, *Down Syndrome Papers and Abstracts
    for Professionals*, that includes a preventive medical checklist
    updated every two years.)

Featherstone, Helen. *A Difference in the Family: Life with a Disabled Child*. New York: Basic Books, 1980.

Kriegsman, Kay Harris, Elinor L. Zaslow, and Jennifer D'Zmura-Rechsteiner. *Taking Charge: Teenagers Talk About Life and Physical Disabilities*. Rockville, MD: Woodbine House, 1992.

March of Dimes Birth Defects Foundation
1275 Mamaroneck Avenue
White Plains, NY 10605
1-914-428-7100

Maternal and Child Health Bureau. *Moving On: Transition from Child-Centered to Adult Health Care for Youth with Disabilities*, 1992. Available from National Maternal and Child Health Clearinghouse, 8201 Greensboro Dr., Suite 600, McLean, VA 22102; 1-703-821-8955, ext. 254.

National Center for Youth with Disabilities
University of Minnesota, Box 721
420 Delaware St. SE
Minneapolis, MN 55455
1-800-333-6293; 1-612-626-2825; 1-612-624-3939 (TDD)

National Down Syndrome Congress
1605 Chantilly Dr., Suite 250
Atlanta, GA 30324
1-800-232-NDSC

National Down Syndrome Society
666 Broadway
New York, NY 10012
1-800-221-4602

National Information Center for Children and Youth with Disabilities
U.S. Department of Education
P.O. Box 1492
Washington, DC 20013
1-202-416-0300

National Organization for Rare Disorders (NORD)
P.O. Box 8923
New Fairfield, CT 06812-1783
1-203-746-6518

Parent Resource Directory for Parents and Professionals Caring for Children with Chronic Illness or Disabilities. Available from Association for the Care of Children's Health, 7910 Woodmont Ave., Suite 300, Bethesda, MD 20814, 1-301-654-6549

SAFE (Stop AIDS Through Functional Education) Curriculum
CDRC Publications
P.O. Box 574
Portland, OR 97207-0574
1-503-494-7522

Spina Bifida Association of America
4590 MacArthur Blvd., Suite 250
Washington, DC 20007
1-800-621-3141

Trainer, Marilyn. *Differences in Common: Straight Talk on Mental Retardation, Down Syndrome, and Life.* Rockville, MD: Woodbine House, 1991.

Videotapes appropriate for teens with mental retardation (available in many video stores): *Strong Kids, Safe Kids,* Paramount Home Video, 1984; *What's Happening to Me?,* VHS C20210; LCA Consolidate, New World Co.

Walker-Hirsch, Leslie, and M. P. Champagne. *Circles,* multimedia curriculum for teaching developmentally delayed people about sexual development, social relationships, abuse prevention, and safer sex. Available through James Stanfield & Co., Drawer P, P.O. Box 41058, Santa Barbara, CA 93140; 1-800-421-6534; or article reprints available from Leslie Walker-Hirsch, RD. #1, Box 37, 935 Hanover St., Yorktown Heights, NY 10598; 1-914-245-3384

ALCOHOL, TOBACCO, AND DRUGS—CHAPTER 12

Al-Anon/Alateen
Family Group Headquarters
P.O. Box 862
Midtown Station
New York, NY 10018-0862
1-212-302-7240

Alcohol/Drug Abuse Referral Hotline
1-800-ALC-OHOL (24 hours a day)

Alcoholics Anonymous
P.O. Box 459
Grand Central Annex
New York, NY 10017
1-212-870-3400
(or check phone book for local chapter)

Center for Substance Abuse National Drug Hotline
1-800-662-4357 (English)
1-800-66AYUDA (Spanish)
1-800-288-0427 (TDD)

Hawley, Richard A. *Think About Drugs and Society: Responding to an Epidemic.* New York: Walker and Co., 1988.

National Clearinghouse for Alcohol and Drug Information
P.O. Box 2345
Rockville, MD 20852
1-800-729-6686
(TDD) 1-800-487-4889

National Cocaine Hotline
1-800-COCAINE

National Council on Alcoholism and Drug Dependence
12 W. 21st St., 7th Floor
New York, NY 10010
1-212-206-6770

National Family Partnership for Drug Free Youth
11159 B South Town Sq.
St. Louis, MO 63123
1-314-845-1933

National Institute on Drug Abuse
5600 Fishers Lane
Rockville, MD 20857
1-301-443-6480

ANXIETY, DEPRESSION, AND SUICIDE—CHAPTER 13

American Association of Suicidology
2459 South Ash
Denver, CO 80222

Bloomfield, Harold H., MD, and Leonard Felder, Ph.D. *Making Peace with Your Parents: The Key to Enriching Your Life and All Your Relationships.* New York: Ballantine Books, 1984.

McCoy, Kathleen. *Coping with Teenage Depression.* New York: NAL/ Dutton, 1985.

National Mental Health Association
1021 Prince St.
Alexandria, VA 22314-2971
1-800-969-6977 or 1-703-684-7722
Information center: 1-800-969-6642

Newman, Susan. *Don't Be S.A.D.:* A Teenage Guide to Handling Stress, Anxiety, and Depression. New York: Julian Messner, 1991.

Nonkin, Lesley Jane. *I Wish My Parents Understood: A Report on the Teenage Female.* New York: Viking Penguin, 1986.

Shapiro, Patricia Gottlieb, for The Children's Hospital of Philadelphia. *A Parent's Guide to Childhood and Adolescent Depression.* New York: Delta Publishing, 1994.

LEARNING AND BEHAVIOR PROBLEMS—CHAPTER 14

ACT Special Testing
Universal Testing
P.O. Box 4028
Iowa City, IA 52243-4028
1-319-337-1332

Learning Disabilities Association of America (LDA)
4156 Library Rd.
Pittsburgh, PA 15234
1-412-341-1515

Bain, Lisa J., for The Children's Hospital of Philadelphia. *A Parent's Guide to Attention Deficit Disorders.* New York: Delta, 1991.

Children with Attention Deficit Disorders (CHADD) National
    Headquarters
499 NW 70th Ave., Suite 109
Plantation, FL 33317
1-305-587-3700

National Center for Learning Disabilities
99 Park Ave.
New York, NY 10016
1-212-687-7211

Orton Dyslexia Society
Chester Bldg., Suite 382
8600 LaSalle Rd.
Baltimore, MD 21286-2044
1-410-296-0232
1-800-222-3123

Colleges with Programs for Students with Learning Disabilities.
    Peterson's Guides, Dept. 5626, P.O. Box 2123, Princeton, NJ 08540

Educational Testing Service (publisher of the SAT)
Admissions Testing Program for Handicapped Students
P.O. Box 6226
Princeton, NJ 08541-6226

REPRODUCTIVE DEVELOPMENT—CHAPTER 15

American College of Obstetricians and Gynecologists
409 12th St. SW
Washington, DC 20024
(Brochures about puberty, menstruation, birth control, pregnancy)

Bell, Ruth, et al. *Changing Bodies, Changing Lives.* New York: Vintage, 1988.

Johnson, Eric W. *Love and Sex in Plain Language,* 4th ed., rev. New York: Bantam Books, 1988.

Johnson, Eric W. *People, Love, Sex, and Families: Answers to Questions That Preteens Ask.* New York: Walker and Co., 1985

Madaras, Lynda, with Dane Saavedra. *What's Happening to My Body? Book For Boys.* New York: Newmarket Press, 1987.

Madaras, Lynda, with Area Madaras. *What's Happening to My Body? Book for Girls.* New York: Newmarket Press, 1987.

McCoy, Kathy, and Charles Wibbelsman. *Growing and Changing: A Handbook for Preteens.* New York: Putnam, 1987.

McCoy, Kathy, and Charles Wibbelsman. *The New Teenage Body Book.*
New York: The Body Press (Putnam), 1992.

National Women's Health Network
1325 G St. NW
Washington, DC 20005
1-202-347-1140

SEXUAL IDENTITY—CHAPTER 16

Hetrick-Martin Institute for Lesbian and Gay Youth
2 Astor Place
New York, NY 10003
1-212-674-2400 or 1-212-674-8695 (TDD)

Parents, Families, and Friends of Lesbians and Gays, Inc.
1012 14th St. NW, Suite 700
Washington, DC 20005
1-202-638-4200
1-800-4-FAMILY

DISORDERS OF THE MALE GENITALIA—CHAPTER 18

American Cancer Society, Inc.
1599 Clifton Rd., NE
Atlanta, GA 30329
1-800-ACS-2345
(Pamphlets on self-examination for testicular cancer)

CONTRACEPTION—CHAPTER 19

National Family Planning and Reproductive Health Association
122 C Street NW, Suite 380
Washington, DC 20001
1-202-628-3535

Planned Parenthood Federation of America
810 Seventh Ave.
New York, NY 10019
1-212-541-7800

Positive Images: A New Approach to Contraceptive Education
A teaching guide for teenagers, 1986; available from Planned

Parenthood of Greater Northern New Jersey Family Life Education Center, 575 Main St., Hackensack, NJ 07601; 1-201-489-1265.

PREGNANCY—CHAPTER 20

Alan Guttmacher Institute
111 Fifth Ave.
New York, NY 10003
1-212-254-5656
(Reports and statistics)

Ewy, Donna and Roger. *Teen Pregnancy: The Challenges We Faced, The Choices We Made (Teens Talk to Teens—What It's Like to Have a Baby)*. Boulder, CO: Pruett, 1984.

National Abortion Federation Hotline
1-800-772-9100

SEXUALLY TRANSMITTED DISEASES—CHAPTER 21

Daugirdas, John T., M.D. *STD, Sexually Transmitted Diseases, Including HIV/AIDS*. Hinsdale, IL: Medtext, 1992.

Herpes Resource Center of The American Social Health Association
P.O. Box 13827
Research Triangle Park, NC 27709
1-919-361-8488
(For information, send self-addressed, stamped envelope.)

National Sexually Transmitted Disease Hotline
1-800-227-8922
(Free information, printed materials, clinic referrals.)

HIV AND AIDS—CHAPTER 22

AIDS Information 24-Hour Hotline of the Public Health Service
1-800-342-AIDS (taped message), or 1-800-342-7514 (questions)
In Alaska and Hawaii, call collect: 1-202-245-6887
1-800-344-SIDA (Spanish)
1-800-243-7889 (TDD)

AIDS Treatment Data Network
1-212-268-4196
1-212-643-0870 in Spanish

American Foundation for AIDS Research
733 Third Ave.
New York, NY 10017
1-212-682-7440

American Red Cross National AIDS Education Office
1-202-737-8300

CDC National AIDS Clearinghouse
P.O. Box 6003
Rockville, MD 20849-6003
1-800-458-5231
(For referrals to data bases and means to access literature)

Hein, Karen, M.D., and Theresa Foy DiGeronimo. *AIDS: Trading Fear for Facts, A Guide for Young People.* Mt. Vernon, NY: Consumers Union, 1989.

Madaras, Lynda. *Lynda Madaras Talks to Teens About AIDS.* New York: Newmarket, 1988.

National Association of People with AIDS (NAPWA)
1413 K St. NW
Washington, DC 20005
1-202-893-0414 or 1-800-92-NAPWA

National Institute of Allergy and Infectious Diseases
National Institutes of Health
Bethesda, MD 20892
(Information about clinical trials for HIV and AIDS, call the AIDS Clinical Trials Information Service: 1-800-TRIALS-A)

SEXUAL ABUSE—CHAPTER 23

Check your local phone listings under "Rape Crisis Hotline" or "Rape Crisis Center."

Childhelp USA National Child Abuse Hotline
1-800-4-A-CHILD (24 hours a day)

Gil, Eliana. *Outgrowing the Pain.* New York: Dell, 1988.

Maltz, Wendy. *The Sexual Healing Journey: A Guide for Survivors of Sexual Abuse.* New York: HarperCollins, 1991.

THE SKIN, HAIR, AND NAILS—CHAPTER 24

American Academy of Dermatology
P.O. Box 4014
Schaumburg, IL 60168-4014
1-708-330-9830

Donahue, Peggy Jo. *Relief from Chronic Skin Problems*. New York:
Dell, 1992.

National Psoriasis Foundation
6443 SW Beaverton Highway, Suite 210
Portland, OR 97221
1-503-297-1545

THE EYES, EARS, NOSE, MOUTH, AND THROAT—CHAPTER 25

National Information Center on Deafness
Gallaudet University
800 Florida Ave. NE
Washington, DC 20002-3695
1-202-651-5051
1-202-651-5052 (TDD)

National Society to Prevent Blindness
500 E. Remington Rd.
Schaumburg, IL 60173
1-800-331-2020

THE LUNGS—CHAPTER 27

American Academy of Allergy and Immunology
611 E. Wells St.
Milwaukee, WI 53202
1-414-272-6071
Physicians' Referral and Information Line:
1-800-822-2762

American Lung Association
1740 Broadway
New York, NY 10019-4374
1-212-315-8700

Asthma and Allergy Foundation of America
1125 15th St. NW, Suite 502
Washington, DC 20005
1-202-466-7643, or 1-800-7-ASTHMA

Cystic Fibrosis Foundation
6931 Arlington Rd., Suite 200
Bethesda, MD 20814
1-800-FIGHT-CF

Gordon, Jacquie. *Give Me One Wish*. New York: W.W. Norton, 1988.
(Story of a teenager with cystic fibrosis.)

National Institute of Allergy and Infectious Diseases
Building 31, Room 7A50
Bethesda, MD 20892
1-301-496-5717

National Jewish Center for Immunology and Respiratory Medicine
1400 Jackson St.
Denver, CO 80206
Lung Line: 1-800-222-LUNG

Steinmann, Marion, for The Children's Hospital of Philadelphia. *A
    Parent's Guide to Allergies and Asthma*. New York: Delta
    Publishing, 1992.

THE HEART AND BLOOD VESSELS—CHAPTER 28

American Heart Association
7272 Greenville Ave.
Dallas, TX 75231-4592
1-214-373-6300, or 1-800-AHA-USA1

THE DIGESTIVE SYSTEM—CHAPTER 29

American Liver Foundation
1425 Pompton Ave.
Cedar Grove, NJ 07009
1-800-223-0179

Crohn and Colitis Foundation of America
444 Park Ave. South
New York, NY 10016-7374
1-800-932-2423, or 1-800-343-3637 (for printed materials)

National Digestive Diseases Information Clearinghouse
Box NDDIC, 9000 Rockville Pike
Bethesda, MD 20892
1-301-468-6344

THE URINARY BLADDER AND KIDNEYS—CHAPTER 30

Ahlstrom, Timothy P. *The Kidney Patient's Book.* Delran, NJ; Great
    Issues Press, 1991.
"Partners in Prevention" (quarterly newsletter about kidney disease),
    P.O. Box 1336, Delran, NJ 08075, 1-800-659-6218.

American Kidney Fund
6110 Executive Blvd., Suite 1010
Rockville, MD 20852
1-800-638-8299

IgA Nephropathy Support Network
234 Summit Ave.
Jenkintown, PA 19046
1-215-884-9038

National Kidney Foundation
30 E. 33rd St., Suite 1100
New York, NY 10016
1-800-622-9010

THE BONES AND JOINTS—CHAPTER 31

Aladjem, Henrietta. *Understanding Lupus.* New York: Charles
    Scribner's Sons, 1982, 1985.

Arthritis Foundation
1314 Spring St. NW
Atlanta, GA 30309
1-404-872-7100

Lupus Foundation of America
4 Research Place, Suite 180
Rockville, MD 20850-3226
1-800-558-0121 or 1-301-670-9292

THE BRAIN AND NERVOUS SYSTEM—CHAPTER 32

American Epilepsy Society
638 Prospect Ave.
Hartford, CT 06105-4298
1-203-232-4825

Epilepsy Foundation of America
4351 Garden City Dr.
Landover, MD 20785-2267
1-800-332-1000

National Headache Foundation
5252 North Western Ave.
Chicago, IL 60625
1-800-843-2256

National Multiple Sclerosis Society
733 Third Ave.
New York, NY 10017-3288
1-212-986-3240
Information Line: 1-800-LEARNMS

THE HORMONAL SYSTEM—CHAPTER 33

American Diabetes Association
P.O. Box 25757
1660 Duke St.
Alexandria, VA 22314
1-800-232-3472

International Diabetic Athletes Association
6829 North 12th St., Suite 205
Phoenix, AZ 85014
1-602-230-8155

Juvenile Diabetes Foundation International
432 Park Ave. South
New York, NY 10016
1-800-223-1138

THE BLOOD—CHAPTER 35

Sickle Cell Disease Association of America
3345 Wilshire Blvd., Suite 1106
Los Angeles, CA 90010-1880
1-213-736-5455 or 1-800-421-8453

The National Hemophilia Foundation
The Soho Building
110 Greene St., Room 303
New York, NY 10012
1-800-42-HANDI

CANCER—CHAPTER 36

American Cancer Society
1599 Clifton Rd. NE
Atlanta, GA 30329
1-800-ACS-2345

Candlelighters Childhood Cancer Foundation
7910 Woodmont Ave., Suite 460
Bethesda, MD 20814
1-301-657-8041
(Youth newsletter; list of local support groups, camps; brochures; sibling
    information)

Leukemia Society of America
600 Third Ave.
New York, NY 10016
1-800-955-4LSA

National Cancer Institute
Cancer Information Service
1-800-4-CANCER

GLOSSARY

Many medical terms are defined in subject-specific chapters. For example, "hematuria" (the presence of blood in the urine) is explained in Chapter 30, The Urinary Bladder and Kidneys. Words like "hematuria" appear in only one chapter that addresses a particular subject. The terms in the following list are somewhat more general and appear throughout the book.

Abdomen. The part of the body between the chest and the pelvis.

Abscess. A small collection of pus, surrounded by inflamed tissue.

Acetaminophen. A pain reliever, in products like Tylenol.

Acute. Sudden, severe, short-term; not chronic.

AIDS. Acquired immune deficiency syndrome; caused by HIV (the human immunodeficiency virus).

Amenorrhea. Cessation or failure of menstruation.

Analgesic. Pain-relieving medication, such as aspirin, acetaminophen, or ibuprofen.

Androgens. Male hormones.

Anesthesia. Loss of sensation, usually produced by medications given before a surgical procedure.

Antibiotics. Medications that destroy bacteria.

Antibody. A substance produced by white blood cells that provides immunity, or protection, from foreign substances.

Antigen. Any substance that stimulates the production of an antibody.

Antihistamine. A medication to control allergy and head cold symptoms.

Autoimmune disease. A disease in which antibodies that attack the body's own tissues are produced.

Benign. Not cancerous, not serious.

Biopsy. Removal of a small sample of tissue for testing.

Cardiac. Referring to the heart.

Chromosome. A unit within each cell that contains genes and determines heredity.

518

Chronic. Long-term, not acute.

Congenital. Of or from birth.

Contusion. A blow to a muscle, a bruise, or hemorrhage beneath the skin.

Corticosteroid. A hormone produced by the adrenal glands; also, medication given to treat inflammatory disorders.

CT or CAT scan. Computerized axial tomography; X-ray study taken from multiple angles.

Cyst. A fluid-filled lump.

Dehydration. Loss of body fluids.

ECG (or EKG). Electrocardiogram; a recording of the heart's electrical impulses, used to assess heart problems.

Echocardiogram. A test using sound waves to assess the heart's structure.

Edema. An accumulation of fluid in tissues, causing swelling.

Electrolytes. Elements (such as potassium, sodium, and chloride) measured in blood and urine.

Endocrine. Pertaining to glands that secrete hormones.

Enzyme. A substance that stimulates specific chemical changes.

Epiphyses. Growth plates at the ends of bones.

Estrogen. A female hormone.

Fetal. Referring to the fetus, or unborn child.

Flank. The side of the body between the lowest rib and the hip.

Flare. An outbreak; the sudden appearance of symptoms.

Gene. The unit on chromosomes responsible for heredity.

Genitalia. Reproductive organs; in females: the vulva, vagina, uterus, fallopian tubes, and ovaries; in males: the penis, testes, and prostate gland.

Glucose. A form of sugar.

Gonad. A sex gland; ovary or testis.

Groin. The junction of the abdomen, or torso, and thighs.

Growth spurt. The increase in height associated with puberty.

Hemorrhage. Loss of blood from the blood vessels.

History (or clinical history). One's record of past medical events, symptoms, or sequence of illness.

HIV. The human immunodeficiency virus, which causes AIDS.

Hormones. Chemicals in the bloodstream that affect many bodily functions.

Hypertension. High blood pressure.

Ibuprofen. A pain reliever or anti-inflammatory medication, as in Motrin, Advil, or Nuprin.

Immune system. The body's defense mechanism against illness.

Immunization. Vaccination; "shots"; protection against contagious diseases.

Immunodeficiency disease. An illness in which the body's immune system is unable to protect against outside infection.

Inflammation. The reaction of tissue to infection or injury, revealed as pain, swelling, redness, or warmth.

Inpatient. Referring to treatment that requires admission to a hospital (opposite of outpatient).

Intravenous. Through the veins.

Laceration. Cut, wound.

Latent. Present but not active or apparent; dormant.

Lesion. A structural change in tissue, such as an ulcer, tumor, or abscess, caused by injury or illness.

Lethargy. Abnormal drowsiness, inactivity.

Lipids. Fats or fatlike substances; i.e., cholesterol, triglycerides.

Localize. To occur in one place; limited, not general.

Lumbar puncture. Spinal tap; a test to evaluate spinal fluid.

Lymph system. The network of channels and nodes (or glands) containing "lymph," a fluid that bathes tissues.

Malignant. Cancerous.

Marker. A sign or degree of measurement.

Mass. A lump; tumor.

Menarche. The first menstrual period.

Metabolism. The body's process of transforming nutrients and fluids into energy and growth.

Morbidity. Illness.

Mortality. Death rate.

MRI. Magnetic resonance imaging; multidimensional picture of internal organs without using X-rays.

Neurologic. Of the brain and nerves.

Nodule. A small node, or group of cells.

Onset. The beginning or early appearance of signs, symptoms, or conditions.

Organic. Having to do with the structure of an organ.

Osteoporosis. Thinning of bone.

OTC. Over-the-counter; medication obtainable without prescription.

Outpatient. Referring to treatment at a doctor's office or clinic without admission to a hospital (opposite of inpatient).

Ovulation. Release of an egg from an ovary.

Pallor. Paleness.

Palpitations. Sensation of rapid or irregular heartbeat.

Pap test. Papanicolaou test; a swab sample of vaginal and cervical cells examined under the microscope for cancer and sexually transmitted diseases.

Pelvic examination. Gynecological, internal examination of the vagina, cervix, uterus, and ovaries.

Pelvis. Ring of bones in the hip area.

Plaques. Patches or deposits on mucous membranes or skin, or inside blood vessels.

Prenatal. Before birth, during pregnancy.

Progesterone. A female hormone.

Prognosis. Outlook, prediction of the future course or outcome of an illness.

Prophylactic. Preventive.

Prophylaxis. Methods to prevent disease.

Prosthesis. An artificial part.

Puberty. The period of sexual development.

Pulmonary. Referring to the lungs.

Regimen. A plan for treatment.

Scan. Diagnostic test, such as ultrasound or X-ray, of internal organs.

Screening. Examination.

Self-limiting illnesses. Those that tend to clear on their own without medical intervention.

Sexually active. Having sexual intercourse once or more.

Spleen. A lymph organ in the left upper part of the abdomen.

Sprain. Injury of a ligament.

STD. Sexually transmitted disease.

Steroids. Hormone medications.

Strain. Muscle pain from overuse.

Sutures. Stitches.

Syndrome. A collection of signs and symptoms which, when they appear together, form a condition or disease.

Tanner stages. Five sexual maturity ratings of puberty based on breast, genital, and pubic hair development.

Testosterone. A male hormone.

Thorax. The chest cage of bone and muscle surrounding the heart and lungs.

Topical. Applied to the skin.

Torso. The trunk, or central portion, of the body, from the neck to the groin.

Toxin. Poison.

Trauma. Injury.

Trial. A course of treatment given for a limited time.

Tumor. Lump, swelling, growth, either benign or malignant.

Ulcer. Craterlike sore.

Ultrasound (or sonogram). A diagnostic test, using sound waves, that gives an image of internal organs.

Utero (or in utero). Within the uterus, before birth.

Vascular. Referring to blood vessels.

Virus. An infectious organism that lives and reproduces in living cells.

INDEX